Awakening to Child Health
I

Holistic Child and Adolescent Development

RAOUL GOLDBERG M.D.

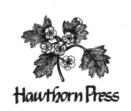

Hawthorn Press

Future books to follow *Awakening to Child Health I*

Awakening to Child Health II – Contemporary Health Disturbances in Childhood and Adolescence

Awakening to Child Health III – Contemporary Therapeutic Approaches to Health Disturbances in Childhood and Adolescence

Awakening to Child Health I copyright © 2009 Raoul Goldberg

Raoul Goldberg is hereby identified as the author of this work in accordance with Section 77 of the Copyright, Designs and Patent Act, 1988. He asserts and gives notice of his moral right under this Act.

Published by Hawthorn Press, Hawthorn House, 1 Lansdown Lane, Stroud, Gloucestershire, GL5 1BJ, UK
Tel: 01453 757040
Fax: 01453 751138
email: info@hawthornpress.com
www.hawthornpress.com

Cover photograph used with the permission of *The Citizen* (*Stroud Life*)
Cover design by Bookcraft Ltd, Stroud, Gloucestershire
Design and typesetting by Bookcraft Ltd, Stroud, Gloucestershire
Printed in the UK by The Cromwell Group, Trowbridge, Wiltshire

First edition published 2009

ISBN 978 1 903458 81 5

Contents

About the Author...*viii*

Preface by Michaela Glöckler.....................................*ix*

Foreword .... *x*

Acknowledgements .... *xx*

1 The Universal Child 1

Universal aspects of the child and adolescent

Idea of the universal child – historical perspectives – modern
perspectives: childhood under attack; childhood resilience –
story of Tobias

2 Meeting the Child 13

New possibilities for meeting the child

Psychophonetics – innovative ways of meeting the child: our own
experience – recollection – four soul functions – accessing original
life experiences through visualization/body awareness/feeling/
gesture/sounding – psyche – empathy – creative resourcing

3 Where Do I Come From? 33

The prenatal journey to birth

Body, soul, spirit – four bodily systems – four
elements – four modes of enquiry – journey down
to earth – male and female principle – the nature of
the cell – the stream of inheritance – the union – the
earthly journey – embryological development – the four
spheres – the fourfold child – the fourfold embryo – the
threefold embryo – life and consciousness in the womb –
core picture and care of the unborn child

4 The Journey: The Three Births of Childhood 70
Cardinal landmarks for the journey ahead

Road map of childhood and adolescence – the fourfold child – three landmark births of childhood: physical birth, birth of the life body, birth of the soul body – the threefold child: neuro-sensory function, metabolic function, rhythmic function – the threefold principle – soul life – body and soul – biographical transformation of the threefold child – two currents of development

5 Citizen of the Earth 95
Arrival on earth: birth experiences

Birth experience – birth options: natural childbirth/home birth/maternity hospital/water birth/Leboyer method – birth interventions: Caesarian section: factors influencing the rising incidence/conventional obstetric viewpoint/midwife viewpoint – effects of Caesarian section on the newborn child – birth by forceps or extraction – three streams – gender – the order of siblings – effects of the environment on newborn – relationship of soul to body – core picture and care of the newborn: caring measures during birth – caring measures after birth – colostrum – vernix – natural feeding vs artificial feeding: breast milk/cows milk/formula milk

6 The Heavenly Years 124
The first three years of life

Road map of early childhood – neuro-sensory system – the will: sevenfold nature – instinct, drive, desire, motivation, wish, intention, resolution – the twelve senses – sense of touch, life, movement, balance, taste, smell, sight, warmth, hearing, word, thought, I – imitation – three human faculties: standing/walking – speaking – thinking; prerequisites: memory, speech, fantasy, play and imagination – neuroplasticity – relationship between movement and speech – between thinking and speaking – core picture and care of early childhood – vaccinations – childhood illnesses – nutrition – environmental impressions – health-giving environment – movement, play, self expression – rhythms and routines

7   The Golden Years 173
The first seven years
Three phases – the physical roadmap – the life/etheric
road map – the sun, moon and planets – the cosmos
within – seven life processes – experiencing the etheric
– the nature of thinking – relationship of thinking to
the etheric – the four ethers: life ether, chemical ether,
light ether, warmth ether – heredity and individuality
– the soul road map – from movement to speech – the
development of feeling – play – toys – stories – from
feeling to thinking – daycare, play groups, nursery school
– repetition and rhythm – synchronization of etheric and
soul streams – physical constitution – three primary types:
head/metabolic/chest – six subtypes: cerebral/sensory –
digestive/muscular – respiratory/cardiac – core picture
and care of the young child

8   The Beautiful, Healthy Years 211
From change of teeth to puberty
The heart of childhood – three divisions – change of
teeth – physical transformation – rhythm – dynamic
transformation – rhythms in homeopathy – rhythm and
life – rhythmic system – Mercury – breathing – breathing
in education – rhythm at school and home – rhythmical
movement: dance, song, music, eurythmy – soul transformation – feeling – the road map: seventh to ninth year
– Waldorf education – stories: picture books, fairy tales,
magic, fables, legends, mythologies – tenth to twelfth year;
pubescence – twelve to puberty – soul life/astral body – balance between body and soul – temperament: four elements
again – melancholic, sanguine, phlegmatic, choleric – four
cardinal organs: lung, liver, kidney, heart – core picture and
care of middle childhood

9   The Youthful and Truthful Years 271
From puberty to adulthood
Three divisions – physical development – male and
female distinctions – metabolic-limb system – liver –
blood – muscles – kidney system – soul development:

desire – sensation – feeling – sympathy /antipathy – emotion – fantasy and imagination – love – sexuality – the secular trend – thinking: concepts, mental imaging, deliberation/judging and concluding – the road map: fourteen – awakening sexuality and the birth of destiny; fifteen – the search for belonging; sixteen – longing, truth and meaning; seventeen – the search for self; eighteen – orientation – first moon node; nineteen – consolidation; twenty – preparation for manhood and womanhood – rites of passage – three thresholds – the character – qualities of colour – the significance of seven – character types: Saturn – individuating type, Moon – imitating, renewing type, Jupiter – thoughtful, organizing type, Mercury – the mobile/connecting type, Mars – the active, masculine type, Venus – the receptive, feminine type, Sun – the harmonious, balanced type – typologies – core picture and care of late childhood and adolescence

10 The Body-Soul-Spirit Continuum in Childhood and Youth 343

Interconnection between body, soul and spirit in childhood and adolescence

Reviewing the journey – interplay of spirit, soul and body – psycho-neuroimmunology – pneumo-psychosomatic factors in child health: neuro-sensory system, rhythmic system, metabolic limb system – the body soul spirit continuum – effects of the body-soul-spirit continuum in the life of the child – soul pictures during childhood and adolescence – experiencing the pneumo-psychosomatic continuum at various developmental levels – soul and body interface – soul and spirit interface – interface of the elements – the vital role of warmth – pathology of warmth and cold

11 Awakening To The I 370

The I nature of the child

Nature of the I – embodiment of the I – mission of the I – recollecting – empathic listening – creative caring – meditative verses – self-knowledge – expression of the I in the journey of childhood and adolescence

12 For Mother, Father and the Universal Child 382

Connecting to the Mother, Father and Child in all parents and all children

Experiencing the universal and eternal relationship that exists between mother, father and child

Notes *388*

Bibliography *411*

Appendix: The Road Map *419*

Index *420*

About the Author

Raoul Goldberg practises anthroposophically integrated medicine in his general family practice in Cape Town.

He has been a school doctor in the Waldorf School Movement for many years and has lectured widely and written articles on many subjects relating to child development and child health.

His primary aim in writing these books is to challenge people to sharpen their natural learning abilities to gain deeper insight into the health and illness of the children and youth in their care as well as into their own childhood and adolescence. Out of this understanding, a rational and intuitive approach to the care and healing of the child within and the child without may be found.

This is a well-written comprehensive introduction to the psychological and physical developmental stages of childhood from the spiritual perspective of anthroposophy.

Dr Michael Evans, Stroud, England

Preface

I have known Raoul and his work as medical practitioner and school doctor for over twenty years, and am very pleased to see the rich fruits of his work published here, the first of three volumes on child health.

Reading this book, one can certainly experience the author's motivating love and concern, and his insight into the real needs of children if they are to grow into capable, secure and active adults.

As he mentions in his foreword, his work was stimulated by questions parents repeatedly asked him in their efforts to gain deeper understanding of their own children.

As co-founder of the Alliance for Childhood, with which Raoul is also affiliated, one of my own central concerns is to encourage initiatives that support and protect childhood. This book certainly aims to do that. It represents many years' work and a great labour of love in helping parents today to provide a solid foundation for their children's future lives.

I therefore hope that all who work with children – parents, teachers, doctors, psychologists and therapists – will turn to this book for support and guidance in nurturing young people in challenging times.

Michaela Glöckler, M.D.

Foreword

This book is about awakening to a healthy understanding of children, and developing effective ways of caring for them.

A growing number of parents as well as professionals in fields such as medicine and education are finding that materialistic explanations of the child's nature no longer satisfy them. While helpful up to a point, they are based on approaches that exclude anything that cannot be measured by physical science. And in the age of quantum physics it has become clear that our science does not yet have the tools, the methodology or even the basic concepts to understand the deep psychological and spiritual nature of children.

Abraham Maslow pointed this out many years ago when, as a student of Prof B.F. Skinner, he declared on the birth of his wife's first baby his realization that 'behaviourism understands nothing about babies!'[1] Since that time, more and more of us have simply outgrown the limited perspective of a purely materialistic science that either excludes the possibility of a soul or spirit, or regards them solely as a product of a human being's physical body.

The impulse to write this book arose out of a question put to me by the parents of a newborn baby: *How can we deepen our understanding of our child through our own personal experience so that we may nurture, protect and enhance his wellbeing to the best of our ability?*

I was struck by this profound question; it touched a deep chord in me that seemed to resound from the covenant that exists between many parents and their growing children: the voice of parents, guardians and carers who consciously or unconsciously feel it their duty to nurture and protect childhood in the best possible way. It was also the voice of parents tired of prescriptive information, who wished to empower themselves to bring up their children in a healthy, creative, wholesome manner. And I also heard in it the voice of the growing child, calling to be understood and cared for and to be given the right time and space to unfold his full potential.

Precisely at this time, destiny led me to two new initiatives.

One was to join a Cape Town working group, affiliated to the Alliance for Childhood,[2] an international association of individuals committed to protecting children. We were a group – teachers at Waldorf Schools, a doctor, therapists and parents – aware of the far-reaching hazards to which children in our time are exposed. We wished to gain insight and skills to help support and protect children.

My work as a holistic medical practitioner and school doctor had, over the past 25 years, brought me close to the world of childhood. I was aware that the basic foundations for physical and emotional wellbeing are established in the first 10 to 12 years of life and that these years play a vital part in an individual's future health. A central part of my family medical practice involved treating children using the integrated medical approach known as anthroposophic medicine, and helping to educate parents using a broad-based approach to their child's health.[3] As a contribution to the Alliance for Childhood, I began to write articles on child health for a wider audience.[4]

The second initiative was Psychophonetics Counselling.[5] Yehuda Tagar, the founder of this methodology, had come to South Africa to deliver a paper at Rhodes University in Grahamstown on sexual abuse and recovery. It soon became apparent that this counselling method had a great deal to offer a holistic approach to medicine; based on a deep understanding of the human psyche, it offered an in-depth training to deepen experience, to open up new frontiers of knowledge and to acquire practical skills in diagnosing and treating illness. I joined the three-year training in Psychophonetics Counselling at the newly established Persephone Institute in Cape Town, where a rich world of experience opened up for me.[6] It was here that I vividly relived and revisited my own childhood, discovering through this training a means of exploring my own past childhood experiences, of developing a compassionate understanding for the different phases of my childhood and of finding new ways to address difficulties I had encountered on the way.

Both these initiatives brought me closely in touch with the spirit of childhood. I realized that the inner being of the child has been a powerful force throughout my medical journey, and was what had inspired me to become a medical doctor in the first place.

I decided to become a doctor while playing at healing animals, as a child. There was never a moment of uncertainty about this choice. My father worked some evenings as an emergency casualty medical officer at the Chris Hani Hospital outside the sprawling African township of Soweto, near Johannesburg; and at the age of eight or nine I would sometimes accompany him on these evening sessions. I witnessed patients injured in car and train accidents or in gang fights and other violence, and in my childlike way I wanted them to get better and tried to help where I could. I seemed in some way to be protected from the blood and gore, for I never felt traumatized by what I saw.

My later medical training at Witwatersrand University ('Wits') in Johannesburg was a time of inner struggle. I was experiencing apartheid – the controlled separation of human beings – at many levels. It was not only politically and socially that I suffered the state-controlled racial separation and discrimination into which I was born; I also struggled existentially with the experience of separation of my bodily nature from my psycho-spiritual one, a duality imposed on my consciousness by an evolutionary process beyond my control. In other words, I fought with the culturally-imposed separation or banishment of the soul and spirit in human life; medically, I rebelled at the narrow-minded materialistic concepts of health and illness imposed on me as a student of medicine by the modern medical establishment. This was a mindset that totally ignored the deeper reality of things, regarding the outer effects, the symptoms, as the only reality.

I was often close to giving up my medical studies, but the child's forces of idealism within me kept me on course. After years of struggling it was an immense relief to discover during my medical internship, in the works of Rudolf Steiner, a science and knowledge of the whole human being that fully resonated with the truth I carried within me. He called this way of viewing the human being *Anthroposophy* taken from the Greek *anthropos* meaning *the whole human being* and *sophia* meaning *science* or *knowledge.* Together with the Dutch physician Dr. Ita Wegman, Steiner evolved a modern holistic system of medicine based on orthodox Western medicine, extending it to embrace the soul and spiritual dimensions of the human being.[7] I felt rejuvenated by a new world of medicine I now discovered, that could become humanized and spiritualized by intuitive knowledge, and where the challenge now was to find the way back from the 'apartheid' of a body sundered from spirit to the authentic unity of the human being.

When one discovers persuasive new insights that seem to provide answers to many of life's riddles, there is a natural tendency to incorporate this knowledge into one's life and profession. One may not have made the original discovery oneself, but one often speaks about it as if one has. How much knowledge does one absorb in this way without testing it oneself? It is often not feasible to check all the facts. We tend readily to believe the expert as an authority on a subject and rely on his judgement. But when we do trust our own independent thinking and original experience, and have the will to test a preconceived idea with our own creative insights, we may often be surprised at the outcome. Let me relate a personal experience to illustrate the point.

It is a commonly held belief that fever in illness should be suppressed. If you ask most people what they know about fever, they will invariably tell you it is part of the disease process that needs to be combated. I was taught as a medical student to suppress fever, yet something in me felt intuitively that this was not correct. Then I contracted tick-bite fever and chose not to take antibiotics or fever-suppressing medication. I let myself experience fever at first hand. It became clear to me, after seven days of fever, that it was my body's natural response to the toxic organisms injected by the tick into my blood. Furthermore, this response was protective and healing, just as the warmth from a father or mother may be protective and healing for a hurt and frightened child.

It was many years later, as my initial contribution to the Alliance for Childhood initiative, that I began to research the role of fever in illness and discovered the scientific validation of my fever experience as a medical student. I found overwhelming evidence to show that fever elicits a powerful defensive and homeostatic reaction in response to provocation.[8] Thus my personal experience gave me an insight into the nature of fever that did not concur with prevailing theory and practice.

Many individuals yearn to access their own intuitive knowledge but, because of perceived limitations, learn to rely on other, outer authorities. Steiner saw no limitations to knowledge and wished to empower his readers to discover higher knowledge themselves. Indeed, before describing the results of his spiritual research, contained in many books and thousands of lectures, he first describes the methods by means of which anyone can come to an insight into higher realities.[9] Through these methods and the exercises described in this book, many of the outcomes of spiritual scientific investigation can be experienced by anyone who applies their mind and will to the process. However, Steiner stresses that one does not need to become a spiritual investigator to acknowledge the fruits of spiritual-scientific research. Anyone who applies a healthy faculty of judgement, free of preconceptions, can become convinced of the truth of certain spiritual communications. Accordingly, in the course of this book, where direct insight and experience in certain matters is not forthcoming, the descriptions offered by Steiner, as an authority in this field, will serve as a starting point. This does not require acceptance of any dogma, but only an open-minded willingeness to sense whether such insights resonate with the reader.

This book rests on the premise that every individual has this fountainhead of knowledge within him which can be awakened and used for his own good and for the good of humanity. Everyone has within him the nature of the child as well as the right means to care for him. And it is the primary intention of this book to awaken to the nature and spirit of childhood and to find worthy ways to protect and care for it.

Every endeavour has been made here, therefore, to access the inner nature of the child and to write out of a personal experience of childhood and adolescence. At the same time, the challenge will be to provide the means by which the reader, given an open and reflective mind and the willingness to employ innate faculties of human experience, can arrive at his or her own inner experience of childhood.

Truth changes all the time according to the position we are in at any particular moment; it grows and matures as we experience life.

What is contained in this book is my experience and my truth, some of which may concur with yours. No doubt, by the time the next edition is due, I shall have many additions and many corrections to insert. My hope is that nothing in this book should be accepted at face value without it being subjected to wholesome, vigorous thinking and independent experience.

Using the rich, raw material of the child's nature, as it unfolds physically, psychologically and spiritually, the full picture of the human being in his totality may reveal itself when the book is taken as a whole.

The Aims of the Book

This book has several objectives, and seeks to meet the needs of a wide range of readers.

- It wishes to awaken a broad-based and in-depth understanding of the healthy child as an essential point of departure for those who wish to offer children their optimum care and protection.
- Those who wish to understand the nature of the human being will acquire a picture of the infinitely vast and rich world of childhood and adolescence culminating in adulthood. The content is validated by knowledge drawn from the natural, humanistic and spiritual sciences.
- Parents and guardians, teachers, and child health practitioners seeking to support the children in their care will find not only a description, but also an experience of this journey that can help them in their caring tasks.
- Others may engage through this journey with the deeper mysteries of the developing child's unfolding life and awakening soul and spirit.
- It also serves as an introductory handbook or work manual for those who seek to know children by exploring the biography of their own inner child. They will find here a methodology through which their journey of childhood to adulthood can be re-experienced.

- Finally, those who wish to know more about themselves, may find here a path of knowledge and a means of exploring their own inner nature.

To facilitate this inner work, introductory exercises are provided in the notes and references sections for each chapter. However, these recommendations should be seen as an introduction to an inner journey that each individual will pursue in accordance with his or her needs.

Getting to know a child well requires us to become a kind of travelling companion on his journey towards adulthood. For this reason the book takes the form of a journey, following the lives of several children from prenatal existence to adulthood. It can become, as it did for me, an inspiring and deeply rewarding experience to travel the voyage through the different stages of child and adolescent development, to the fully-grown adult at twenty-one; and to witness then the birth of a potentially free individual into the world.

This foreword and the first two chapters prepare our meeting with the child and provide a framework for experiencing the journey ahead. Each of the seven following chapters describe the journey itself. There is imaginative content to help adults re-experience childhood, a description of physical and psychological development, a road map of each year and a core picture as basis for a rational approach to optimum supportive care. The advice given should be seen as recommendations rather than recipes, to be tried and tested by each individual. The final three chapters draw the currents of childhood and youth together and place this journey in a healing context. An attempt has been made in each chapter to balance the qualities of 'head, heart and hand' into an integrated, whole picture. The case histories of all children described are drawn from my life and clinical practice and are given with the kind permission of their guardians. All names have been changed.

This book deals with healthy childhood and adolescent development. A second book is planned as Part 2, which will cover in much greater detail the illnesses and disturbances that children experience today. Part 3 will deal with a contemporary therapeutic approach to these conditions.

In a book of this kind it is very tempting to include more than seems necessary. I have justified the inclusion of certain content because I believe it will be required for a fuller understanding and experience not only of this book but of the books that follow.

Living in all children is a reality that unfolds according to developmental laws that are true for us all. This is the prototype, the human child's living 'design' whose universality embraces the individual variations and potential that distinguish each child. Like any living being it has phases of inception, gestation, birthing, growing and maturing that span the best part of twenty-one years. Faithfully and predictably, these universal laws express themselves in the growth and development of every child, and have done so since time immemorial. We can discover the science and the laws governing this universal nature of the child with healthy thinking, feeling and perception. I have chosen to call this reality, manifesting so uniquely and beautifully in each individual child, the *universal child*.

This universal spirit of childhood has the right to be heard, understood, cared for, nurtured and protected by trustworthy custodians; it wishes to unfold into adulthood in accordance with its true human potential.

It is vital that consciously aware people in our time awaken to the reality of childhood. *Children are the life substance of our humanity, a healing power that is desperately needed to balance the life-destroying materialism of our age.*

Notes and References

1. A. Maslow, *Religions, Values and Peak-Experiences,* Penguin Books, 1964, 1976.
2. **Alliance for Childhood**. This international association promotes policies and practices that support children's healthy development, love of learning, and joy in living. Public education campaigns bring to light both the promise and the vulnerability of childhood. The Alliance acts for the sake of the children themselves and for a more just, democratic, and ecologically responsible future. The work of the Alliance is carried out by its **board and staff** (www.allianceforchildhood.org.uk) in consultation with its **partners** (http://www.allianceforchildhood.net/pdf_files/board). The Alliance's work is

funded by grants and donations from foundations and from hundreds
of individuals.

3. **Anthroposophic medicine.** This system of medicine which takes its
    name from the Greek word *anthropos,* meaning *whole human being,*
    was developed by Rudolf Steiner and other medical collaborators in
    the early 1920s. It provides a deep and broad understanding of the
    human being as a living body, soul and spirit. Health is conceived
    as a condition of balance between body, soul and spirit, ill health
    their imbalance and healing the re-establishment of the balance. This
    holistic picture can be attained by one's own personal experience when
    one learns to observe oneself in health or ill-health. Anthroposophic
    medicine describes the specific relationship that exist between the
    world of nature and the human being, enabling the specific substances
    and forces within minerals, plants and animals to be harnessed and
    used rationally and individually in therapy. Illness is thereby treated
    at a far deeper level than can be achieved by symptomatic treatment.
    Transformation and self-empowerment is actively supported as part of
    the healing process.

    Anthroposophically integrated medicine is an extension of
    conventional western medicine. It forms a broad medical framework
    into which other therapeutic systems such as homeopathy, naturopathy
    and acupuncture can be integrated. A great many other therapies may
    be used in this integrated medical system to assist the healing process.
    Some include: therapeutic counselling, art therapy, therapeutic
    eurythmy, nutritional therapy, rhythmical massage, hydrotherapy,
    and crafts and trades applied therapeutically.

4. R. Goldberg, series of articles published in *The South African Journal
    of Natural Medicine* (2001 to 2007).

5. **Psychophonetics Counselling**. Psychophonetics is a method
    of personal transformation and self development, life coaching,
    counselling, consultancy and psychotherapy based on Rudolf Steiner's
    anthroposophy and psychosophy and developed by its founder
    Yehuda Tagar. It acknowledges the living body, soul and individual
    spirit as aspects of an integral human constitution with a potential
    connection to vast resources of vitality, creativity, intelligence,
    compassion, intimacy, expanded awareness and spirituality. As an
    expression-based counselling modality, it extends the client-centred
    conversational approach to psychotherapy with non-verbal expressive
    modalities of *body sensing, gesture and movement, visualization* and
    use of the *sounds of human speech.* This allows rapid access to deep
    psycho-emotional layers of experience. It is a short-term counselling-
    coaching process, that encourages people to take responsibility for
    their own healing, transformation and development. It supports real
    development of relationships, sexuality, parenthood, vocation, creative
    and artistic expression and spirituality. It facilitates effective recovery
    from addiction, depression, anxiety, trauma, abuse and dysfunctional
    behavious patterns, complementing holistic and anthroposophic

medicine in healing a range of physical, psychosomatic, psycho-emotional, psycho-spiritual and psycho-social conditions.

6. **Persephone Institute of Psychophonetics** is an international educational, consultancy and research institute based in Cape Town, South Africa, with branches in the United Kingdom and Australia, specializing in professional training based on psychophonetics and psychosophy. It is dedicated to the integration of personal, spiritual, professional and artistic development

7. R. Steiner and I. Wegman, *Fundamentals of Therapy An Extension of the Art of Healing through Spiritual Knowledge,* Rudolf Steiner Press, London 1983.

8. R. Goldberg, 'Fever – A Gift for Health', *South African Journal of Natural Medicine*, issue 4, 2001.

9. R. Steiner (1894), *Philosophy of Freedom* also known as *The Philosophy of Spiritual Activity,* Rudolf Steiner Publications Inc., New York 1963; R. Steiner (1904), *Theosophy. An Introduction to the Supersensible Knowledge of the World and the Destination of the Human being,* Anthroposophic Press Inc., New York 1961; R. Steiner (1904/1905), *Knowledge of the Higher Worlds. How Is It Achieved?* Rudolf Steiner Press, London 1969; R. Steiner (1910), *An Outline of Occult Science,* Anthroposophic Press Inc., Spring Valley, New York 1972.

Acknowledgements

I am indebted to many individuals for the creation and realisation of this book:

All the children I have met throughout my life who have helped me to shape my understanding of childhood and adolescence.

Rudolf Steiner, one of the foremost spiritual researchers of our times who opened up new frontiers of knowledge and experience, affirming for me what was living as truth within me.

Yehuda Tagar, who gave me the tools to explore my hidden nature and spirit and my creative potential, making it possible for me to open up and experience the inner world of the child.

My wife Katherine, who sacrificed a great deal to give me the space and the time to write this book.

Martin Large, who placed his trust in me from the beginning of our work together and never wavered because he recognized the importance of a book of this kind.

Matthew Barton, who took on the daunting task of editing this book and sensitively helped me to mould it into the finished product.

Michaela Glöckler, who found the time in her incredibly busy schedule to write the introduction to this book.

Anya Kotzuber, for the personal and animated illustrations.

John Button, who, through his efficiency, made the typesetting and proofing so easy for me.

Stan Maher, for his support and encouragement in the initial stages of writing this book.

To others who gave guidance, support and advice along the way: my daughter Karen, Elina Komorova, Michael Grimley, Batya Daitz, Mary G Hauptle, Keriesa Botha, Jenz Eggers, Joan Sleigh, Julian Sleigh, Hanna Hack and David Auerbach.

CHAPTER I

The Universal Child

I am the Quintessence of Childhood. Know Me and You will Know Your Child

In whatever role we support children – as parents, guardians, health professionals, caregivers or advocates – our general picture and idea of childhood will inform our understanding of each individual child, as well as the caring that follows from this. In other words, we start from a sense of what is general or universal in every child. We may have acquired this picture from our own experience of childhood, and by observing children. It can also be amplified by studying and researching the nature of childhood. This universal picture allows us to know something about the child, however, without ever having lived or worked with children. It can exist in us fairly unconsciously and pre-verbally, or we can become more fully aware of it.

Parents expecting a child, with this basic feeling for childhood, may have some idea of when their child should sit up, crawl, stand, walk and talk. They will have to wait until their own child arrives, however, to experience the joy of observing exactly how and when she[1] does this. There is an inexorable law underlying child development: every stage of the growing child unfolds with such precision and synchronicity that it is possible to trace normal development according to highly predictable parameters. The study of embryology gives an awesome picture of a dynamic developmental process that unfolds according to exact laws of growth and development. Almost all children stand at about 9 or 10 months and walk by 12 months; and second dentition very usually begins in their seventh year.

Once we know something about this generalised *universal child*, we can then apply this idea to each individual instance, also allowing the reality before us to infuse and inform the picture we carry within us. A mutuality is at work here, an interaction between our universal picture and the specific child in front of us.

Getting to know this picture within us of the universal child, standing behind and archetypally representing every individual child and adolescent, can give us deep insights that are fruitful for nurturing actual children. This picture is like a deep pattern or template, working from time immemorial, against which present reality can be gauged.

In this chapter, therefore, we will explore the reality of this universal picture, comparing it with various historical perceptions of childhood. The chapters that follow will then connect us more deeply with specific stages of child development, applying this more universal knowledge to understanding particular, diverse children, and caring for them.

The Archetype of the Child

We connect to this whenever we refer to, or think about, 'the child'. You may recall a decision to bring a child into the world, or perhaps you remember wanting to learn something more about a child. What picture comes to mind when we reflect on the joy or innocence of childhood, or when we speak about street children or abused children in a general way? Here we do not have the picture of an individual child in mind, but something larger, grander, representing all children in general; we have in mind the *idea* of the child.

Ideas have reality, and the power to inform our feelings and actions. The idea of the child lives powerfully within us: in our thinking about children, in our deep feelings for them and in the deeds that we accomplish for them. It was this idea that inspired me to write these books. The universal child embraces the epoch of human existence stretching from conception to adulthood, during which we can witness the perfection, exquisite beauty, absolute harmony and integration of healthy development through childhood and adolescence, but also the abnormal development, ill health and disease that involve pain and hardship for all concerned.

Our picture of the child will naturally vary greatly in accordance with our own personal experience and we will generally relate to children according to this personal view. One person will devote her life to serving children; someone else will be indifferent to them or avoid them as far as possible; another may hate children or actively abuse them. The way in which the idea of childhood has found expression throughout the ages is dictated by the personal experiences, or perceived ideas and prejudices, of the custodians of childhood. This may also be shaped by the voices of leaders and authorities who express the subconscious will of the people. The collective social or cultural voice will then determine how children are regarded and cared for. They are to a great extent at the mercy of their custodians. Cultural perceptions of childhood may be more or less in harmony with real universal laws inherent in child development.

The Child Through History

We can broaden our understanding of the universal or archetypal child by examining how children have been regarded and treated throughout history, and what conceptions of childhood dictated this. The influence of society on children is nowhere better described than in the book, *The Disappearance of Childhood* by Neil Postman,[2] and my comments below draw heavily on his analysis.

Our ancestors had very different attitudes to children. The Greeks practised infanticide and were severe disciplinarians; at the same time they were passionate about education and were the first culture to establish schools. This shows that they were aware of childhood as a distinct and separate phase of life, with its own laws, and that they wished to impart to children knowledge or skills that would turn them into adults.

The Romans had a more advanced sense of childhood, as reflected in the depiction of young, growing children in their art, and a description in their literature of the need to protect children from adult secrets. Postman postulates that the idea of shame and the need to protect children presupposes a conscious awareness of the special nature of childhood. The first known law prohibiting infanticide came into effect in the last years of the Roman Empire. With the empire's collapse in the fifth century AD, literacy and education faded away, along with a sense of the differences between child and adult.

Well into the Middle Ages, an oral tradition prevailed and exerted a great influence on the concept of childhood. Childhood was thought to end when the child began to communicate like an adult, at around the age of seven. There was no conception of further childhood development, no idea of education and no awareness of differences between child and adult.[3] Nor, therefore, was there any perceived need to protect children from activities that we today regard as exclusive to the adult domain, such as caring for others, earning a living, social relationships, sexual activities, marriage, violent conflict and so on. The medieval child was thus exposed to every facet of the adult world. Breughel's paintings depict children unashamedly engaged in excessive drinking and lustful scenes with adults. Children were to all intents and purposes miniature adults. High mortality rates amongst children must also have influenced attitudes towards children, either making adults more protective or, if they did not wish to become too attached to their offspring, less so.

Then, in the middle of the 15th century, the revolutionary invention of the printing press led very quickly to a rapid culture of literacy, and gave rise to a new conception of childhood. Literacy and the world of knowledge that this opened up became an exclusive right of adults. Thus the idea of childhood was born again and in the course of the sixteenth century clear distinctions between children and adults became evident. Children were regarded as human beings with natures and needs that differed from those of adults, and required special attention. As part of the requirement to move illiterate children towards literate adulthood, schools were inevitably established, and this undoubtedly had a powerful influence on child development. Children were dressed, and addressed differently from adults, and were seen to speak and act in a distinct way. They were once again excluded from a range of adult activities that were considered inappropriate for their age. Strict discipline and shaming were introduced as a way of controlling the untamed and wild forces of child nature. Self-control was regarded, in contrast, as a characteristic of mature adulthood.

The works of Locke in England and Rousseau in France contributed greatly to the Age of Enlightenment and helped to cultivate the idea of childhood. Locke regarded children as unformed human beings to be moulded into refined adults by literacy, proper education and right upbringing. Rousseau, on the other hand, respected the child's unique nature of pure innocence and joyful spontaneity and wished to protect it from the harmful effects of literacy, formal education and adult manipulation. Though divergent in principle, both views voiced the need for adult care and guidance.

By the mid-19th century the concept of childhood had become social reality. Even the industrial revolution, which brutally exploited cheap child labour in mines and factories, could not destroy the idea of childhood that had taken root in the middle and upper classes of the western world. This gradually filtered through to the lower classes and across national boundaries, not least through great works of literature such as those of Wordsworth, and somewhat later, Dickens. By the end of the 19th century, illiteracy had virtually disappeared in Europe and America, governments took responsibility for the welfare of children, and parents adopted a more humane approach to their children. In 1899, important works by Sigmund Freud and John Dewey were published which provided the fundamental paradigm for mainstream contemporary thinking and psychological research on childhood in the 20th century.[4] The work of Jean Piaget and most other researchers is founded on the premises laid down by Freud and Dewey, that the constitution of the child has its own specific structure and laws of development which must be nurtured and protected by adult custodians. In the scientific frame of reference of Darwinism and reductionism prevalent at that time, childhood was seen as a distinct *biological* entity, and no longer merely a product of culture, social class or education.

At roughly the same time as these two radically influential works appeared, Rudolf Steiner was formulating a view of the human being that extended the idea of childhood into whole new dimensions. In the first quarter of the twentieth century he wrote many books and delivered hundreds of lectures in central Europe and England in which he offers a compelling picture of the universal child and the latter's interconnected physical, psychological and spiritual development from pre-natal existence through to adulthood.[6] In 1921 he founded the first Waldorf School in Stuttgart where his insightful educational principles were put into practice for the first time. Waldorf schools now exist in many countries. These principles drew not only, however, on a preconception of what childhood *should* be, but also, decisively, on precise and careful observation of human stages of development. To practise such observation Steiner extended contemporary scientific methodologies with what he called 'spiritual science': a mode of enquiry and research into spiritual realities alongside physical ones. He saw physical and spiritual worlds as being profoundly interconnected and mutually influenced, and held that human life in general, and child development in particular, could not be fully understood without the originating spiritual dimension.

During the first half of the twentieth century, the special status of the child as an innocent and relatively helpless being who required nurturing and protecting, took root in the collective psyche of the western world. Laws were passed, and attitudes changed in family, schools, and society in general, contributing to a progressive sense that childhood needed care and protection. In 1924 the Geneva Declaration of the Rights of the Child affirmed the need to extend particular care to the child. In 1959 the Declaration of the Rights of the Child was adopted by the General Assembly of the United Nations.

Today there is worldwide support for the dignity and protection of children. In the Universal Declaration of Human Rights proclaimed in 1989 by the United Nations, childhood was granted a status entitled to special care and assistance. All countries have charters, campaigns, and support and focus groups that actively work to safeguard the vulnerable nature of childhood. The Alliance for Childhood is one such international organization that is committed to supporting and protecting the wellbeing of children.[7] In South Africa, Nelson Mandela, the first democratically elected President of South Africa and a world-renowned leader of legendary status, is an active patron of children.

Childhood Under Attack

At the same time however, other forces were and are at work, impacting powerfully on children's wellbeing. These forces are rooted in a materialistic conception of the human being and the world, and have been evolving for many centuries as humanity gradually lost its intuitive, harmonious connection both with the natural environment and with deeper spiritual realities. By the mid-nineteenth century, science had emerged as the new religion because it could provide the quantifiable proof and justification for its sense-based materialistic worldview. It became the authority in which people increasingly placed their complete faith and trust. What could not be perceived or quantified was not thought real. To put this radically, since only material things could be perceived, psychological and spiritual realities had either to be dismissed, or assigned to and subsumed within the fields of biophysics, biochemistry or biogenetics as an – albeit more refined – extension of matter.

Inevitably as a natural consequence of this paradigm shift, the rampant material conquest of the world and the human being began. At the same time as greater respect and care is accorded to children, paradoxically we see the ideas of Darwinism gaining ground, propounding the view that the human child is simply a higher animal engaged in a fight for survival. We see the industrial age passing into the age of technology, and launching a new assault on the universal child in the form of electronic media and entertainment increasingly devoid of the human element and antagonistic to self-directed play and the life of the creative imagination. With the invention of photography, telephone, gramophone, cinema, radio and finally television, which became entrenched in American homes by 1950, communication became so modified that the picture and sound byte took over from the word as the dominant means of communication.[9] When we consider that the average child watches four hours of TV daily and that in the USA one-third of children, from babies up to six years of age, live in homes where the TV is on almost all the time, we can expect a significant impact on the life of the child. With the development of computer science, technology's inexorable advance is having ever stronger effects on children's body and psyche; the intrusion of computer games, internet, and mobile phones strike at the most intimate areas of their life, overlying as it were the subtle, nuanced inner growth of imaginative perception with an irresistible array of powerful images imposed from without. We can well ask where things will go from here ...

What we see here, playing itself out both on the global stage as well as in the life and soul of each individual child, is the struggle for the freedom of the universal child to manifest in a healthy way. On the one hand there is a groundswell of support and respect for the archetypal nature of the child to express itself in a free and healthy manner; but on the other there is a lack of awareness, or even ruthless disregard, for the vulnerability of childhood. Such disregard militates against the healthy unfolding of general laws inherent in child development, leading to widespread disorders and disruption of this development.

Children today face a minefield of potential hazards that threaten every phase of their existence. Prenatally, already, the life of the growing embryo may be terminated when parents or other stakeholders regard this new life as too burdensome for it to be allowed to continue to live and be born. In the womb, the baby is at the mercy of the mother's internal nutritional, chemical and psychological environment. Though the embryo may be well-protected within the mother's body, it can still be harmed by external influences.

From the moment the child is born, she may be exposed to the rigours of a harsh external environment: immunization, chemical medicines, industrial pollutants, nutritional stresses, violence and abuse in the home and society; also the legal but harmful drugs caffeine, nicotine and alcohol, and a wide range of illicit chemical substances. And last but not least, computer technology and mass media that modify and control her perceptions.

Many excellent books have been written on the toxic environment of children, such as Sue Palmer's *Toxic Childhood*[10] Garbarino's

Raising Children in a Socially Toxic Environment[11] and Oliver James's *Affluenza.*[12] *Set Free Childhood* by Martin Large provides a survival guide for parents to cope with computers and TV.[13] Any number of documented studies exist of child neglect, abuse and exploitation in every country, both in the developed and the developing world.

Part 2 of this book examines childhood disorders caused by, among other things, environmental factors of this kind.

The Resilience of Children

In the face of all the dangers and difficulties, the survival capacity and resilience of children remains immense. They may be vulnerable and relatively helpless, yet hidden within their fragile bodies there is a tremendous will to live, a huge capacity to adapt and an immeasurable vitality and healing potential. Many children have been abused in the most vicious ways, yet manage to carry on with their lives, with hopefulness and even cheerfulness.

One such example is 'Sarah', who by the age of three had experienced physical and emotional abuse at the hands of an unstable mother and her live-in partners. She was frequently looked after by relatives yet remained relatively untroubled by her very insecure circumstances.

Naturally these experiences will impact on her life at some time in the future, but at this stage in her life, she finds from some resource within herself the innate resilience to carry on living a relatively normal life.

We learn as small children to deal with our life circumstances by adapting and responding in the best way possible, in accordance with our own nature. No one teaches us how to do this; we do it intuitively and without outward assistance. One child, for instance, when faced with violence, will disassociate or withdraw her conscious awareness so she does not perceive what is going on around her; another child in the same situation will become shy and withdrawn or even autistic; a third child will become hyperactive or aggressive and may begin to imitate the violence. We can only feel awe for the ingenuity with which each child, according to her nature and resources, discovers the best means of survival and adaptation to meet the most difficult circumstances.

The Universal Child: the Spirit at Work in the Genome

Notwithstanding individual differences – the specific nature of each child – there appears, then, to be a universal wisdom, integrity and lawfulness that reveals itself in the constitution and biography of every child, as we observed above in relation to embryological development and subsequent milestones. Contemporary medical science ascribes this to the genome – the genetic makeup of the child – believed to regulate every aspect of the child's life. Yet even if this genome is a biochemical blueprint of the child's physical and physiological characteristics, it does not explain the intelligence that created it. There must be a universal but individualized prototype, a blueprint as it were at work in every individual child. This unseen wisdom and intelligence is really what I mean by the universal child, and it is something we will return to frequently as we seek ways to nurture different stages of childhood in the best possible way.

As we explore the voyage of childhood from conception to adulthood this creative paradigm will come more clearly into focus: we will accompany the universal child from prenatal existence to physical birth, through early childhood and the pre-school years, the junior school years of mid-childhood and finally through adolescence to adulthood. Clearly, whole textbooks can be written on each of these phases, and of course a vast literature on them exists. Our focus, however, will be on the essential elements of each period of development, and the way each gradually gives way to the next. By grasping the signature of the genius at work at each stage of development we can come to form a tangible sense of the guiding, creative force that runs as a living thread through the lives of all children, in all phases, both in health and illness.

The Journey of Tobias

There is a beautiful account in the biblical Book of Tobit that relates the journey of Tobias in his passage from childhood to manhood.[14] His blind father sends him on a mission to retrieve money owed to him in a distant land. He is accompanied on this journey by a companion who turns out to be the archangel Raphael, who guides him on his journey and instructs him in the art of healing. He learns the secrets of the human body and how to heal it; when a fish jumps out of a river into his hands, he uses its heart and gall bladder as healing substances to cure his father's blindness. He is also shown the mysteries of the soul and spirit, enabling him to drive out demons from his prospective wife, and find union with his feminine counterpart.

In this story Raphael guides the development and destiny of Tobias towards manhood and his life tasks as a physician and healer. Raphael is able to guide Tobias because he understands the mystery of human development – specifically the mystery of the universal child. The more we deepen our understanding of the archetypal laws at work in childhood, as a deep pattern of health and development, the greater will be our capacity to guide, protect and heal the actual children who need our help.

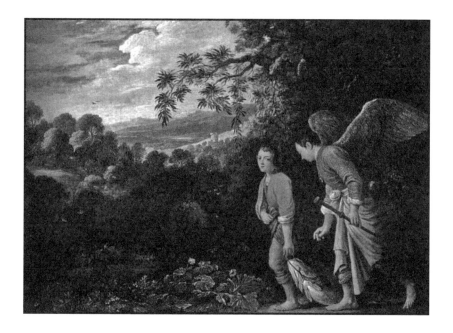

Raphael Leading Tobias

You are the universal representative of all children;
From time immemorial children embody you.
Your universality is the measure of each individual;
Within your time and space children unfold their existence.

You mark the journey they travel from conception to
adulthood
And through the laws of growth and development you
unfold your reality;
We wish to understand these laws and know your
mysteries,
For you will then reveal to us the wonder of every single child.
We wish you to teach us how to invoke you
For this will create strong and healthy adults who will take
humanity forward into the future.
We wish to learn how to protect you
For when we fight to protect you, our sons and daughters
will be safe.
Are you just an idea or concept, or a figment of my
imagination?
You remain silent and invisible, hidden in each child.
Yet I can conceive you, thereby create you and can
therefore understand you.
And this makes you a living reality –
For how, without my conception of her,
Could I recognize a child?
You are the universal child and I will seek to know you.

CHAPTER 2

Meeting the Child

Will you Hear Me and Listen to My Story?

To begin with the inner world of childhood is a closed book. The gestational period of 280 days in the womb is almost completely hidden, apart from sporadic movements felt by the mother, the heart beat picked up by a stethoscope, and perhaps a couple of ultrasound scans that may reveal the gender and general shape and size of the foetus.

When he is born we meet the child face to face for the first time, with wonder and joy at this new being about whom we know so little. Who is he? Where did he come from? It is a common experience that the newborn infant is not entirely of this world.

We wish to get to know the child. What kind of child is he, who will he become? For the first nine months we listen and watch as the child expresses himself through movement, gesture and sound, unable to tell us in words how he feels or what he needs. An attentive mother who watches and listens closely will learn to understand her child's needs intuitively rather than rationally. As the body grows and the organs mature, immense developmental processes are taking place completely hidden from view.

The child learns without anyone teaching him how to crawl, stand, walk and talk. One day, usually at some point in his third year, we become aware that Jonathan is no longer calling himself by his name but has discovered another way of naming himself and henceforth refers to himself as *I*. By doing so he triumphantly declares *I am here!* As parents or carers we have nothing whatsoever to do with these changes: we simply watch the wise intelligence at work in the growing process. Sometimes words of profound wisdom can surface from hidden depths: My godson Uriel, aged four, spontaneously informed his parents that 'when I listen to music from the cello my heart goes away from me and only comes back to me when the music ends'. Where does such a comment come from? There are times in early childhood when a child is more expressive, times in later childhood, in puberty and adolescence when the child is more silent or inward; but mostly the inner life of childhood is a world closed to us. This book explores innovative ways of penetrating the hidden world of childhood.

Starting from Our Own Experience

In this journey of exploration let us start from a place we all have in common, that of our own personal experience.

The idea of the general or universal child outlined in Chapter one offers an underlying context for insight about the particular children we meet in life, as their parents, guardians, relatives, friends, teachers, health professionals or other caregivers. Children themselves are usually our best teachers. We generally base our understanding about parenting on our personal experience and specific interactions. As first-time parents we are usually unsure at the start, but quickly gain confidence as we get to know our child better. We may seek advice from someone with more experience; we try it out: sometimes it works, sometimes it doesn't.

We may also acquire information about childhood from other external sources, by reading popular or academic books, from the internet, from talks and courses and by studying the works of great educationalists. While this information may be satisfying intellectually, it remains borrowed information until it is digested by our own life experience, through working and living with, and caring for children.

These are the two common and generally accepted ways of gaining knowledge of childhood, both of which are entirely valid.

But there is another way of understanding a child: from within, through recalling and reliving our own inner journey of childhood.

If we had no contact with children or access to information and we suddenly came across a child, we would undoubtedly recognize in this young human being something known and familiar, for we have all taken the path through pre-natal existence, childhood and adolescence. We have all been a tiny seed embryo that developed through foetal stages to become a newborn child. All of us have lived through every phase of being a child – infant, toddler, preschooler. Each of us became a pubescent child, teenager and adolescent, passing these milestones on our inexorable march towards adulthood. While these were human experiences common to all, they were also experiences unique to ourselves. For eighteen years we move through childhood to adolescence, one phase merging into the next, like an artwork that requires a certain given time to be shaped; then follow another few years before we take possession of the key to adult life – traditionally at twenty-one. The stages of development are not arbitrary but evolve through three predictable and precisely defined cycles of seven years, which we will examine in subsequent chapters.

The Inscriptions of Memory

In one sense the job is done when we enter adulthood and we can now step forward into the next chapter of our life. Yet when we review what we know about these twenty-one years, when we try to recall what happened in this quarter of a lifetime, we actually know very little indeed. The first year of life is completely veiled and most people remember very little of the first three years; we may know less of our own childhood than we do of the children in our care. Yet the script has been recorded somewhere in our memory: we can call up certain memory pictures through conscious effort, and others rise up spontaneously through some association or trigger stimulus. These memory pictures are usually like still photographs imbued with a very personal, dreamlike quality that rises up from hidden depths. We know that all these memories belong to the same person and that somewhere within us our own life narrative is present; we can trace it in a more or less sequential time frame, even if sporadic and discontinuous, with many gaps.

If only we could remember more about our childhood and adolescence we would know a great deal more about this journey.

The fact that memories can and do resurface shows that our early experiences are indelibly transcribed in a hidden archive, allowing us to remember our childhood. There is a vast body of research which validates this claim. All forms of regression therapy rest on the premise that deep memories from all phases of development exist in the subconscious and can be called into conscious awareness through a variety of techniques.[1] Psychophonetics, for example, is a psychotherapeutic modality that may consciously awaken this hidden memory right back into the embryonic period.[2,3] It is this methodology more than any other that has enabled me to explore the hidden world of childhood and adolescence more deeply. The experiences acquired in this way are characterized in the following pages as an example of how our earlier experiences can be remembered.

Some readers may object that this is a realm of the subconscious that should be left undisturbed. It is their freedom *not* to go there just as it is someone else's freedom to do so. This book describes ways of exploring the realm of childhood at many different levels, and each reader will decide the level at which he wishes to experience this: as a reader, as an observer of children wishing to understand childhood better, or as an inner participant on a voyage we have been on before, one that can deepen understanding of our own childhood and of the children in our care.[4]

Original Experience

Our past experience is present within us as a body of memory which can in some measure be consciously accessed. It has unique value as our personal recapitulation of the human developmental process, offering us the means to know something unique about childhood and adolescence from the inside.

How have we acquired this experience? If we consider the channels through which our life experience comes to us we discover four different human activities: perceiving, feeling and thinking the world, or acting in the world. The child perceives the outer world of sense impressions as well as the inner world of sensations, and mental pictures. He also has feelings, thereby acquiring rich and personal experiences of life. When the child become active in his thinking, he acquires experience by understanding and giving meaning to what he perceives and what he feels. And finally the child enhances his experience by actively engaging and interacting with the world. However conscious our experience, whether of a bodily, emotional or cognitive nature, we cannot deny that it is real, that we are its authors, and that this content has been and is being received by some aspect of ourselves which makes use of this experience every day of our lives.

As we have seen, much of human experience is unconscious and forgotten, submerged in the subconscious from where its inner content continues to affect us. As a child we learn a wide range of physical, mental, psychological and social skills which are stored in us forever, to be summoned when we need them. Once we have learned the skills of riding a bicycle or of reading and writing, we never lose them. Nothing learned by experience is lost. Like the annual rings of a tree, we carry all our ages inside of us. Furthermore, our negative experiences – our fears, doubts, distrust, disappointments and so on – are also stored inside, to be triggered again when a familiar situation arises.

But where is the body's memory? Where are all these experiences stored? This is a question that continues to elude science. There are of course areas in the brain that can be stimulated to evoke a memory, but this does not show where or how memory is stored. I do not believe medical science will ever find memory – just as it will never discover where mind or psyche are located as long as it searches for it in the physical body, using a mode of investigation predicated on sensory investigation alone.

Mind and Matter

This is because every molecular part of the physical body, including the memory-designated part of the brain, is mineralized chemical substance that is completely recycled in every seven-year period. But this recycling of chemical substances does not erase our life experiences, which remain stored somewhere, somehow in our body.

You can test this by recalling a particularly unpleasant event that occurred many years before: if you observe closely, you can often sense it in a specific location in the body. I remember shooting a bird with my pellet gun at the age of nine, and every time I recall this event I feel a twinge around my heart.

So if memory is not to be found in the brain or in fact anywhere in the physical body, where does it reside? We shall return later to this intriguing question.

From Object to Subject

Thus experiences of which we become aware form our store of practical wisdom. But nowadays by far the greater part of conscious experience for most people is knowledge acquired through observation and awareness of the outer world. The focus in contemporary science is almost exclusively on the external object. It has to be kept completely separate from the observing subject by such means as double-blind studies, so that the subject cannot influence the object. The observing subject is mostly left out of the picture.

People study every possible subject under the sun and beyond and apply themselves diligently to become an authority in the field. Yet very few will study themselves and their own human experience and become an authority on their own self. There are many reasons why this is so; there appears to be a greater interest in outer things and little inclination or interest for self reflection. Some people may be wary about 'muddying' the apparent clarity of objectivity and others find it uncomfortable getting to know themselves.

Yet in the same way that we can study any phenomenon in the outside world – say a crystal on the table in front of us – it is possible to focus our attention on ourselves and explore the nature of our human experience. The only difference is that here I am both subject and object: both are always present and it takes only a slight shift of focus to make my subjective experience the object of my study.

When I examine my own experience on my inner laboratory table, what do I discover? A content that derives from **three sources**:

- *from my body*, mainly through sensations and reflexes, mediated by sense organs and bodily impulses;
- *from my inner life* through memories, mental images and thoughts, feelings and emotions, reactions and impulses;
- *from the outer world* as direct sense impressions that are acquired through perception and may be stored inside me as sensations and memory pictures.

I further discover that I gain access to this content essentially through **four inner activities**. An everyday encounter with a child will illustrate the experience: I see a child, I hear him cry. Firstly I make use of *sensory* or *perceptive* awareness to perceive the child that stands outside me. I notice as well that the outer impression has an effect on my body; I tense up and my ear drums vibrate with the high pitched cry. Next I observe that I am feeling sad and anxious and realise that this activity of *feeling* is not dependent on the body. Then I discover that I have thought about the child: he is crying. Why is he crying and what can I do to help him? I discover that *thinking* is required to make me aware of what I have perceived or felt. I may *visualise* a mental picture of myself when I was a child, I may *reflect* on what is causing the child to cry or I may deliberate on what I should do to help. Finally, I notice that I act on my perceiving, feeling and thinking by *doing* or *willing* something: I may *react* impulsively or *wish to do something* or *say something or take the child into my arms*.

I thus discover that all experience involves one or more of these four activities: **sensing**, **feeling**, **thinking** and **doing** or **willing**. They are the natural experiential tools we make use of throughout our life to learn about ourselves and the world. And throughout this book we shall be consciously working with these activities of experience to understand the journey of childhood and adolescence.

Childhood experiences, as we have seen, are often not readily accessible. Some conversion process must have taken place for them to be stored and packed away; and they must have been written in a form that our body at least can access, and by an intelligence largely hidden from us. This memory code can be deciphered: like an archaeologist I can bring to light childhood experiences that are locked in my body.

In the course of writing this book, I needed to understand more about the tenth year of childhood. I observed a number of children in their tenth year. One of these nine-year-old children was going through a difficult time. I tried to understand him and help him by listening and speaking to him. I read what I could about this stage of childhood and discovered that it is often a challenging time for children. The literature told me that this is when the child feels his childhood paradise fading away; and that many children become aware of another world around them that is dark, unknown and terrifying. I recalled that both my children had death premonitions in their tenth year.

Having trained as a psychophonetics counsellor, I decided to complement the information thus gained by seeking to discover something about the tenth year in my own personal biography.

> I begin by focusing on this period in my life and try to remember any detail that reminds me of this time. I recall the Oris watch with the red date hand that my parents gave me for my ninth birthday. I find myself clearly visualizing myself as a small child taking great comfort from the watch with the red date hand. This visualization is for me a very accurate picture of an event that took place fifty-odd years ago. As I allow my mind's eye to rest on this picture, I am aware of suddenly **feeling** very sad and lonely; I am deep inside the experience of surging feelings, as if I am **dreaming**, with a feeling of sadness and loneliness. I now notice that the feeling gives way to a specific sensation of tightness and constriction in my body. I **sense** a very unpleasant, tight sensation, especially around the chest, that connects me powerfully to the tense and lonely experience of the nine-year-old child. Suddenly I am aware of wanting to run away and hide; I am terrified of something and am **reacting** in a reflex manner towards the cause of the fear.

By focusing one's attention on inner, subjective experience, by learning to distinguish between the faculties of visualising, sensing, feeling and reacting, and by observing oneself in these different modes, it is possible to access fresh and vivid mental imagery of personal childhood experiences. The ability to observe ourselves and to think clearly and rationally about what we perceive, allows us to become conscious of inner experiences that usually remain hidden.

Modes of Experience

To begin with one becomes aware of the activity of **visualizing** or conjuring up a clear memory picture of the tenth year. Visualizing is a natural perceptual ability that calls up pictures living in our unconscious memory, something we do quite normally and mostly half-consciously all the time. It can be refined by mental concentration to become fully conscious, readily available and a rich means of communicating with our past experiences. We may notice that these mental picture images are imbued with a sense of the past.

With **feeling** and **sensing** the experience becomes immediate, deeper and more intense, arising from hidden unconscious depths. Feeling and sensing are similar experiences and are sometimes used interchangeably. We often say 'I feel the rain on my skin' when we actually mean 'I sense the rain on my skin'. In feeling we are completely in the present and free of the body; when feeling sadness or joy I experience myself, but not my body; in sensing, however, I experience myself in relation to my body or the external world, using sensory organs to perceive sense impressions coming either from inside or outside the body. For instance, we have an internal sense that enables us to perceive our bodies' wellbeing so that we notice when we are hungry, thirsty or tired. We can detect fine areas of tension in many muscles, nerve endings and connective tissue areas; we can tell when we feel healthy and when we feel ill.

You can try to sense what is happening in your body right now. In the act of sensing, I go to meet a sense impression, intensely interested to know what is out there. I want to know all about this sense impression so that I can decide whether it is something I like or dislike. In sensing we connect with the world and integrate it into us, into our own experience of whether we like it or we don't.

In the activity of **reacting**, deeply unconscious experience wells up from hidden depths expressing itself in some reflexive action. We will include this realm of experience in the sphere of activity or of will inasmuch as the will has to do with human actions and reactions. One reacts in a reflex manner towards the cause of emotional hurt, in a way not much different to an irritation on one's leg that is relieved by scratching or by reflex movement of the leg. In the one instance it is an emotional issue, in the other a physical-biological one that triggers the reaction.

We can only become conscious of the four modes of experiences – visualizing, feeling, sensing and reacting – when we can observe ourselves in these activities. This is a conscious reflective activity that allows us to observe our own inner activity. In reflecting about something we are always removed from our previous experience, but usually we are not aware we are doing this. By consciously standing outside oneself in this mode of observing inner experience, one opens up a doorway to higher faculties of sensory perception.[5]

Psyche or Soul

This inner life of experience may be designated the psyche or soul in keeping with familiar terms. By experiencing the activities described above, soul life comes alive as an expression of one's own personal and intimate being. We thus find that these four basic activities constitute the psyche: thinking (all cognitive processes), sense activity (perception and sensation), feeling (including sympathy and antipathy) and will (all volitional processes in which we engage actively with the world).

In his *Model of Experience Literacy*,[6] Yehuda Tagar identifies four modes of actively exploring experience, by means of which every aspect of it can be expressed and communicated. He has developed a methodological process of entering an inner experience, staying there long enough to become acquainted with it, then making it visible by a gesture so that, when one lets go of and exits from it, one is able to observe where one has been. He calls this expressive process

Enter-Exit-Behold. You enter the experience by focusing awareness on the memory of an event and on the mental picture that rises up (visualization); you can then intensify the mental picture so that a bodily sensation, feeling or reaction arises. These are the stages we have described above. The process continues by trying to find a gesture, movement or sound that embodies the inner experience; next you move consciously out of the experience, even physically out of the gesture you have created, so that, from outside, you can observe in imagination the after-image of the experience. A simple example is recalling eating a lemon.[7]

The two modes of 'experience literacy' – gesture/movement and sound – enable us to penetrate inner experiences and express them more deeply. Together, in summary, the four modes are:

- Visualization
- Body awareness/sensing
- Gesture/movement
- Sounding.

Let us return to the experience of the anxious child – sensing the tightness in his body, feeling his fear or reacting to something unpleasant. I allow my body the freedom to authentically express these experiences in movement or gesture, like an actor or mime artist who uses the body to dramatize an inner condition. The feeling and bodily sensation brings about a corresponding bodily response, firstly in the form of a tight, constricted posture and then when the experience passes into reaction, in a movement of withdrawal away from something fearful.

I need only hold the reactive position for a few seconds, then move physically aside and observe or visualize my previous posture or movement as if seeing an after-image on the mind's inner screen. In my awareness I preserve the after-image of the terrified child trying to get away from something.

As I allow the picture to play before my mind's eye, another dramatic picture rises up in my consciousness: a nine-year-old child is standing under a tree aiming his pellet gun at a dove perched on a branch a few feet above his head. The dove is completely motionless and serenely peaceful as the boy pulls the trigger. The bird drops at his feet. He picks up the dead bird, holds it in his hands and is overcome with grief and guilt for what he has done. He flees in terror at the cruelty he has witnessed in himself and is unable to share this experience with anyone. For days he is inconsolable, deeply remorseful, and prays for forgiveness; he has had his first experience of death and has no one to share it with. In his sadness and loneliness he vows to be respectful of life ever after.

All the expressive arts, such as drama and dancing, draw on our capacity to give outward expression to inner experiences. The body as a whole, as well as every single part – the arms, chest, fingers, eyes, even the eyelids – can dramatically express the nature of experience. The fine nuances of expression, posture and gesture in fine art are likewise an external portrayal of what lives deeply within. Everyone understands the language of **movement** and **gesture** – babies, illiterate people and academics alike; we all know from our own inner experience what a gesture of joy or sadness means. In the same way, inner experience can be expressed outwardly in speech, in a verbal approximation that gives voice to a deep inward impulse or emotion.

> In the vow to be respectful of life, which later culminated in fulfilling his dream to become a doctor, the nine-year-old child was **speaking** his truth.

Finally the power of **sounding** can be used to enter the experience on an even deeper level.

> From the child's pain there emanates a sound – an inconsolable cry of deep remorse, giving deep expression to his experience at this age.

Sound is resonance or vibration. A violin string produces a particular sound according to its rate of vibration or resonance. The sound will depend on who plucked it, what was living in him at the time, the way it was plucked and so on. Is it possible that every soul experience vibrates the musical strings of the body, resulting in resonating frequencies that are stored and never forgotten in a vast sound-memory bank that lies close to the cellular organism?

Are we close to the mystery of memory here? Is it stored in us in resonance? If so, we may then understand why, according to Rudolf Steiner, memory is stored in that patterned, resonating, organized system of life forces known to traditional Chinese medicine as chi and to Indian Ayurvedic medicine as prana. Rudolf Steiner calls it the life or etheric body, or body of formative forces. He once described the life body as the synthesis of all the sounds of human speech resonating together.[8]

We shall be speaking a lot more about this universal and human life principle in the forthcoming pages.

In using the sounds of human speech – the consonants and vowels – we can therefore access the true sound of human experience and enter its deepest, vibratory level. From the sounds of the human voice and of human speech, of course, come the language and music through which you and I communicate with each other.

Conscious application of the normal faculties of the human psyche therefore make it possible to open up our personal inner experience of a particular time in life, firstly by observing inner phenomena of memory (visualizing), then by re-living the experience (sensing and feeling), subsequently seeking movements, gestures and sounds that give outer expression and form to resonant inner states, and finally by stepping away from this gesture to observe it as an after-image.

As we trace the journey of childhood unfolding in this book, or listen to the narrative of children entrusted to our care, it is possible at the same time to consciously shine the inner torch on our own experience. This makes exploration of childhood more meaningful, vividly personal and interactive. Our own personal experience begins to tell us what the tenth year was really like and illuminates an aspect of the universal child common to every child. The books and experiences of others will then merely confirm our own experience.

It needs to be said here that this means of meeting the child, through the child within each of us, requires a particular focus and the development of new skills that are usually acquired through coaching and practice. A good deal of patience may be needed before we start actively remembering original experiences. We will have many opportunities in the course of this book to try and access the inner world of childhood (the word 'remember' of course, literally means 'reintegrate'); and we may only connect initially with a small fraction of the original experience. But we should know that it is there within us and that we are making use of it all the time, consciously or unconsciously.

Mothers consult me who have received no training in childcare, yet know intuitively how to handle and speak to their children, even in the most difficult situations. Where does this intuition come from other than through their own original experiences? This is a fund of unconscious knowledge of which we can gradually become more aware.

There are many books on inner child work that deal with a range of these aspects.[9] The essential thing is to establish the relationship with our own original experience as a living, resonant reality.

In my own case I discovered something new about the nine-year-old child. From here, a new awareness, a deep feeling of love, empathy and compassion may unfold for the child. And through this connection one is more able to develop the capacity to empathize with every nine-year-old and his struggles. The insight this gives enables us to know what is needed to accompany a child through his difficulties.

Empathy

The capacity to remember and relive past experiences leads quite naturally to a second level of human experience that can enhance our insight into the world of childhood: this is the faculty of empathy.

Although empathy as a human capacity has existed since the beginning of time, it is only since the middle of the 19th century that empathy as a concept found its way back into the mainstream of human consciousness. In 1858, the German philosopher Rudolf Lotze introduced the word from the Greek *empatheia* meaning *to feel into* or *with something*. In 1903 the German word *Einfühlung* was translated into the English word *empathy*, and the word to *empathize* was coined in 1924.

This probably indicates that this soul faculty is still very young in humanity's collective subconscious soul life. In our time it seems to have become something of a buzz word much used by psychologists, philosophers, journalists and even politicians. There is probably no single faculty of the human psyche that could offer a more effective counterweight to the misfortunes that have befallen our planet and the human race than that of empathy. If a critical mass of human beings develop a conscious awareness and application of empathy in their lives, it seems fair to say that this could make a significant contribution to evolution; it might even be the single most important factor in rescuing the planet earth and the human race. For our purposes in this book, empathy is vital for reaching a deep understanding both of the child within us and the child in our care.

> Proceeding further with an inner experience of the remorseful nine-year-old, we find that this opens up a new level of awareness. With an open heart we listen to the deeply troubled child, heavy with the pain of guilt and remorse, and allow ourselves to enter into his suffering. This evokes an intense feeling of compassion for what he went through. We know what he has undergone because we feel our way fully into his experience. Through this powerful identification with his experience we can meet the child at a different level – that of empathy. To have someone whom the child feels can understand what he is going through is a special gift for him: he is no longer alone.

Empathy takes us beyond our own personal experience. It moves from 'me' to 'you'. If I delve deep enough into my own layers of experience I will discover that in my universal being you are in me and I am in you. This is an experience many are familiar with when they fall in love; and in fact, loving perception of the other is what is called for. Having found you within me, I can rise out again towards you with the will to find out something about you – to understand, feel and act in a way that can help you. And when I do this I experience an uplifting power that enhances my human potential.

How can we invoke empathy so that it begins to work its wonders for us and our children? Some will say you either have it or you don't, but this could also be said of someone who has not yet learned to write or to think logically. Before acquiring the skill one will be blind to its potential. Empathy is a capacity of the human spirit that can be developed and trained like any other.

Of course it is true that some people seem to have more empathy than others; some seem to be born with it, others to acquire it through a life of struggle or service. Almost every mother knows what empathy is. We have all been touched by it as babies and young children; some of us have been parents; many of us own pets; we have felt deeply for the street children and the AIDS orphans. Some of us have listened with empathy to our own inner, hurt child. Empathy begins with interest for oneself, which then moves towards interest for the other. The more you learn about yourself, the more you will know about the child in your care, the more you will be interested in him, the more you will wish to do the very best for his life as if it was your own; empathy teaches us *to do unto others as we would wish them to do unto us.*

When empathy flows unhindered towards a child, he feels understood, trusted and respected. You may not know exactly what he has experienced, but he will know that you have been there, present with him, and this will make him trust you. It will open up the space for a healthy relationship and the maximum opportunity for support and protection.

The example of re-invoking one's own experience as a nine-year-old illustrates how empathy can connect us in a unique and vibrant way with our childhood journey at any age. In the chapters that follow we will explore many opportunities for practising empathetic skills.

Creative Resourcing

The faculty of empathy leads us to a third level of enhancing human experience: this is the capacity that Tagar calls *invoking or resourcing*, which I choose to call *creative or innovative resourcing*. This is a faculty that can help us discover and provide what is needed in the child's life to resolve difficult issues.

Every human being is a wellspring of creativity. We may not regard ourselves as being creative yet a closer look will reveal that our very nature is intrinsically creative.

Biological and Psychological Creativity

From the moment of conception we are immersed in a biological creative stream that unites the forces of heredity with an organized system of living processes to guide and regulate the development of the child through to adulthood. In the next chapter we will explore the extraordinarily creative developmental processes of the child in the mother's womb. In subsequent chapters we will examine how the child's biological nature unfolds creatively as it grows downwards to 'grasp hold of' the neuro-sensory system, then the cardio-respiratory region and finally the metabolic-limb system over a period of twenty-one years. The highly organized life processes interacting together, guide and regulate physical and chemical substance to create a living body which grows through sequential stages of development.

The accompanying psychological stream of creativity becomes visible to us from birth as the child begins to unfold and elaborate his inner life. We notice first the high degree of sensitivity and reactivity to many sense impressions – a touch will evoke a bodily movement, an outer sound will elicit a certain reaction. Later, the life of feeling will become apparent as the child makes known his likes and dislikes in no uncertain terms. Thinking and reflecting become independent faculties only later in the soul's creative life.

In accordance with his specific soul nature and the environment he finds himself in, the child will use his soul faculties of sensing, reacting, feeling, reflecting and expressing to construct a particular personality that bears within it a variety of personality types or personae.

Let us say that an infant experiences that his mother, for whatever reason, is emotionally distant from him. He desires her warmth and love but senses that these feelings are not accessible to him; he reacts by crying a lot, waking constantly, feeding inconsistently and therefore not thriving. This aggravates his mother's difficulties because she is even less able to provide her baby with what he needs. The child's needs are not satisfied and he carries within himself, as a reaction, a constant feeling of anxiety and uncertainty that shapes his personality. He becomes a shy, anxious and nervous child. At the same time, he may learn to find comfort in a fantasy world of imaginary beings and enjoy hours of pleasure living in this world. Thus he is also a highly imaginative and artistic child. In this way he creates out of his inner experience an internal group of different personae that he discovers work best for him.

The world of the psyche is vast and infinitely varied, and in accordance with inner and outer environment and specific life needs, the developing soul will create a personality from its vast potential.

Working Creatively

What, you may ask, has all this creativity to do with understanding and caring for children?

Through our experience of reflecting, sensing, feeling, reacting, observing and expressing ourselves as outlined above, we become aware of a highly active and creative force weaving and working through every dimension of our existence. We may sense this as a stream of intelligence guiding our existence at every level: biological, psychological and spiritual. And it is part of our essential nature to express this creative world in creative deeds.

Some people are more consciously in touch with creativity, born with a natural gift for creative expression and an ability to express their innate creativity. Yet everyone has this as an inborn quality, and we can all nurture and develop it. It is similar to the empathy that we do not access until we become conscious of our deeper nature, discover our ability to feel with others and learn to make use of it in life.

If we learn to trust our creativity and look for ways to express it, we begin to open up an immense potential that we never dreamed existed. What percentage of your human potential do you think you are using? Most of us will admit that we are using only a very small portion of our creative possibilities.

Using Creativity to Resolve Problems

We saw in the example above that personal experience and empathy can bring us to deep insight into a child's situation. Following from this, *creative/innovative resourcing* enables us first to see and then do what is needed to offer further help. Here a process is set in motion to facilitate a deeper connection with the tenth year of childhood. How does this work in practice?

Above we saw that the child of all ages is always present in us like the rings in the tree trunk, and if we wish we can go there and rediscover him. When we find him we can do something to set the problems right. We can take up the task of restoring and redeeming for the child (ourselves) what his circumstances at that time did not permit. We have only to overcome the unfamiliar experience of communicating consciously with another part of ourselves, something we are in fact doing continuously and mainly unconsciously all the time. For the psyche finds innovative ways to cope better and frequently guides and instructs us how to do things more efficiently.

> Until recollection of this experience, there was no one the child thought could possibly understand his grief and remorse and so he suffered in his isolation. This grieving child is still present within me. But now there is someone – the person (myself as adult) who is taking the trouble to observe and understand the child; this person realizes that the child is today still hurting and that what he needs to heal his hurt and loneliness is a trustworthy, understanding, adult friend and guide. And this I myself can become for him! The child needs this so that he may overcome his hurt, mistrust and isolation.

This is an aspect of the self that can be invoked by imagining such an empathic friend, feeling our way empathically into him, sensing this person physically, becoming him in gesture and action and speaking out of him; to begin with this is enacted in the way the director of a play will assign a specific actor to play the role of a certain character exactly as the script demands. Later, when one knows the part it can be played invisibly within one. One can then create a partnership between these two parts of oneself – the hurt child and the trustworthy adult friend – just as one would help and support a nine-year-old child who was going through difficult times. In regular inner dialogue and interaction one can bring about deep healing of old soul wounds.

In the same way, new partnerships can be created with the actual children in our care, based on active, creative/innovative resourcing. When we sense what a shy child needs to help overcome his shyness, we can become the very character that can best build up his confidence – unconditionally loving, trusting, reassuring, protecting and praising. Though we may be assuming a role here, which the child needs, this does not imply any lack of authenticity on our part: we put our whole self into it.

In Summary

Our point of departure was our own human experience which opens a path to the inner world of childhood and adolescence. In travelling through the bodily experiences of sensing, mental imagery and physical expression in sound and gesture to our own original experience, we go back to the past. Through feeling and compassion we arrive at a soul experience of empathy that brings mindfulness into the immediacy of the present moment. Through observing and thinking we discover new insights and creative resources that can open the spirit to possibilities for the future.

This experience leads us to an awareness of our own full being and that of the child as a foundation for further exploration of child health. The body is the instrument that enables me to experience the outer world of matter; the psyche or soul is the inner life of experience itself, and the spirit is the part of my being that connects me to a higher spiritual reality, allowing me insight into higher truths.

Equipped with these tools for tapping into inner experience, we are ready to embark on a fruitful journey into the world of childhood and adolescence.

I bear hidden within you the wisdom, the life, the creativity of the past. There is so much that I can teach you if you will remember my story. It is present inside of you; you only need to re-experience it. Will you picture it, sense it, feel it and express it? There is so much that you can help me with if you listen with an open heart. Then you will know who I am, what I am missing and how to set me free. Then I will grow to become who you are and together we will discover your great potential. There is so much to learn, together.

CHAPTER 3

Where Do I Come From?

From a Faraway Star I Enter the World and Fashion a New Life

Does the prenatal life of a child begin at conception, or before? We do know with some certainty that the earthly existence of the child begins with life in the womb, but, like life after death, existence prior to conception is a mystery that crosses thresholds into other dimensions. We have no way, to begin with, of knowing anything about these pre-earthly conditions; and even the embryo's development is shrouded in uncertainty, for instance about when we should regard it as human.

Many young children ask, *Where do I come from?* What honest answer do we give them? The way we deal with this challenging question will affect our attitude to ourselves, our fellow human beings and life in general, for there is a world of difference between having a solely material or also a spiritual origin. If we originate entirely from the fusion between the material substance of an egg cell and a sperm cell, our whole being depends on this union alone. All our thoughts – such as this very question *Where do I come from?* – and feelings, for instance those evoked by the answer to this question, are then also a material product of the biochemical make-up that develops from this solely physical union.

Is our self-awareness a physical impulse, a neuro-chemical secretion that somehow lights up our consciousness? Or does it arise from a non-physical, supersensible organization that exists both independently of and interdependently with the physical organization? Is the specific personality and unique individuality of the child just an expression of the child's biochemistry or genetic constitution, developing somehow from the union of the father's sperm cell and mother's egg cell? Or does some kind of spiritual essence as an independent entity connect at some moment with the physical body and establish mutual interdependence with it?

As we embark on our exploration of the world of childhood, we need to establish from the outset a view of the human being that forms the basis for our deliberations. This investigation is one we can pursue experientially, as in the previous chapter, through our own independent thinking and our conscious experience.

Four Bodily Systems

Our culture and upbringing have taught us the importance and reality of the body. Through our physical senses we observe earthly objects in the form of minerals, plants, animals and the human body itself. Our bodies are composed of the chemical materials of the outer world; they therefore belong to this world, revealed to us only through our sense perception. We can observe the texture and shape of our own body, its form can be weighed and measured, its constituent materials can be analysed. The body's solid matter – teeth, bones and nails are the hardest and most rigid; cartilage and tendons are firm but not as hard as bone; skin is soft and elastic; hair is fine and silky – is relatively easy to investigate. The inner organs likewise have their various forms and textures: for instance a kidney is firm and compact whereas a liver is firm and pliant. All these materials belong as a compact, organized *solid* system to a human form that is uniquely different from the animal forms.

One may also notice without much effort that the body consists of fluid substances: there are secretions of different kinds, perspiration from the skin, blood and lymph that course through closed circulatory systems and internal fluids that permeate every cell of the body. We can visualize all these different fluids streaming, pulsating and mingling in continuous flowing movement as an organized *fluid system* largely contained within the contours of the solid organism.

With further observation and reflection, we can become aware that the body contains aeriform or gaseous substances: oxygen-rich air from the external atmosphere is continuously inhaled into the lungs, from where it enters the blood and is carried to every cell; carbon dioxide-rich, oxygen-poor air is then transported back to the lungs and breathed out again into the atmosphere; hollow cavity organs such as the stomach and bladder, and cavities like the sinuses are always filled with air. A volatile, highly mobile picture of an organized *aeriform system* can be imagined, which actively connects an inner with an outer world.

Finally, without too much additional effort, we can experience a fourth component as an innate part of our physical nature, namely our 'body' of warmth. A different grade of warmth can be experienced on the body's surface compared with its interior. A sensitive thermometer will reveal a difference in temperature between the skin, armpit, mouth and anal cavity. The internal organs likewise have their distinct warmth differences: for instance the temperature of the blood is 37°C whereas the temperature of the liver is 40°C. Every human being has her own very distinct, organized and differentiated *warmth system* which is singularly able to permeate all other physical matter – solid, fluid and gaseous – and is regulated to a large degree from within.[1]

These four bodily systems are complex and highly organized, and each functions according to very different laws. These are the same laws that govern material substance in the natural world. Let us now examine these laws.

Different States of Matter and Elemental Forces

The substances of nature are either in a solid, liquid or gaseous form and can be transformed further into finer states of matter and energy such as warmth and light. Each state of matter has distinct characteristics. Solid substances are clearly different in character from liquid or gaseous ones. All solids are compact, have contours and are fairly immobile, whereas liquids have less firm boundaries and, given the right conditions, tend to flow until equilibrium is achieved. What gives ice, water or steam their specific nature? They are all composed of the same chemical elements, hydrogen and oxygen, in the ratio of two to one. Yet they are all so very different in character. What is it that creates the difference? Besides the substances involved, there must be something else present in the different states of matter which endows each with its special nature.

Some kind of force is present in solid physical substance that brings about the character of solidity, contour and structure. All mineral substances such as salt or sand have a rigid and generally well-defined or even crystalline structure; we experience solid substances as objects which are quite separate from us, foreign and lifeless. Their earthly solidity also makes them the most impenetrable.

The elemental force working in fluid substances such as water or milk, is completely different, providing the character of watery fluidity and flowing form. Because they are not fixed and structured to the same degree, fluids can move and flow, continually adapting to the environment in which they find themselves. Their fluid, flowing nature also allows them to connect substances with each other, so that they mix, mould, merge, blend, dissolve and combine – all processes which are indispensable for life itself.

The forces living in the air permeate and connect with substance to a greater degree than those which act respectively in solids and fluids: the air stirs up the dust, dries out the sand and penetrates our food to provide us with aromatic fragrance; it is always present around us and we cannot live without it for longer than a few minutes. It is highly mobile with an enormous ability to disperse and expand into the widest spaces and, under pressure, to condense and shrink into the smallest confines. In our air-borne breathing and speaking we connect directly with other human beings. The element of air also allows other things to manifest and be experienced by us: sound becomes audible and light is made visible in the form and colour of things; the starry sky is clearest when the air is clean and pure.*

---

* It is not generally known that light is invisible, and can only be seen when rendered visible by a surface of some kind.

Although we do not conventionally regard warmth as a state of matter, its presence in fire tells as that it is a force existing in its own right. Apart from this natural phenomenon we either experience warmth as a quality present in the other substances of matter, or as an element integral to our own nature. Warmth is all-pervasive, capable of penetrating all natural substances: it warms the stone and creates the warm wind, and permeates every aspect of the human being – not just bodily tissues, but also, in its non-material aspect, our feelings and thoughts, our highest ideals and actions. It is also the force that brings all things into activity, transforming solid ice into liquid water and then into gaseous steam, germinating the seed and ripening the fruit. Warmth generates energy and drives all processes, and as such it is an all-powerful and indispensable activating force in the universe.

Four Modes of Enquiry[2]

Solid Observation

Modern, materialistic science is not wrong in its attempt to observe the physical world in physical terms, although this mode can only be of use in relation to the 'earth' element of solid substance. Here we can stand separate from the object and observe it without entering into it more deeply than noting its outer form, structure and composition. We can describe all details objectively with fixed concepts and descriptive references. This mode of observing is static and relatively rigid, confined as it is to the separate objects observed, such as the cells kept fixed and static under a microscope or anatomical specimens in preserve jars. This may be called solid or earth-bound observation. In this world of solid substance, the scientific tools of weighing, measuring and quantifying are entirely appropriate.

Fluid Observation

With a little effort, however, we can mobilize our thinking and imagine living objects as if they were in the process of developing and changing. For in reality living things are not static but constantly moving and changing. We can observe the transformation of living things though usually not instantly or continuously. We can watch a plant growing from a seed into a seedling and then into the mature plant through various stages in time. We can observe the plant, or the developing embryo – as we will shortly – at any stage, and imagine the unceasing growth that is taking place as long as it is alive. In this mode of observation, we need a kind of thinking and visualizing that is alive and fluid. As a young medical student I had the good fortune to study living chick embryos and to observe a sphere of life activity so powerful and vigorous that the transformation of embryonic forms happened almost visibly before my eyes. This mode of observation has a fluid nature to it; it is mobile and in constant flow and may be regarded as fluid observation in line with the living nature of fluidity that sustains life-imbued matter.

Aeriform Observation

In both the earthly and fluid modes of observation, the world of matter is always outside the one observing and belongs as described above to the realm of the body. Yet the moment we begin to notice how this world impacts on our inner being we find a very different perspective. Watching in awe as the chick embryos changed their form within the hour, I remember the feeling of joy and exultation I experienced, and a physical sensation of warmth and expansion which moved me to exclaim at the wonder of my experience and to share it with my colleagues. This is an experience of my own creative power. Whereas we can designate as body only what can be observed as an object outside of us, our own inner reality is one we ourselves create. This is a dimension completely independent of and distinct from the physical realm. The centre of my reality now becomes my inner experience. The world of embryological development becomes *my* affair; I connect it to my inner experience and I construct this world out of my own personal inner activities of feeling (joy and exultation), sensation (warmth and expansion), willed action (reaction, exclamation and the desire to share) and cognitive awareness (mental pictures, evaluation and concepts). These are the activities constituting the dimension we have named in the previous chapter the psyche or soul, which the human being creates herself, and which will be a major subject of exploration and experience throughout the book. Resembling the outflow and inflow of air in breathing – since it actively expands to connect with and penetrate the world, and contracts back into its inner centre with a new world of experience – this is a mode of experience which we can term aeriform observation.

Warmth Observation

We can enjoy the world of the soul for the pleasure and joy it gives us and keep it as our personal experience; or we can go beyond this and open ourselves to a further dimension. The joy I experienced in observing the growing embryo is present only as long as I am observing or recalling the experience. But my experience calls up something within me that wants to know what it is in the growing and changing forms that fills me with such awe. What is this force of life that moves and transforms matter so vigorously with an intelligence so precise and perfect that every part and every living function are so exactly synchronized with every other part and function? Here I begin to reflect on a mystery hidden in the outer world of nature, an inner law that governs the living world; and I deduce that in the vigorously growing embryonic cells there must be some kind of system of dynamic forces that guide and actively transform material substance. This invisible force is one that my activity of thinking discerns. Whether we call it chi, prana, life or etheric forces, it reveals itself to me as hidden law working through the external world. Here I am looking at things from a completely different perspective, no longer concerned with myself, with my own feelings of wonder for example, but deducing a significance that encompasses all living things. In my thinking, in other words, the world of nature can speak about itself, reveal its secrets, connect me with the essence of all things and thus bring insight, order and coherence into life. This is the dimension that may be called the spirit, to which the conscious soul opens in thinking. It is likewise a dimension completely independent of and distinct from body and soul.

Warmth is the element capable of spanning between body, soul and spirit: we can physically warm ourselves in front of a fire, we can feel emotionally warm towards someone or we can become fired up by an exciting idea. When I discovered the reality of this dynamic life force at work in embryos, my body instantly glowed with warmth. The mode of awareness in which warmth inwardly activates and warms my thinking to connect me to universal laws may therefore be called warmth observation.

Deepening Experience

The four ways of observing described above can be combined with the modes of experience literacy described in the previous chapter to gain a deeper experience of all aspects of life.

Let us say we wish to learn about an interesting plant in the garden. We begin by thoroughly observing its outer form and various parts, perhaps reading up about its inner structure and function and other interesting botanical facts; in this way we make use of our earth-bound sensing and thinking, connecting with the plant's *physical nature.* Next we observe the plant as it grows from seed to flower and fruit, and inwardly, with *fluid thinking,* visualize the plant growing and changing dynamically through time. Here we connect with the etheric nature of the plant, its living dimension.

Then we can pursue our observations further into inner experience in two ways: we can connect through deep empathy with the plant as it strikes our senses, and experience the effect it has on our inner sensing and feeling. We can find an appropriate gesture for the sensation. We can also focus on our inner mental picture of the plant and let this image work on us through sensing and feeling to form the gesture. The first focuses on an outer perception, the second on an inner perception or mental image. In *aeriform observation* we connect inwardly with the plant's inner nature, experiencing the plant's living processes and the forces of nature working on it.

Entering the fourth mode described above, we can now detach ourselves from the subjective feelings of the experience and, with the objectivity of *warmth beholding,* discover the inner law and 'being' or true nature of the plant. Here we connect with the creative forces and universal laws in which the plant is embedded, and through which it exists.

In this way we can also come to an inner experience of the four elements – of solid, liquid, air and warmth – as well as the four systems of the body in which each element chiefly works.[3] And in the same way we can observe our own inner child, or an actual child in front of us, and come to a deeper insight into her nature.

Body, Soul and Spirit

Through conscious awareness and conscious experience we can thus arrive at independent insight into the nature of the human being. And what we discover is that, in our totality, we do not consist solely of material substance, but of three fundamental qualities or characteristics that can be designated as body, soul and spirit. In all our further considerations we shall regard the growing child as comprising of these three constituents that connect her to three universal dimensions:[4]

The **body** is the part of the child that belongs to the given world of matter and can be perceived by the physical senses as an outer object. It provides the physical foundation, the vehicle and instrument for the soul and spirit to exist and function within the earthly dimension. The solid, physical part that provides form and structure is the physical body. The **life or etheric body** is the dynamic, flowing part that sustains all the life processes: that vibrating, resonating system already referred to above and in Chapter two.

The **soul** is the child's inner experience which she creates for herself as her own inner world. This provides the vessel within which the spirit can work, and expresses itself through cognitive activities, feeling responses, sensations, and willed actions.

The **spirit** is the aspect of the child which belongs to a higher spiritual reality and universal laws, to the realm of the true and good.

Each constituent appears to be connected to one of the four elements and can be directly experienced by a mode of observation and experience that is related to that element.

Physical body	solid system	solid substance	earth observation/ experience
Life body	fluid system	fluid substance	fluid observation/ experience
Soul	aeriform system	air substance	aeriform observation/ experience

| Spirit | warmth system | warmth substance | warmth observation/ experience |

For many years I was intrigued by the question: If the soul and spirit are independent entities existing within the body, where do they come from and how do they connect with the body and make it their earthly home? While the origin of the body as the product of the union of an egg and sperm cell is well known to contemporary science, the origin of soul and spirit is a subject that even contemporary religion has difficulty in explaining and for the most part ignores. I found the keys to understanding these questions in embryology – the science of prenatal human development from fertilization to birth – enlivened by an inwardly experienced approach to phenomenology, and illuminated by a spiritual-scientific view of the world.

The Journey to Earth

It is generally accepted that conception or fertilization is the moment when human development begins. It is also likely that this is the moment when the soul-spiritual dimension connects with the physical. But what takes place before this seminal moment? How do soul and spirit arrive at this point of entry into the material world? In most cases our conscious experience does not stretch back far enough to allow direct insight into these questions. The best we can do is read with an unbiased mind the accounts of those who profess to know about these things. In doing so we can create pictures of these events in our minds, then allow this imaginative experience to resonate through our soul and try to see if it strikes us as true.[5] Steiner, an accomplished researcher in the spiritual realm, gives us a detailed picture of prenatal experience, describing the preparation that is necessary before the momentous event of conception takes place.[6] As a working hypothesis let us consider Steiner's description of the prenatal journey and its culmination in the moment of conception.

He describes how, at a certain point in the child's spiritual history – in an earthly timeframe perhaps several hundred years after a preceding death – the eternal core of the human being, the human I[7] – makes a free decision to return to the earth after a long spiritual sojourn. It must return since it is only here that the I, by passing through earthly experience, can continue its transformational development through many lives or incarnations. This return is like the contraction in consciousness that occurs when one descends from a high mountain: at the summit the whole surrounding countryside can be seen; as one descends, the originally expansive and radiant view of the world becomes progressively constricted and dimmer. The human individuality, with help from cosmic beings, begins to fashion for itself the spiritual foundations for a future earthly body. Steiner calls this the 'spirit germ', which is the physical body's prototype contained in every human being.[8] Is this the origin of the universal child? He describes it as majestic and huge as the universe itself, becoming ever smaller and more contracted as the spiritual individuality moves towards birth.

How can we imagine this process? We can possibly gain some idea of it when we try to recall our experience of some event in our lives and find that all we are left with is the contracted picture of the event in our memory. One might also think of a contracted seed containing the whole potential for a new plant within it. The spirit germ has to compress within it a memory of the universe which comprises the whole human being for, as Steiner informs us, there are no mountains, rivers and forests in the universal spiritual world, only the human being in the company of other spiritual beings.[9] This descent passes through seven distinct spiritual spheres of the cosmos, each of which provides the human individuality and spirit germ with new and different qualities. Whereas the I passes on imperishably through many incarnations, the spirit germ is created anew prior to each new incarnation. In proximity to the earth, the united human I and spirit germ gathers up the soul body of the newborn child much like a magnet draws iron filings together in ordered and regular form. It is in this sphere too that the stream of inheritance and the future parents are chosen. Influences are brought to bear on the mother and father to come together. This spiritual nexus now consisting of the I, soul body and spirit germ awaits fertilization. Consciousness has narrowed down, the memory of the descent through spiritual spheres has become dim, but the will to be born escalates as the hour of conception approaches.

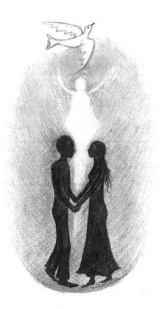

The folklore myths and legends of many cultures depict this pre-birth process with pictures of birds, often white birds, that bring the child's spirit down to earth. The white stork that brings the baby to the mother is a modern remnant of this ancient pictorial wisdom.

Male and Female Principles

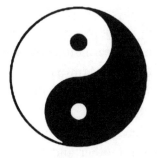

The details of the physical development of egg and sperm in the reproductive organs of the ovary and testes are well documented by medical science. The phenomena associated with these reproductive elements reveal a striking polar contrast between the male and female sexual components that appear to complement each other to create a complete whole. This is depicted in the ancient universal symbol of yin and yang.

Let us consider some of these physical polarities.

- The testes descend from inside the body to their location at birth in a sac outside the body; the ovaries are located deep inside the body, floating freely in body fluids.
- The male organ of procreation is a limb-like organ comparable to a sword, whereas the female organ is a receptacle that resembles a sword sheath.
- A healthy fertile male constantly produces mature sperm cells from puberty onwards into advanced age and will have two to three hundred million sperm cells available at all times for fertilization; a healthy fertile female will liberate one single mature egg cell for fertilization once a month at ovulation time, until her periods cease.
- The sperm are tiny, contracted, finely structured and highly mobile cells – the smallest cell in the body – consisting essentially of a light-refractile, bullet-shaped head and a fine, flagellating tail;

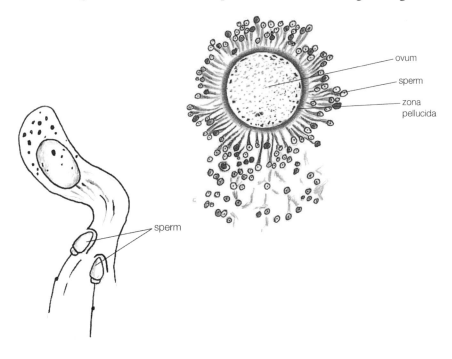

ovum

sperm

zona
pellucida

sperm

the ovum – the largest cell in the human body – is thousands of times larger, round and full, relatively simple in structure and immobile and enclosed in a thick light-reflective membrane.

- Within the reproductive organs, the male and female sex cells undergo a complex developmental maturation. As they mature, the sperm cells get progressively smaller in size while the ova get progressively bigger.

We can complement these observations with our experience of the masculine and feminine principles: the male principle tends towards heaviness, coarseness, hardness, physicality and activity – characteristics that are associated with the earthly dimension; the female principle in contrast tends towards softness, pliancy, spirituality and receptivity – qualities associated with the cosmic dimension. We may conclude that the male principle embodies forces specifically oriented towards the earth, towards vigorous, goal-directed activity and towards a form and structure that is hard and contracted, whereas the female principle provides cosmic universal forces that work away from the earth, and expresses its nature through the soft, warm, nurturing and yielding powers of spiritual, imaginative and intuitive processes.[10]

The Nature of the Cell

The cell is the basic organized unit of life, ranging from unicellular organisms like amoeba to the highly complex multicellular organs in the human body. Cells are grouped together, become differentiated and form the five different tissues of the body: surface tissue (epithelium), connective tissue, sclerous or skeletal tissue, muscular tissue and nervous tissue. These tissues are organized and differentiated further to become the various organs of the body. Thus all the tissues and organs are composed of billions of interconnecting cells, all of which originate from the female germ cell, the ovum, after it has been fertilized by the male germ cell, the sperm.

The cell consist of a semi-fluid colloidal material called cytoplasm contained within a surrounding semi-permeable cell membrane.

Cells vary greatly in size and form, and all contain various internal organelles, vacuoles and granules. The largest and most prominent component is usually the nucleus that contains the 23 pairs of filamentous chromosomes, whose specific sequences of molecular components (proteins, nucleic acids) constitute the genes. Every cell has the remarkable capacity of reproducing itself by replicating every component part of the cell. Thus one cell divides into two cells and so on. This function of cell division is the fundamental biological process of procreation, development and maturation of organ systems. As all cells have a limited life span and die off constantly, this function is also the means whereby organ systems are maintained. Yet this function of replication is only one of many other vital processes that take place continuously within the living cell. The cell has a life of its own and will continue to grow if removed from the body and provided with all its biological needs. It also breathes in oxygen and carbon dioxide, circulates fluids, transports nutrients, such as salts, sugars, fats and proteins, digests and destroys substances, secretes others and maintains a specific level of warmth. One can only marvel at the way in which all of these complex cellular activities are so perfectly regulated and sychronized with one another. Contemporary science explains this very precise functional and structural organizing capacity by attributing it to the command structure of the brain centre of the cell – the nucleus – and its chromosomal genetic material. The entire coding sequences of the chromosomes known as the human genome have now been fully deciphered and decoded, and are believed to regulate the form and function of every human capacity including thinking and feeling. The genome certainly appears to determine physical and chemical characteristics such as the colour of hair, size of the body and composition of chemical substances; but non-physical or non-chemical attributes such as musical virtuosity or a compassionate nature have never been proven to be induced in this way and cannot be attributed to the physical-chemical make-up. Only a materialistic conception of the human being must necessarily assume this. The moment soul and spirit are accorded their own independent reality, the genome's significance is limited to the biological realm of the human being.

Cell Structure

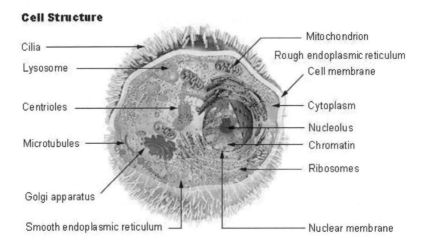

Medical science also conveniently overlooks what governs and directs the brain centre: there must be some power that organizes, regulates and directs the genetic material. We have already discerned an intelligence that governs and regulates life – the life or etheric body weaving and pulsating ceaselessly through all living activities. This works within all cellular activities and determines the ordering and functioning of all living chemical structures including the human genome.

The Stream of Inheritance

Both male and female germ cells contain only 23 chromosomes or in other words half the full complement of genetic material. The sperm contains the genetic material of the father who carries in all his body cells the combined genetic material of his father and mother, and so on back through endless generations. The ovum contains the genetic material of the mother who likewise carries the combined genetic material of her father and mother, back though the generations. With the union of ovum and sperm at fertilization, the genetic material of father and mother are mingled to create the full complement of 23 paired chromosomes, in other words 46 chromosomes, which are henceforth present in every body cell except for the sex cells. These undergo a specialized cellular replication where only half the chromosomes are produced. Thus every cell of the body will carry the combined genetic material of both father and mother. It should be emphasized again that this genetic material is composed of chemical substances which belong only to the realm of the physical/etheric body.

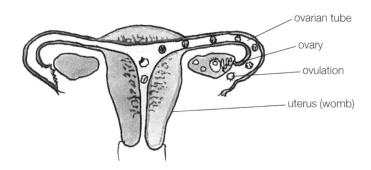

The Union

When the sublime moment of conception is close at hand, we may imagine that the spiritual complex of the child's I, spirit germ and soul body, is in a cosmic sphere close to the earth.

At ovulation, the mature ovum is liberated from the ovary into the sea of the abdominal cavity where it is drawn towards the open funnel-shaped end of the ovarian tube by sensitive, waving, anemone-like fronds guarding the opening of the tube; it begins to travel down the tube towards the mother's womb.

At the opportune meeting of the potential father and mother, millions of sperm cells enter through the mouth of the uterus and move chemo-magnetically towards the single ovum in the ovarian tube. The ovum is viable for only 48 hours and only one of the 200–300 million sperm cells will bring about fertilization. No human being has ever witnessed a live fertilization and the best live observation we have of this event is fertilization conducted under artificial conditions. Under the microscope, thousands of light flashes can be seen radiating towards the single light-haloed ovum, as the myriad of light-studded sperm rush to be the chosen partner to fertilize the mother cell. A beekeeper may be lucky enough to witness an event of a similar nature, namely the fertilization of the queen bee by thousands of male drones: the queen bee bejewelled by the light of the midday sun, flies out of her hive, soaring higher and higher to test the endurance and strength of the best of the comparatively armoured drones that rush after her like shining knights.

A number of sperm approach the ovum but only one is able to penetrate the radiant outer membrane – the so-called 'zona pellucida' – and enter the inner sanctuary. It is in this decisive, life-creating moment of union between sperm and egg, that the spirit germ descends to unite with the physical, fertilized germ cell substance provided by mother and father. We can see this extraordinary moment imaginatively as the shimmering dove of spirit descending to and connecting with the earth.

This moment of conception triggers a series of remarkable events.

- Sperm and ovum lose their discrete separate contents and identity and fuse into a new whole. One can observe under the microscope a moment of blurring where nothing can be clearly visualized. The fertilized ovum appears to be in a state of chaos out of which a new world can come into being, for out of chaos new beginnings can arise. Steiner describes the fertilized material as completely pulverized and able to surrender itself to the cosmic influences because of its physical disintegration.[11]

- Steiner informs us that the whole universe pours into this chaotic moment, imprinting the forces of the stars and planets on the exquisitely sensitive living substance: an influx of forces which determine the horoscope of conception.

- In uniting with the physical germ, the spirit germ is sundered from the complex of I and soul body to which it was initially connected, leaving in its wake a very powerful feeling of loss. This acts like a vacuum and draws together etheric life forces from the universal ether to form the child's future etheric body. Perhaps we can imagine the empty feeling of losing something very precious and desperately needing to fill the gap with something just as precious. The complex composed of I, soul and etheric body hovers invisibly in close proximity to the region where fertilization took place.

- All further growth of the germinal human being is initiated, and embryological development as we know it can now begin.

Embryological Development

Throughout the following description one should endeavour, using fluid thinking, to imagine this dynamic process in three dimensions and in continuous movement, so that one developmental process works synchronously with a multitude of others.

The single united cell, with single united nucleus and single set of 46 chromosomes, will cleave after about 30 hours into two cells, each with a nucleus and a set of 46 chromosomes. Each cell will

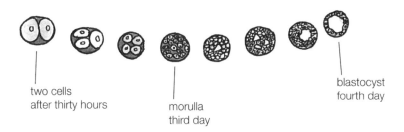

two cells
after thirty hours

morulla
third day

blastocyst
fourth day

replicate itself until 12–16 cells develop on the third day to form a compact, spherical, mulberry-shaped clump of cells known as a morula. This cleavage of cells advances rapidly as the developing embryo enters the uterine cavity at about day four. Now fluid percolates between the cells creating a confluent fluid area on one side and a concentration of dense cellular matter on the other, the embryoblast, the whole surrounded by a thin cell wall, the trophoblast. The embryoblast has an internal part, the internal cell mass which will become the embryo proper and an external part,

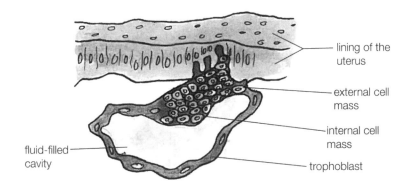

lining of the
uterus

external cell
mass

internal cell
mass

fluid-filled
cavity

trophoblast

the external cell mass which will become the future placenta. The embryo resembles a tiny bubble and is called a blastocyst.

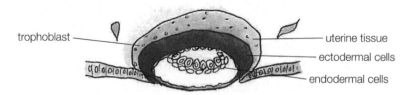

trophoblast ——————————— uterine tissue
——— ectodermal cells
——— endodermal cells

The trophoblast cells covering the embryoblast begin to grow into and penetrate the lining of the uterus, thereby anchoring the blastocyst to the wall of the uterus by about the sixth day.

At the end of the first week we see a pinprick-sized embryo firmly implanted in the mother's womb, governed perfectly by activities set in motion by the conceptual union. What, we may ask, directs these complex and precise activities and where does the impulse for growth and division of the cells come from? The events that take place in the second week give us the answer to this question.

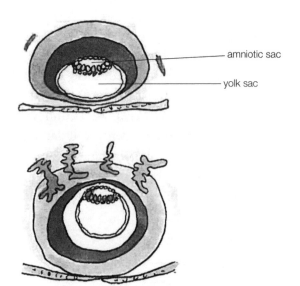

——— amniotic sac
——— yolk sac

During the second week, the embryoblast will differentiate into a two-layered disc structure – like two adherent coins of different thickness, suspended in a fluid cavity. This consists of a layer of flat (ectodermal) cells connected to the innermost layer of the trophoblast cell structure and a taller layer of attached (endodermal) cells. The ectodermal cells soon become separated by fluid-filled clefts, which coalesce to form a fluid-filled tiny sac, the amniotic sac. At the other pole, the endodermal cells will proliferate in the next

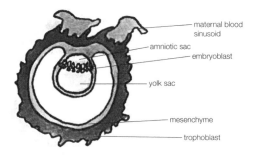

few days to surround a new sac filled with thicker viscous fluid, the yolk sac.

However, it is the growth of the trophoblast which is dominant during this period, actively growing and differentiating into different layers surrounding the embryoblast and penetrating ever deeper into the uterine wall. At this interface between embryo and maternal body, a communicating system of fluid-filled spaces will rapidly break through to connect with the maternal blood circulation, thereby establishing the nutritional lifeline and the future placenta.

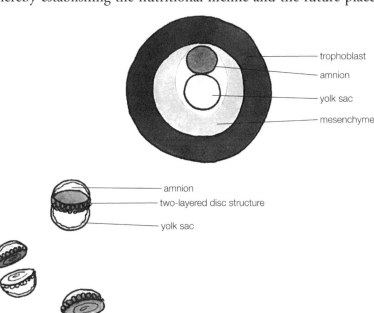

Towards the end of the second week, a new embryonic tissue called the mesenchyme will appear to line the inside of the trophoblast and surround the amniotic sac and yolk sac.

At the end of the second week, the germinal human being is the size of a pea and consists of a two-layered disc structure each connected to a globe-like sac; the upper ectodermal disc layer forms the floor of the hemispherical amniotic sac, the lower endodermal sac forms the roof of the hemispherical yolk sac. Surrounding this entity are the two other tissue layers, the mesenchyme and the trophoblast. There is as yet no resemblance to the future human being. In essence there are four spheres surrounding the embryonic bi-laminar or two-layered disc structure as shown below.

The Four Spheres

It is a remarkable and undeniable fact that these embryological events occur precisely in this way in every human being, as if guided by some invisible force, unchanged, one presumes, over aeons. What, one may ask, guides these events so exactly? Secondly, why are these four spheres formed *before* the development of the embryo proper, which lags strikingly behind? And thirdly, why do these four sheaths develop in the unique way they do, in their specific spatial orientation, in their particular sequential order and in their different composite tissues? It is only after these four spheres have been completed that the embryo surges forward in growth and differentiation in the third and fourth week. In the biblical story of creation, the heavens are created before the earth. Only then can the earth come into existence. The embryological phenomena reveal the same creative order: first the circumference comes into being, only after which the centre begins to develop. Embryological development may be seen to recapitulate mythological stories of the creation of the world and the human being, and several authors have cogently described these connections.[12] Steiner gives us a detailed description of the evolution of the earth in four cosmic evolutionary phases starting with a warmth phase, which he calls the Saturn epoch, followed by a light/air phase – the Sun epoch, passing into a water phase – the

Moon epoch, and finally attaining our current solid condition –
the Earth epoch.[13] König attempts to connect Steiner's description
of earth evolution with the maturation of the egg cell in the female
ovary prior to fertilization.[14]

To try to find answers to the three questions formulated above,
we will need to look more closely at these four sheaths and to
examine their relationship to the whole human constitution.

Through progressive branching, the trophoblast grows further
into the tissue of the womb; it develops to become the chorion,
which completely envelops the embryo and the other three sheaths,
protecting them and connecting them with the nutrients and
warmth of the blood from the maternal nurturing system. The
chorion actively takes what it needs from the maternal blood and
actively gives up to it what the embryo excretes. It will also become
the central organ of the embryonic blood system. The chorion tissue
over the implantation site of the embryo will become the future
placenta. The trophoblast /chorion appears closely connected to the
warmth element.

The mesenchyme layer that lines the embryo proper is the
connecting layer between the outer chorion and the inner life of the
embryo. The region where mesenchyme attaches the amnion and
embryonic disc to the trophoblast/chorion is the forerunner of the
future umbilical cord. It later connects with an outgrowth of the
yolk sac known as the allantois; together this mesenchymal/allantois
sheath has a strong connection to the forces of the air element.
In reptiles and birds it functions as an organ for breathing before
hatching.

The amnion is the watery sheath that directly surrounds the
embryo and is filled with a pulsating, circulating fluid containing
protein and salt.

The yolk sac contains a viscous physical/chemical substance that
nourishes the embryo in its early stages of growth.

The Fourfold Human Being

Let us now look at the human constitution from another point of
view, one we have touched on earlier – the physical body, etheric

body, soul and spirit – and then try to relate these aspects to the developing embryo.

Physical and Etheric

We have already noted that the physical body is made up of all the chemical substances of earthly nature, and provides the physical foundation for bodily structure and function. Experience readily informs us that there is a major difference between a dead body and a living body. At the moment of death, a living body, be it plant, animal or human, will begin to break down and disintegrate into its component chemical elements. This does not happen while it is alive. Something to do with the living organism holds together the integrity of form and function through a number of self-regulating life processes. These same processes are dynamically at work in the growing embryo. In Chapter two, in seeking the source of memory in us, we referred to the vibrating, resonating organization of life forces as the human life or etheric body. Above, likewise, we discovered this inner force through the activity of thinking described under 'warmth observation' above.

We can visualize the physical body as completely interpenetrated by this vibrating energetic system, which extends slightly beyond the physical body. This transforms the lifeless mineral constituents of the body into living substance capable of growing, reproducing, carrying out all biological processes, maintaining and repairing the human organism. Life is only possible when water is present. Water is the element that maintains life and, through its connecting and flexible nature, is most suited as the substance medium through which the life body can fulfil its functions. Is this the force that sprouts the seed and grows the plant? Is this indeed the organizing force, working through the element of water, that drives the physical developmental processes of all living beings in an unalterable pattern, directing the extraordinary synchronicity of every phase of development?

Soul or Psyche

We have also traced our own life of inner experience and discovered faculties that we characterized as psyche or soul. A sleeping person manifests very little of the psyche other than in her dream life, whereas the life processes are all highly functional during this state. The psyche comes alive in the dreaming state, and when we wake up and become conscious of the surrounding world. We can try to imagine these soul activities permeating every element of the physical and the life body, and extending as an aura perhaps an arm's length beyond the physical body. The soul faculties enable us to be sensitive and aware of our environment, as well as to develop an inner life expressed through reflective, emotional and volitional activities. Sensitivity and feelings are finely reflected and embodied in the organs which carry the air through the human body. The breathing system registers every change in our emotions. Indeed, the Greek word for psyche, 'psùkhè' is also the word for breath. The air's highly mobile and volatile nature is most closely connected to the psyche, and can thus act as its intermediary. As the wind shapes and forms a wave, so the force of the psyche, working within the element of the air, forms and shapes all developmental processes.

The I

Awareness of our inner experience directs us to our various soul experiences: we can be inwardly reflective, we can dive into sense impressions of the outer world, we can notice our experience of feelings or emotions, or we can become active in our will nature in different ways, and realize our aims and intentions. We can discover all kinds of personality types that we act out in the course of our everyday life: the mother, wife, daughter, child, the controller, the frightened person, the career woman and many others. So who actually am I? There must be someone who integrates all these different parts of my being. I act very differently depending on whether I am more focused on using my body, my soul or my spirit nature. Who is it who chooses to read this book, who decides to explore the inner nature of childhood and is able to observe the various aspects of soul experience? This capacity of self-awareness is only possible in the attentive wakeful state. Yet I am also present in the sleeping and dreaming states of the body and soul. The core of myself, my higher self, is a hidden, mysterious human power that never shows itself outwardly, but works selflessly through all my human experience. From around the age of three onwards, every person expresses this immense power through the most commonly used word in our vocabulary, the tiny, most humble, yet most powerful word – 'I'. It is the only word I can use to refer to myself. Through our self-awareness expressed through the word I, we realize we are beings completely separate from and independent of all others. This has something to do with the core centre of our truly human existence. This I or higher self is the unique individuality of the child that makes her different from every other person, shapes and develops her potential and directs her life journey in a unique and special way. It is this eternal individuality that we have described above that makes the decision to return to earth and that draws together the spirit germ, soul and life body of the child on its journey towards incarnation into the physical realm. It is this power and entity that determines and chooses our destiny. I choose to name it 'the I' because this is how we designate this truly human aspect of our being in daily life.

This third and governing power can also be visualized as penetrating every part of the human being and radiating for a distance of several feet from the centre of the heart. Just as the etheric body requires the mediating substance of water, and the psyche requires that of air to work into the world of matter, so the human I requires warmth to penetrate into all other realms. In its ability to penetrate all other states of matter and to generate energy and activity, warmth is the element most closely connected with the nature of the human I.

The I lives in the sheaths of body and soul, and belongs to the world of spirit that may live in it.[15] To the extent that the spirit lives in it, the I is eternal; to the extent that it lives in the physical, etheric or soul life, it is subject to the laws that govern these dimensions. For instance, the forces that live in the soul, such as fear, guilt or rage may be so overwhelming that the forces of the I submit to its dominance. In my work I constantly encounter human beings whose I does not manifest through spirit but through soul and often a very disturbed soul – for instance in addiction, abuse or depression. In the addictive personality the I is submerged in the addictive soul nature and subjects itself to these laws. It is inactive in its true realm, it simply makes a choice to be dominated by the lower soul forces.

The Fourfold Embryo

With this as a background, let us return to the grand picture that stands before us at the end of the 14th day of embryonic life: The spirit germ gives to the physical germ substance with which it has united, its universal human form. The rudimentary embryo is encompassed by four well-developed sheaths – the chorion, allantois, amnion and yolk sac – while the human I, soul and life body still hover above.

We see that the character of the four embryonic sheaths and the fourfold human constitution reveals compelling correspondences that may indicate some specific relationship between them. We may also find strong connections between these fourfold relationships and Steiner's four evolutionary epochs of the earth.

Chorion	**Saturn**	**warmth**	**human I**	**attentive awareness**
Allantois	**Sun**	**air**	**psyche or soul body**	**dreaming awareness**
Amnion	**Moon**	**water**	**etheric or life body**	**sleeping, living body**
Yolk Sac	**Earth**	**earth**	**physical or mineral body**	**lifeless corpse**

It was Karl König, in 1965, who first suggested that the four embryonic sheaths serve as the respective embryonic homes for the four human sheaths of body, etheric body, soul and I in this first phase of human development.[16] It is a plausible idea that becomes more persuasive the more one enters into the reality of the fourfold human being and the nature of the four embryonic sheaths.

The spirit-filled I, soul, and life body are present in the wider circumference of the developing embryo. They have not yet connected with it and will need to unite at some point with the physical organism. Each member of the human constitution will require a tissue-appropriate sphere within the growing organism from where it can carry out its special functions and activities. For this reason it seems that the appropriate embryonic sheaths must first be created to house the I, soul and life body before the embryo itself is formed, allowing these supersensible aspects to work into the embryo, and mould and shape it from a closer vantage point. Once the embryo has developed to a point where it can accommodate these supersensible forces, they will be able to enter the embryo itself and act from within it.

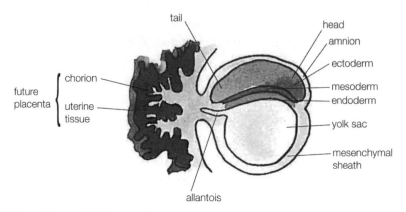

The Threefold Embryo

During the third week of embryonic development, dramatic events take place. First of all the embryo acquires a three-dimensional orientation. One end of the embryonic disc grows more rapidly, becoming wider, and indicates the later head region. The head-tail axis is created. Then cells from the ectodermal disc change their character and migrate into the space between ectoderm and endoderm creating a third middle layer called the mesoderm. The ectodermal layer becomes the back region, the endodermal layer becomes the front. The front-back axis is established. And into this third layer a thicker cord of cells appear in the midline to form the notochord, the primitive vertebral column, designating the midline axis, thus forming the left-right axis.

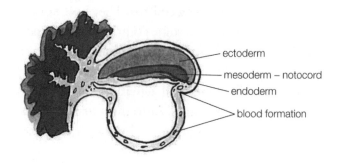

By the 17th day, three essential elements have been established within the embryo as prerequisite for a further union of the spiritual human being with the physical.

1. Orientation in three dimensions has come about: there is a distinct front and back, left and right, and above and below.
2. The primitive vertebral column provides the intention of upright posture.
3. The mesoderm has developed between the layers of ectoderm and endoderm to create the third germinal layer where – in coordination with the chorion – the embryonic blood will be formed. The blood is the carrier of warmth, which, as we have seen, is the element through which the I connects with the physical organism.

Steiner tells us that on this day or soon after (up to the 21st day), the supersensible nexus of human I, soul and life body unites with the physical body:[17] it is tempting to assume that the life body unites with the watery amnion sheath, the soul connects with the aeriform mesenchyme/allantois sheath and the I enters the warmth sphere of the chorion. The physical body has its foundations in the yolk sac.

In ancient legends, the 17th day appears to be an auspicious day. The Great Flood begins on the 17th day of the 2nd month (Genesis 7: 11), and the Ark came to rest on Mount Ararat on the 17th day of the 17th month (Genesis 8: 4).

Although there is as yet no closed blood circulatory system, there is nevertheless a very clearly visible pulsating stream of tissue fluid moving from head towards the tail. At about day 18 or 19, cell clusters appear at various points in the streaming fluid. It is unclear whether these clusters arise through densification and slowing down of the tissue fluid or develop out of the mesenchymal tissue. These clusters fuse to form cords of cells which canalize to create tubes that connect together to establish, within a few days, a closed, connected system of blood vessels. These convey the streaming fluid from head to tail.

Only towards the end of the third week do cell clusters appear on either side of the head pole, indicating the origin of the primitive heart. The developmental sequence of the blood circulation is very significant: we first see a pulsating stream of tissue fluid, then a closed blood vessel circulation develops and only then does the heart appear. This points to the fact that the tissue fluid and bloodstream do not require the heart to drive the blood circulation, as is postulated by contemporary medical science. If there is no physical pump, what moves the blood in this organized way? The answer again lies in the invisible etheric forces. Like the power of the sun which drives the cycles of nature, these forces weaving dynamically through the blood drive the circulation.

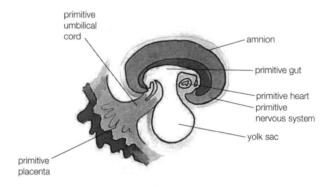

The embryo is now growing very rapidly. As the embryonic disc increases in size, especially in the head-tail axis, and the amniotic fluid cavity progressively grows, the embryo bulges into the amniotic cavity and folds progressively forwards and backwards until it gradually lifts off from the yolk sac. This results in important changes.

1. Part of the yolk sac is pinched off to form the primitive gut.
2. The heart cell-clusters come together in the midline and fuse to form a thickened heart tube that descends into the chest region.
3. The amnion gradually encloses the embryo.

By the end of the third week – after just 21 days – the early placenta is formed, the three-layered embryo has found its spatial orientation and has lifted off from its nutritive base, and the primitive heart and blood circulation, and gut and nervous system, are all in place.

We may visualize the child's I, soul and life body now united with the physical body and working through their respective embryonic sheaths throughout the rest of life in the womb.

The three germinal embryonic layers will form the foundation for the future human organism.

In later chapters we will describe three principal constitutional systems of the human being to which the structure and function of all individual organ systems can be assigned.

- Neuro-sensory system – the information-receiving system that provides the biological basis for psychological functions of thinking, sensing and all cognitive learning.
- Cardiovascular-respiratory system – the archetypal rhythmic system that provides the foundation for all biological rhythmic functions, in turn providing the dynamic basis for our life of feeling.
- Metabolic-motor system – the system that generates metabolism and movement and provides the foundation for all will-based functions.

All the tissues and organs contained in these three constitutional systems are derived from the following three germinal tissues.

- The ectoderm will form the tissues and organs of the neuro-sensory system.
- The mesoderm and endoderm will form the tissues and organs of the cardiovascular-respiratory system.
- The endoderm and mesoderm will form the tissues and organs of the metabolic-motor system.

The embryo at this stage (three weeks) is about the size of a small pea and resembles a tiny watery spherical globe attached to the inside of the mother's womb.

The period from the 4th to the 8th week of development is known as the embryonic period, at the end of which all the major features of the external body, including face, eyes, ears, nose and limbs can be recognized. In the 4th week, the three germinal embryonic layers of ectoderm, mesoderm and endoderm will begin to differentiate in uniquely specific ways to form the foundations of all the individual organ systems. During the 5th week the brain begins to expand much faster than the rest of the body, generating more than 250,000 brain cells per minute! By the 6th week, these organs are virtually completely formed and separated into their different parts, perfectly guided in

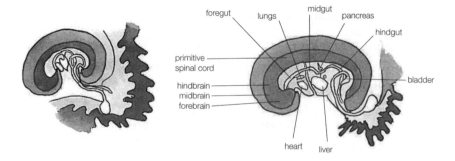

exquisite synchronicity. For instance, the heart has folded, cleaved into four chambers, with internal heart walls and valves. The digestive system has divided in the most complex fashion into all its different sections.

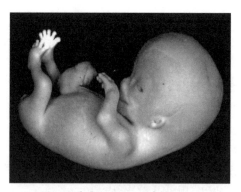

8-week human embryo

The finely structured nervous system with its sense organs has been formed and is already functional; and the limb buds have appeared. It has taken approximately forty days for the basic structure of the human being to be formed and the first spiritual-physical equilibrium to be established. Stanley Drake points to this period of forty days as the period during which the soul-spiritual nature of the child can adjust to physical earthly reality.[18] This period of forty days as an adjustment period between different states of consciousness is reflected in ancient mythologies: Noah waits for forty days before opening the window of the ark; Christ fasts for forty days in the wilderness; there is a period of forty days between the resurrection of Christ and his Ascension.

This exquisitely formed human being is suspended in its ocean of living, form-shaping fluid, embedded in its air-sensitive mantle and its warmth-protective sheath

The subsequent period of life in the womb, the foetal period, from the 9th week onwards, is characterized by rapid growth of the body. The head that was one-half of the body length is about one-third at 20 weeks and about one-quarter at birth. By 12 weeks the face becomes human-like, hair begins to grow and the sex can be determined. Between 16 and 20 weeks, foetal movements are first detected by the mother.

Life and Consciousness in the Womb

From the perspective of a spirit-based science, a life and consciousness that belong to the embryo itself are present by the end of the 3rd week. Organ systems are formed and functional by the 6th week. One may assume that a stable equilibrium exists between this soft, pliant, vigorously growing body and what dwells within it as soul and spirit. As will become evident in subsequent chapters, there is a master plan unfolding from the moment of conception throughout the development of the child and adolescent, whereby the three supersensible members connect themselves sequentially with the body and penetrate it ever more fully. The first stage of this incarnation process unfolds in this gestational phase in the womb.

Although the developmental activities of the foetus progress independently of the mother, it is nevertheless highly dependent on the environment of the nurturing mother for all its biological needs, conveyed to it via the placenta and umbilical cord. At the same time, it is protected by the organs and tissues of the maternal body – such as liver, kidneys and immune system – and by the placenta, from many potential hazards in the maternal environment.

The unborn child awakens progressively to her own experience.

When does she begin to sense and feel her environment? When does she begin to react to outer and inner stimuli? Four-dimensional foetal imagery shows foetuses at 12 weeks appearing to stretch and kick, at 18 weeks to open their eyes and at 26 weeks to scratch, 'smile', 'cry', hiccup and suck. They can react to various sensations such as temperature, sound, colour, light, smell and taste. Are these reflex or purposeful reactions and movements? Are the quickening foetal movements in the 4th month, the first felt by the mother, an outer sign of this awareness and reactivity? During the 5th month, movements become stronger and the mother feels them forcefully. We know that the eyes are fully formed and mobile by the 6th month and the eyelids open and close. By this time the development of the foetus has attained a level of independence that allows her, under optimum conditions, to survive outside the womb. By the 7th month most premature babies survive.

By connecting empathically with the life of the foetus, we can awaken to an awareness and experience of the unborn child in the womb.[19]

Core Picture and Care of the Unborn Child

- A mother and father each offer one single germinal body cell as two halves of the inherited substance that will provide the physical-chemical substance for the future physical body.
- This provides the physical substrate for the higher members of the child to enter the realm of earthly embodiment or incarnation and to begin a new journey on earth.
- At conception the spirit germ that may have something to do with the universal child unites with the fertilized physical germ.
- Four embryonic sheaths are first created into which the four higher members enter in the third week; from here they direct the gestational development until physical birth takes place.
- The first 280 days of this life take place in the hidden, nurturing and protective confines of the mother's womb.
- The vast majority of pregnancies produce normal babies. The causes of 40 to 60 percent of all birth defects are unknown. Genetic factors are responsible for about 15 percent; environmental factors for approximately 10 percent and a combination of the two for about 20 to 25 percent.

In order that the growing embryo and foetus receive optimum care and protection in an extremely vulnerable period of existence, their future custodians should be aware of the following potential dangers.

- There are generally greater maternal and foetal risks for teenage pregnancies and women over 35 years of age. The teenage mother is physically, emotionally and socially less able to support a healthy pregnancy: physical immaturity, poor eating habits, alcohol, drugs, lack of partner support are some of the factors that increase the risk of having a baby with health problems; these include low birth weights, organ weaknesses, prematurity, foetal alcohol syndrome and many others. Older mothers have a much greater risk of stillbirths, miscarriages, ectopic pregnancies and congenital abnormalities as a result of tissue ageing and chromosomal aberrations.
- A healthy and balanced diet containing proteins, vitamins, mineral and other essential nutrients is essential to prevent foetal risks and abnormalities.
- Exposure to X-rays and other types of radiation that may affect the unborn child adversely should be avoided since actively growing cells are highly vulnerable to radiation. Other medical interventions during pregnancy such as ultrasound investigations and amniocentesis (amniotic puncture) should be limited to those that are essential for optimum care of mother and child.

Diagnostic ultrasound uses very high frequency sound waves to scan the foetus in thin slices and creates a picture of the foetus by reflecting repetitive ultrasonic beams onto a monitor screen. It has been in clinical obstetrical use since the late 1950s mainly for diagnozing and confirming early pregnancy, determining the age and size of the foetus, pelvic size, the position of the placenta, malformations, multiple pregnancies and a host of other information that has greatly reduced the risks for mother and child. Research over the past three decades has examined five controversial endpoints where ultrasound may be a risk factor: these are childhood cancer, dyslexia, non right-handedness, delayed speech development and reduced birth weight. There is controversial evidence with regard to the latter three endpoints but most medical authorities and institutions claim there is no unequivocal evidence of adverse effects and that the sensible use of diagnostic ultrasound far outweighs the risk that may be present.[20] Since it is probably impossible to fully exclude the possibility of harmful effects, it is better to err on the side of caution when deciding whether to expose the unborn child to these high-frequency sound waves.

Amniocentesis is a procedure in which a small amount of fluid is withdrawn from the amniotic sac by a needle inserted through the abdomen and uterine wall that is guided by an ultrasound picture. It is used mainly to screen for genetic abnormalities which can produce conditions such as Down's syndrome and neural tube defects such as spina bifida. There are low risks associated with this procedure, which include leakage of amniotic fluid, injury to the foetus, infection and rarely miscarriage, although the statistical risk of losing the child is quoted as 1 in 200.

- Excessive physical exertion, exposure to extreme heat or cold, continuous loud noises or vibrations, and long periods of travelling, especially air flight, should be avoided as far as possible.
- Diseases such as rubella (German measles), AIDS, syphilis and genital herpes can be transmitted from mother to child. An effective rubella vaccine is available but it must be administered at least 90 days before pregnancy commences to be safe for the growing child. An HIV-positive mother can pass on the virus to the foetus, either in the intra-uterine period, during the birth process or via breast feeding. Treatment with anti-retroviral medication can reduce transmission. Syphilis can be detected and treated effectively. Most babies contract the herpes virus during birth and due to the high morbidity and mortality associated with this should be delivered by Caesarian section. Mothers with diabetes or hypertension should be carefully treated to prevent foetal abnormalities.
- Sanctioned drugs such as alcohol and nicotine, all recreational drugs such as heroin, amphetamines and cocaine, and medically prescribed drugs such as antibiotics, sedatives, antihistamines, the birth-control pill (some women continue to take the pill

not knowing that they are pregnant), hundreds of others, are potentially dangerous for the foetus. Even certain herbal remedies may be harmful. The golden rule is to use only drug and medicinal substances that have been well-documented as safe for use in pregnancy.

- It is well-documented that the emotional state of the mother has an influence on the unborn child. Maternal stress has been linked with spontaneous abortions, premature births, low birth weights and difficult deliveries. Every effort should therefore be made to reduce emotional stress in the mother and to create an optimally supportive environment for mother and child.

If we enter actively into the rich inner and outer phenomena that the embryo and foetus present to us, we can form a vivid imaginative picture of life in the womb.

My delicate, expansile body floats weightlessly in the pulsating fluid that passes freely through my transparent body; I feel part of a greater whole; I hear celestial sounds; I feel the warmth and light of the sun's pulse. My tissues expand and grow in vibrant activity. As my body grows bigger, the space around me becomes smaller. I cannot move as freely. My head draws me gradually downwards; I feel the weight of gravity; I lose my mobility as I begin to outgrow my first earthly habitation. The will to be born becomes ever greater. I sense the time is near and signal to my earth mother that she must prepare for my arrival on earth.

CHAPTER 4

The Journey:
The Three Births of Childhood

My Journey Spans Three Births and Three Cycles of Seven Years

This chapter will give an overview of childhood through to adulthood, as a clear route map for each phase of the journey we will be exploring in more detail in subsequent chapters.

The child, somewhere in his nature, bears an irrepressible will to engage with life on earth. Where does this will come from? It cannot come from the child's physical-material nature but it is far more plausible that it comes from his soul and spirit, endowed by prenatal existence. We have witnessed how conception sets in motion an unstoppable developmental process that culminates in the birth of the child. This is the beginning of his journey on earth.

As we travel on our exploratory voyage we will see how the developmental process continues with the same resolute determination over the next two decades: an infallible developmental law unfolds, manifesting in all the predictable growth phenomena of every healthy child. The child finds his way into a new physical body that will serve as his home and vehicle. He will need to get to know this body, transform it and make it his own.

We may infer from this that all the phenomena we experience during the voyage of childhood, all the developmental milestones and changes we observe as the child travels through the different stages of childhood and adolescence, express the way in which his soul-spiritual nature increasingly penetrates and connects with his physical-material body. In fact, the entire developmental process from childhood to adulthood is the story of the embodiment or incarnation of the soul and spirit into the child's material nature.

Let us try to perceive this deeper reality at work behind the outer phenomena of child development.

Three Landmarks

Three major landmarks in the developmental terrain of childhood and adolescence stand out so clearly that they cannot be missed. The first one is the **physical birth** of the child, the second is the **change of teeth** in the seventh year and the third is **puberty** which takes place around the fourteenth year. These milestones occur approximately every seven years, signalling a transitional stage where one life phase has been completed and the next begins. Each of these may be regarded as a kind of birthing event that announces a certain level of developmental maturity.

> I have worked hard to complete this leg of the journey. Now I can relinquish one particular dependency and move on towards full independence.

These three births and the three seven-year periods that connect them are the road map we wish to follow in our exploration of the child's journey towards adulthood.

The Road Map of Childhood and Adolescence

These three landmarks divide the journey into four sections, as illustrated in the Road Map on page 94:

- The first period from conception to physical birth was explored in some detail in Chapters one to three;

- The second period of early childhood, spanning approximately seven years from birth to the change of teeth, will be covered in Chapters four to seven;
- The third period of middle childhood, also approximately seven years from the change of teeth to puberty when adolescence begins, will be explored in Chapter eight;
- The fourth period of late childhood and adolescence spans the time from puberty until adulthood. Although this begins tentatively at the age of about 18, it only comes fully into its own at 21, again a period of approximately seven years. We will cover this period in Chapters nine and eleven.

The Fourfold Child – Three Births

In previous chapters we examined in some depth the four principal constituent aspects of human nature: a physical body made up of the chemical elements of the mineral world, a life organism that vitalizes the physical body in all its many biological functions, a soul organization that provides this living body with awareness and sensitivity, and an inner core nature which makes each of us into a unique, self-aware individual.

The only birth which is generally acknowledged as such is the birth of the physical body. However the other three, non-physical or supersensible aspects likewise undergo a process of development to a certain stage of maturity and then also come to birth. Each of these 'supersensible bodies' then continue to grow and develop further throughout life.

Birth, one can say, is the emergence of a growth process that has attained a certain level of maturity following a period of inner containment and often unseen development. Writing this book came to birth only after much inward reflection and preparation. A civilization, an initiative, or a child who is born, emerges out of a developmental process only once it has matured to a sufficient level. And this usually occurs in a confined and hidden place, like a seed that requires the right conditions before it will germinate. The flower blossoms like a new birth after the leaves have unfolded, and the butterfly emerges from the cocoon after a time of inner growth and transformation. In the course of development, living things go through cycles of gestation and birthing. Thus human development is the chronicle of birth, growth, transformation, gestation and further birth again at different levels of maturity. We can look back to our own repository of original experiences to recall gestation and birthing experiences of various kinds.[1]

Physical Birth

The development of the physical body from conception to physical birth was described in Chapter three. As the embryo grows we saw at a very early stage how the four embryonic sheaths make their appearance in order, it would seem, to provide a home by the end of the third week for the child's higher members to engage in the developmental process. From the protective peripheral shelter of these sheaths they are then able to direct the growth and maturation of the physical body for the remainder of the gestation period. The outer embryonic sheaths – the chorion and mesenchyme/allantois – give rise to the placenta and the umbilical cord that together serve as the mediating organs between mother and foetus.

The placenta is a discoid, cake-like organ that belongs jointly to mother and child. It is made up of a foetal portion formed by the chorion/mesenchymal sheath and a maternal portion formed by the innermost layer of the uterus; each develops its own independent blood system that connects back to its respective blood circulation. A placental barrier is created that prevents the mixing of maternal and foetal blood.

The primitive umbilical cord arises also from the embryonic sheaths, at one end of the embryo where the mesenchyme connects amnion and chorion. It becomes progressively constricted with folding of the embryo and elongates progressively to become a spirally tortuous cord measuring 50 to 60 cm at birth. It is the lifeline connecting the foetus with the placenta.

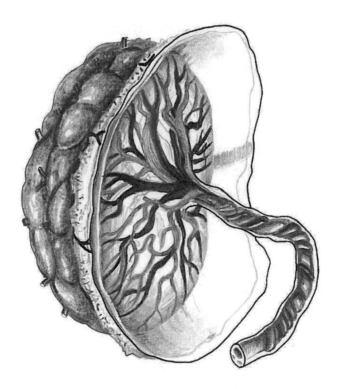

The placenta is a most remarkable organ which, as we have seen, is created by and for mother and child, in that it provides for the interchange of material substances during intra-uterine life. It simultaneously performs a number of life-sustaining tasks, functioning as:

- a lung that brings oxygen to the foetus and takes carbon dioxide away
- a digestive organ that transports nutrients such as water, salts, sugars, fats, amino acids and vitamins to the foetus
- a liver that builds up nutritional substances (carbohydrates, proteins)
- a kidney that excretes urine containing unwanted metabolic substances
- an endocrine organ that synthesizes hormones (oestrogen, progesterone and human chorionic gonadotropin – HCG) which maintain the pregnancy
- an immunological and protective organ that acts as a barrier to pathogenic organisms and harmful substances.

Let us imagine the following:

> The physical body of the embryo is unfolding dynamically within the protective and nurturing embrace of the embryonic sheaths, deep within the womb which itself is deep within the mother's body. The placenta lies between mother and foetus as a life-supporting organ for the foetus. The latter is entirely dependent for its survival on its connection via the umbilical cord with the placenta and thence the maternal organism. It requires 280 days for the physical body of the child to mature to a level of independence where it can free itself from the support of its protective sheaths. During this time the mother offers unconditional nurturing and protection until the child is mature enough to exist separately in the world, as an autonomous entity.

In the momentous process of giving birth, the child breaks out of his ensheathed space, becomes separated from his mother when his life cord is cut and emerges as a separate physical human being who henceforth can live an autonomous existence. He has arrived as a physical human being in the physical material world. We will examine this birth in greater detail in the following chapter.

Birth of the Life Body

The newborn child is brimming with life. He cannot grow and develop without the force of life working through him. Physical material such as sand or rock cannot sustain life, and all biological functions such as cell division and metabolism, maintenance and repair are only possible because of the organized system of active life forces we have chosen to call the 'etheric'. It is this system of forces that gives life to the child and drives the growth and transformation of the child's physical body.

At birth this physical body is predominantly an inherited body, a developmental product of the unified physical substance of mother and father. But these original inherited cells are constantly being replaced over the next seven years by the child's own actively functional life processes. The child himself, we can say, is transforming and remodelling this inherited body into a body he can call his own, that is suitable for his further life journey. This bio-organic transformation process has, like the gestational development of embryo and foetus, a highly organized mode of action. Working its way sequentially through the body's systems, it acts first on the neuro-sensory system, then on the system of rhythmic processes and finally on the metabolic system. It takes the best part of seven years for the growth of the neuro-sensory system to be completed, after which time a remarkable event occurs.

In his seventh year the child begins to shed his first set of teeth, and the first of a new set erupt. He does not shed his skin like a snake or drop a finger or a toe like a tadpole shedding its tail, but instead his teeth drop out! Why the teeth and what does this signify? Whereas all other tissues including the hard bony skeleton have been replaced by new cells, perhaps many times over, by the seventh year, the cells of the milk teeth are just too hard and dense to dissolve and replace like other cells. The only way is for them to be cast out. Thus the emergence of the new teeth is the signpost announcing that a point has been reached in the child's development when the entire inherited body has been completely transformed.[2]

> My second body has been born. I carry with me now not one single cell of what I inherited from my parents. I have transformed this inherited body and I have fashioned my own new teeth, just as I have fashioned the rest of my body.

What is it that creates these new teeth and transforms the old inherited body into the child's own new body? Behind the complex biophysical and biochemical changes that we see taking place in the growing child, stands the architect and enlivener of the physical body, the etheric genius: bringing about this transformation, it works steadily through this gestational period of seven years to change every living inherited cell into one that now has the stamp of the body's own life forces. Only when these life forces have attained a certain degree of maturation can the etheric body come to birth.

Just as the physical body of the child is protected in the embryonic physical sheaths provided by the mother's body for nine months while he develops his own autonomy, the etheric body of the child also needs a gestation period during which it grows and develops within a protective etheric sheath for the best part of seven years. This sheath is provided primarily by the etheric life forces of the mother and to some extent by the father and close family members.

How can we picture this process? There is an ancient myth I once heard many years ago, depicting the growing child connected by a silver life cord to a golden sun which resonates with the cosmic sounds of the life-supportive universe. This points to the invisible connection so tangibly present between a mother and her child. One may observe, for instance, how the nutritive or emotional ill-health of a mother can impact on the health of the child; a depressed mother frequently has to deal with a recurrently ill child.

The first milk tooth that falls out is met with great excitement. The whole family and of course the child in particular, senses the importance of this event. It is indeed a cause for celebration, for it is the child's second birth. A significant milestone has been reached and, with instinctive wisdom, we wish to reward each tooth that falls out, since it brings him closer to the completion of his own body. This process occurs over several years as the child attains his full second dentition.

With the emergence of the child's own permanent teeth we see changes taking place in the child's mental and cognitive processes; he begins to think differently, becomes able to think more abstractly and his memory becomes more continuous and expansive. Thus, with the birth of the etheric body and the completion and conclusion of certain organic functions, other functions become active. It is as if a part of the etheric life force is liberated from its organic activities, becoming progressively more available for other activities. This means that the same formative life forces which previously facilitated the growth of cells and guided their integration into the physical organs, now allow mental life to 'grow' and to flow into developing soul structures or 'organs'.

Steiner describes this transformation precisely.

> The forces that prevail in the etheric body are active at
> the beginning of the human being's life on earth and most
> distinctly during the embryonic period; these are the forces
> of growth and formative development. During the course
> of earthly life, a part of these forces emancipates itself from
> this formative and growth activity and becomes the faculty
> of thought – those forces which in ordinary consciousness
> produce the shadow-like world of human thoughts. It is
> of the greatest importance to know that the human being's
> ordinary forces of thought are refined formative and growth
> forces ... And this force of thought is only a part of the
> human formative and growth force that works in the etheric.
> The other part remains true to the purpose it fulfilled at the
> beginning of the human being's life.[3]

Thus this change of teeth signifies a certain degree of completion
of the dynamic process of remodelling the inherited body, and
dramatically announces the birth of the etheric body.

This second birth of childhood – the birth of the etheric life
forces – frees the child from his parental etheric sheath, thereby
permitting a further measure of independence. This birth can be
recognized by many changes that occur at the time. Morphologically,
the child loses his round chubby form, becoming relatively slimmer
and contoured. Physiologically, the activity of heart and lung as well
as all other rhythmic functions in the body become a new focus of
development.

Corresponding psychological changes are also seen. The child
moves from experiencing the world mainly through imitation and
creative activity to experiencing it through feeling. The full range
of emotions – joy and sorrow, love and hate – are felt more deeply
than before, colouring thinking and behaviour. The child's thinking
becomes less directed by sense perceptions and more imbued with
imaginative pictures that arise out of his own creative faculty. But
the change of teeth is the most powerful image of this second
birthing process.

School Readiness

Only now is the child ready for primary school because the faculties needed for thinking and memorizing in a school-appropriate way are available through freeing of the formative life forces. If we call on the child's abstract thinking and memory prematurely, we will be drawing forces away from essential, formative biological activities. This leads to a weakening of the body's organic foundations. Children entering the Waldorf School[4] are for this reason carefully assessed for school readiness, an important indicator of which is the change of teeth.

Enlightened educators in other systems, in Scandinavia for instance, have also observed that children from the seventh year are much more ready to learn than younger children. They are also less vulnerable since the birth of a more autonomous etheric body provides them with greater resilience. One has the feeling that they now have their own 'etheric skin' delicately protecting them.

Birth of the Soul Body

From a very early age the growing child has an inner life that allows him to be conscious of and sensitive to the impressions of his inner and outer world. This is due, as we have seen, to the presence of his soul that governs all drives, impulses and desires, and the soul functions of sensing, feeling and all volitional activities. When these soul forces engage with the physical-etheric body, a sentient or soul body comes into being.

The soul body, like the physical and etheric bodies, follows a similar process of development: it has a pre-birth gestational phase, a birthing process and a postnatal developmental phase. The gestational phase takes place over a period of approximately fourteen years, during which it is growing and developing within a soul-protecting sheath.

Initially the developing soul body of the child is ensheathed by the soul activities of his close community; these include all the soul qualities of his parents, but also the collective voice of the community: the customs, religious convictions, the manners and morality of the social group in which he finds himself. The child therefore relies heavily on the guidance and protection of parents, and of the community in which parents find themselves. Later on, as the child finds his own community of friends, this embraces and contains him. This is why the group psyche – as it manifests in the gang, fashions and fads, best friends etc. – will feature prominently in the child's soul life, representing as it does the psyche of the primary school child until he comes of age.

The unprotected soul life of a child is therefore especially vulnerable to psycho-emotional impressions. Whereas the physical-etheric body takes the brunt of environmental assaults in the first seven years, it is the different aspects of the developing psyche which can be directly injured in the second seven-year period.

During the first seven years, this soul activity works most powerfully through the life of the senses and the activities of will (drives, desires) and is intensely involved in the development and the healthy function of certain organ systems, finely shaping them and developing their inner sensitivity. The infant's tongue, for instance, is sensitive to the chemistry and consistency of the milk that enters his mouth. Watch how his whole being senses the flow of milk deep into his body.

Likewise, all the inner organs develop an 'organo-awareness' sensitizing them towards their respective functionality; thus the secretions of the digestive system are highly sensitive to the nutrients that come to meet them: the salivary glands secrete a different glandular composition for proteins or starches; fat that enters the digestive tract immediately induces a flow of bile or pancreatic enzymes which break down fats; the liver is highly sensitive to the different breakdown products of digestion as well as to many toxic substances; the heart is sensitive to the blood content, the lungs to the composition of the air. All the organs and tissues of the body owe their sensitivity to the developmental activity of the soul body in the first seven years of life.

Then, from the beginning of the change of teeth in the second seven-year period, the forces of the soul body begin to metamorphose and become active in the rhythmic functions of such organs as the heart and lungs. We will see later how these rhythmic processes provide the physiological basis for the psychological function of feeling. By working on the rhythmic processes of the body – the rhythms of the heart, the breathing, digestion, of sleep and countless other rhythms – the soul is developing the life of feeling in the young child. With maturation of these organ systems, the soul body will then become more active in metabolic and limb development. At this stage the sexes differentiate properly, accompanied by growth in the larynx, chest, muscular and skeletal system as well as in the development of the sexual organs.

The soul, moving through these organs, brings about powerful physical and emotional changes reflected in the surge of hormones, increased muscle mass and bone growth. The soul or sentient body has a powerful investment in the urogenital organs which, as we know at first hand, are closely linked to our sentient life. With the maturation of the sexual organs which takes place at puberty, the soul forces conclude their work in the reproductive sphere and are available for other functions.

At puberty the soul body is born and becomes free of its protective sheath. This is a major threshold when the child takes another huge step forward in his development. Just as the change of teeth expresses the closure of one developmental period and the liberation of growth forces for other faculties such as memory and imagination, so puberty testifies to the conclusion of a second life epoch and the awakening of 'postnatal' soul forces.

At this third birth – the birth of the soul body – the child's organism is now developed to such a degree that he can begin to direct his attention to the outer world in a new way and gain a greater measure of control over his environment. This is possible because the psyche has begun to loosen itself from its activity in building up the organs, becoming free for individual soul expression. He now has the beginning of a soul skin, a self-contained life of feeling and awareness, which allows him to open himself more safely to the outside world.

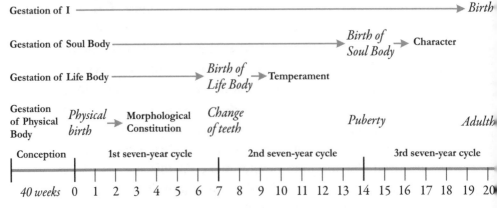

The Road Map (see Appendix for a fuller version)

The three births are the three transitional stations in three seven-year periods that span the development of childhood and adolescence. These seven-year cycles provide a foundation for a deeper understanding of the developing child. To gain insight into these cycles of childhood and youth, we will need to have a working knowledge of the threefold child.

The Threefold Child

We have discovered through our own experience that a human being, and thus naturally a child, consists of the three fundamental dimensions of body, soul and spirit. The body belongs to the world of nature and comprises both physical and life bodies. The soul is the inner world of the child and encompasses the experiences of thinking, sensing, feeling and will activities. The spirit is the aspect that connects the child to higher spiritual dimensions. This view is like looking at the human being from a high vantage point. When we descend from these high altitudes we can discover other essential elements of the child's nature.

Let us begin by looking phenomenologically at the morphology of the human body.[5]

Firstly, as obvious as it may seem, the human body always appears to us a specifically human form: it always has a head with a face in front, attached to a chest and trunk; upper limbs are connected to the chest, lower limbs are connected to the trunk and so on; in the form of every child, we see a human archetype coming to expression.

Secondly, when we look at this human form in a fresh and unprejudiced way, the distinctive features are: a **head** region which is the upper section of the body, is round in shape and is relatively immobile apart from the movement of the jaw. Then a **middle section** comprising the **chest region** which is barrel-shaped, connects the head to the **lower section** of the **trunk** and has movement limited to the action of the lungs and diaphragm. Finally we have a lower region comprising the **abdominal–pelvic area** and the **lower limbs**, which are the most mobile parts of the body and have a distinctly radial and linear character.

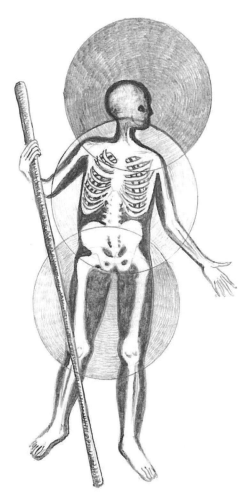

Head   **– upper section**
Chest   **– middle section**
Abdomen/pelvis/limbs – lower section

There may be other ways of representing the human form but as we shall see below, this threefold division offers a sound basis in our further explorations of the human constitution.

Looking in more detail, above and beyond overall morphology, we notice that the head houses the brain behind a wall of solid bone, and the main sense organs of sight, hearing, smell and taste. The brain has its extension in the spinal cord and in the fine network of nerves that issue from the brain and spinal cord and course throughout the body. These **neuro-sensory organs** are finely formed and generally have a symmetrical structure; for instance there are two eyes and ears, two fairly similar sides of the brain and bilateral nerve pathways, all with very finely formed parts.

In contrast the abdominal-pelvic area houses the **metabolic organs** – including the digestive organs, liver, spleen, gall bladder, pancreas, kidneys, and hormonal and reproductive organs. These organs are generally not as finely shaped and are non-symmetrical: there is only one liver, one spleen and one uterus.[6]

The **limbs**, like the metabolic functions, are built for movement and comprise muscles, bones, joints, and tendons. Deep within the bony substance the bone marrow produces the various blood cells which form an essential part of the metabolic-limb system.

Within its rhythmically spaced bony rib cage, the middle section houses the **rhythmic organs** of the heart and lungs, which are somewhere between the other two sections in terms of their symmetry, their fine structure and their mobility.

Neuro-Sensory Tissue Function

We can probe further into the body by examining the microscopic and physiological nature of these three systems. Neuro-sensory tissue is finely formed and has a poor capacity to grow, multiply and regenerate; nerve cells are formed in the embryonic stage and do not readily regenerate when injured.

Certain components of this system, such as the white matter of the brain, nerve tissue, and the lens and cornea of the eye, contain relatively little blood. The neuro-sensory system functions as a central information-receiving system of the body, gathering information from outside and leading it towards the brain. Its direction is centripetal, towards the centre, which is the spherical head. One can experience this dynamic directly by imagining oneself as the neuro-sensory system drawing sensory information centripetally towards one's centre.

Metabolic Tissue Function

The metabolic tissue, in stark contrast, has enormous transformative and regenerative capacity. For instance, the cells that make up the lining of the intestinal tract are replaced every three days and a damaged liver that still has an intact structure can grow back to its normal size. The metabolic organs all have to do with metabolic activities that move, generate or remove substances dynamically in a centrifugal direction, from the body outwards, utilizing functions such as absorption, transport, secretion, excretion, etc. The movement here is essentially from a centre outwards, namely centrifugal. Again, if one imagines oneself as a metabolic centre, the dynamic moves from the centre to the periphery.

Rhythmic Function

The primary rhythmic organs of heart and lungs exhibit continuous rhythmic activity in their alternating mobility and immobility. You can feel how your chest expands, pauses, contracts, pauses, expands, pauses; and continues like this throughout life. Through the rhythm of contraction and expansion, systole and diastole, these organs transport and circulate the blood and respiratory gases in the body.

Developing tangible awareness of our own bodily processes can give us an inner imaginative experience of these three dynamic functions.[7]

The Pervasive Threefold Principle

We notice further that this threefold principle is present on a smaller scale in every part of the body. Thus in the **head** itself, it is the round upper rigid part – the skull and the forehead containing the compact rounded brain – that is most head-like in nature. The middle part contains the nose which is the entry and exit point of the rhythmic breathing system, and the part of the face that lends us greatest facial expression – the eyes, nasal region and mouth. The lower part of the head is the most mobile and can be regarded as a modified limb by virtue of the presence of the jaw joint. If you examine a skull carefully, you can hardly fail to notice the similarity between the jaws and the limbs: the two upper jaws like metamorphosed upper limbs contain 10 upper milk teeth like ten fingers, the two mobile lower jaws like modified lower limbs contain 10 lower milk teeth – ten toes.[8]

The **heart** has its own nervous tissue and nerve-conducting system; in its systolic and diastolic function it is the archetypal

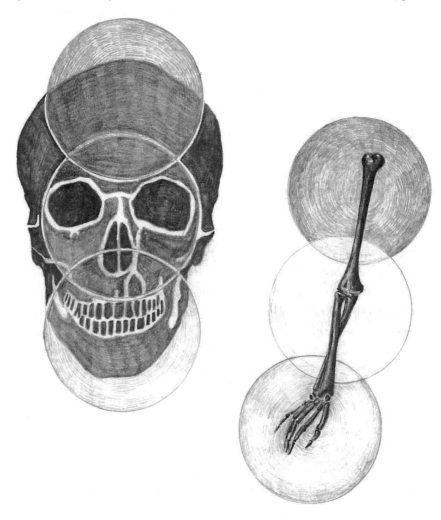

rhythmic organ. It also contains valves that open and close, and specialized muscles that move rhythmically.

The **hand** or **foot** has a compact round heel part, a central palm or arch and a more mobile and radial part, the fingers or toes.

The Threefold Cell

Every single cell in all tissues exhibits these three divisions: the round nucleus containing the genetic coding material is the brain of the cell; the mitochondria are the organelles responsible for cell respiration; and other components, like the diffuse tubular limb-like systems of the endoplasmic reticulum, Golgi apparatus and other granular structures, have distinctive metabolic function (see diagram of a cell on page 48).

This principle of the whole always represented in the part – the macrocosm always contained in the microcosm – was well known to our ancient forefathers and was called the 'law of correspondences' by alchemists. This shows us that although the neuro-sensory system is chiefly contained in the head region, it is spread throughout the whole body; and the same is true of the other two systems.

When we now observe the other aspect, our inner life, we discover other interesting phenomena. By experiential means we have already found soul life to have the following characteristics:

- Experiences of thinking such as reflection, reasoning and mental picturing as fully conscious activity in waking life;
- Experiences of feeling as a partly conscious activity similar to dreaming;
- Experience of will as an unconscious activity similar to sleeping.

Here too, therefore, we discover a distinct threefold division in the constitution of the human soul.

There is nothing more real for the human being than his own experience. If we are true to our experience and acknowledge it as real, with its own independent reality, we will have to conclude that the soul is a self-contained, independent entity and that its faculties constitute our experience.

As a self-contained entity independent of the body, we posed the question of the soul's origin. In Chapter three we explored imaginatively its journey towards, initial connection with, and progressive union with the physical body.

If we wish to be consistent with this picture of the soul, we will have to ask the second age-old question: Where does the soul reside? Through what parts or processes of the body do the soul activities of thinking, sensing, feeling and will connect and unfold their function?

The Brain Soul

Ancient cultures regarded the heart, liver or breathing as the seat of the soul. Contemporary biomedical and psychological thinking, based on a materialistic world view, sees the seat of the psyche in the brain and substantiates this conclusion through a wide spectrum of evidence-based research that claims to link soul activities to neurological function. In the following chapters the relationship between body and soul will be explored in greater depth and an attempt will be made to validate the specific correspondences. For now, let us simply assume that the physical body's correlation with the cognitive and sensory psychological functions can be observed in neuro-sensory processes and their extension into the sense organs.

When I form a mental picture of a tree or remember a past event, I presuppose a previous sensory experience when I first saw the tree or experienced the event. Senses are all specialized parts of the nervous system and are connected to the brain by nerve fibres. Conscious thinking requires the instrument of the healthy brain for its active function. A great deal of scientific research substantiates this connection.

The Feeling Soul

However, when we examine modern research phenomena factually and without preconceived ideas, we find that feeling- and will-based experience are connected with organ processes other than the brain.

Observe a child in deep feeling and see the subtle changes in the blood circulation and the respiration. Anger or shame will immediately cause a child to blush as blood fills his face, before mental activity is activated; fear will cause pallor through movement of blood from the periphery to the central vital organs; joy, delight and enthusiasm will create a pleasant warm sensation as blood circulation becomes harmonious.

Feelings always affect the breathing in some way, making it go faster, slower, suspended, more regular or irregular, deeper or shallower.

It appears, therefore, that the life of feeling is somatically linked with the respiratory and circulatory systems, those organs connected to the rhythmic system of the body that provide the basis for all biological rhythmic functions.

The Will Soul

When a child activates his will through some drive or desire, his body will always be seen to be in movement, and the organs most active will be those of the locomotor system – muscles, bones joints etc. – and those of the metabolism. We can discover that the unconscious activities of will are supported by the complex processes of metabolism, whose generating activities and ramifications again extend throughout the entire organism.

Body and Soul

It was Rudolf Steiner who, in 1917, after 30 years' research into human nature, first made these revolutionary discoveries about the threefold nature of body and soul, and their connection.[9]

There appears to be a close correlation between the three principle systems of the body and the faculties of the human soul that make use of these three systems to express themselves.

If we compile all the above phenomena we find that the human being has a distinctly ordered tripartite nature, in which each 'realm' functions according to specific laws and principles. For the sake of clarity we can put this into a schematic summary to illuminate the distinct differences between the three spheres:

Neuro-sensory system	thinking/sensing experiences
Rhythmic system	feeling experiences
Metabolic-limb system	will experiences

HEAD	CHEST	LIMBS
Neuro-sensory system	rhythmic system	metabolic-limb system
Round	round – radial	radial
Immobile	semi-mobile	mobile
Symmetrical	intermediate symmetry	asymmetrical
Finely structured	intermediate differentiation	undifferentiated
Non-regenerative	intermediate regeneration	regenerative
Receiving information	rhythmic functions	energy and substance-generating
Centripetal tendency	centripetal/ centrifugal	centrifugal tendency
Consciousness pole	mediation pole	life pole
Cold/death	intermediate warmth	warmth/life
Contraction/systole	systole/diastole	expansion/diastole
Thinking/cognitive activities	feeling activities	will/volitional activities

Underlying these outer phenomena is the overarching threefold principle of body, soul and spirit. Experience of the nature of the body will tell us that the neuro-sensory system's cold, compact and contracted quality, its centripetal tendency, immobility and relative lifelessness, is ruled by the laws of the body; the metabolic-limb system's warm and expansive nature, its centrifugal tendency, mobility and life-sustaining nature can be experienced as governed by the laws of the spirit. The rhythmical and mediatory nature of the rhythmic system places it in the realm of the soul forces which mediate between body and soul.

Psychologically, however, this polarity is reversed: the neuro-sensory system, as the pole of waking consciousness and thinking experience, is ruled by the laws of wakeful cognitive awareness; the life of the will belonging to the metabolic-limb sphere can be experienced as actively connected with our sleeping nature; for the will as we have seen is completely hidden from our conscious awareness; and between these two, feeling life corresponding to the rhythmic system resides in a dreamier form of consciousness.

This is the threefold picture that the universal human being conveys to us. We will apply these principles to our exploration of the child's biography through successive phases of childhood.

Biographical Transformation of the Threefold Child

The child's developmental journey, as we have seen, proceeds in a systematic and unalterable manner, following ordered laws of development. Here I will give a brief overview of this biographical process, and this will be expanded in subsequent chapters.

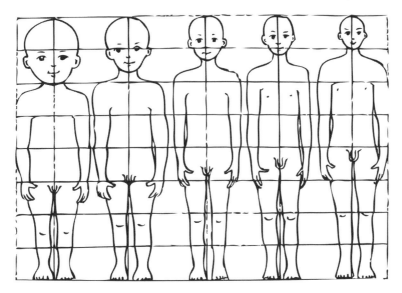

Diagram illustrating scheme of body proportions (according to Stratz)

In the first period of intra-uterine development and the first seven-year period up to the change of teeth, the head and neuro-sensory system are formed first and grow fastest, reaching almost full development at about the seventh year. This is well illustrated by the head size and weight at various ages: at birth it weighs 1/6th of the entire body weight, compared to 1/10th at 10 years and 1/35th in adult life.

At the same time the soul is powerfully active in the life of the senses and will, whereas feeling and thinking life are less prominent. When the young child is awake he is constantly moving and absorbing sense impressions through every sense organ.

In the middle period of childhood, biological development focuses intensively on the regulation and maturation of the cardiovascular and respiratory functions. The chest sphere now predominates. It is only by the 14th year that the circulation and lungs become fully developed. Because feelings are intimately connected with rhythmic processes, the soul is working particularly in feeling life during this period.

The last period of childhood, from puberty onwards, is characterized by the development of the metabolic and motor systems; we see a powerful growth spurt where the limbs, metabolism and sexual functions begin to develop more actively. Hormonal organs and the limbs are only fully developed by 18 to 21 years. This is the period in which the faculty of thinking is consciously developed.

Two Currents of Development

Two distinct but simultaneous and synchronistic streams of development may be discerned in the phenomena presented above. The one is biologically driven and determines form and function; the other is psychologically guided, and comes to expression in soul functions. In terms of the interplay between body and soul nature, they develop from opposite poles:

- In early childhood the *neuro-sensory system* and *will experience* develop together
- In middle childhood, the *rhythmic system* and *feeling experience* unfold. In late childhood the *metabolic-limb system* and *thinking experience* come to maturity.

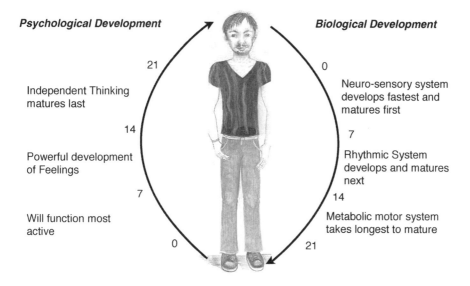

Psychological Development   *Biological Development*

21   0

Independent Thinking
matures last

Neuro-sensory system
develops fastest and
matures first

14   7

Powerful development
of Feelings

Rhythmic System
develops and matures
next

7   14

Will function most
active

Metabolic motor system
takes longest to mature

0   21

Synchronistic biological and psychological development
(From: *Enhancing Your Child's Potential*, R. Goldberg 2002:
Dreamcatcher Publications)

The formative forces proceeding from the life/etheric body start
in the head region, work their way through the chest region and
complete their organic growth tasks when the metabolic limb system
matures in early adulthood. They operate through three periods of
seven years.

The awakening soul forces working through the soul body start
in the will sphere of the metabolism, penetrate upwards through the
feeling realm of the rhythmic system and complete their work when
the thinking activities of the neuro-sensory system have matured
in early adulthood. They likewise work through three seven-year
cycles.

Childhood can only be understood when these two developmental
currents are properly grasped, for all the phenomena we observe
in the growing child are an expression of the way body and soul
unfold in the growing process. This key developmental model will
be explored in greater depth in following chapters. As we try to
understand the interconnecting law of body and soul development
unfolding in three cycles of seven years, we will once again recognize
the archetype that belongs to the universal child underlying the
biography of every individual child.

In the beginning I am active in my will.
When my body is ready I am born into matter;
My perceptions unfold as I build my nerves and senses;
With wonder I discover the world,
Both the sun and the earth.
When my life forces are active I am born into life;
My feeling awakens as I develop my rhythms;
With the pulse and beat I can feel the world,
Both the light and the darkness.
When my soul body begins to flower I am born into soul;
My thinking strengthens as my limbs grow strong,
With my empowered will
I can step into the world
Both in my power and in my weakness
As an independent person.

CHAPTER 5

Citizen of the Earth

I Arrive on Earth as a Unique Individual in a Unique Body

For most parents, the physical birth of a child is a momentous event, never to be forgotten, and celebrated at every birthday. It is the culmination of nine months of the most careful work of growth and development that takes place completely hidden from our gaze. We may have seen a two-dimensional scan of the foetus, but we know virtually nothing about the unborn child. We wait with great suspense and expectation to see for ourselves who this person really is. And her emergence into the physical world is one of the greatest joys we can experience. The anticipation, mystery, and transcendant, other-worldly nature of the newborn child fill us with awe and reverence. Something about the newborn child is different from anything else we know. And it is less what we see visibly in front of us that gives us this feeling, but rather what we cannot see, what we sense lives in the future of the child, still unborn yet present in seed form. This soft, helpless body will grow in time into a strong, mature adult and allow the individual to unfold her human potential.

From the perspective of the child who has elected to be conceived and to be born, physical birth is a decisive and wilful act to leave the safe confines of the mother's body and to enter a new and strange environment. We have considered (as a hypothesis) how the child's soul-spiritual nature descends through cosmic spheres to make its first prenatal connection with the earthly, material world by uniting towards the end of the third week with the embryonic sheaths. From this peripheral shelter and safety the soul and spirit guide and regulate foetal development in the womb. During the gestation period of 280 days, the growing child is protected from earthly influences by the dwelling her mother provides. A new life is unfolding in the sanctuary of her mother's body; a child is growing through the unconditional biological support of the mother's life processes. This is an awesome picture. An incomparable intimacy is created that underlies the unique kinship between mother and growing child: a bond which exerts an immense influence on the wellbeing of the child, especially in her first seven years of life, and will continue throughout both their lives.

In the final weeks of pregnancy we can sense how the call to enter the world becomes ever more powerful as earthly influences become stronger. At a certain moment the child knows she is ready to move forward on her journey: she has to let go of a warm, nurturing shelter and face the rigours of a potentially harsh environment. And she has to negotiate a relatively small, dark and narrow passage to find her way into the outside world.

As the labour of birth begins, our creative imagination can picture this descent into earthly reality.

> My head descends into the vortex of the womb, drawing me down towards the portal of the earthly world. I approach the birth canal, it slowly yields and expands to my urging. I enter the gateway, propelled forward by my headstrong will, and squeezed onward by the muscular, massaging will of my maternal partner. My earthly drive becomes ever more powerful until the mantle of celestial water that protects me can no longer bear the pressure, and the membrane ruptures. The life-sustaining water drains away and I feel my earthly weight as the pressure of gravity presses down powerfully on my head and body. My heartbeat increases rapidly; I am forced downwards, squeezing painfully through the tight, dark and narrow space; and then, with a final thrust, my bruised head emerges into the fresh air and light-filled space.[1]

At this auspicious moment of birth, the child emerges for the first time from the maternal sheaths and announces her arrival in her own unique way. This first image of the child, the way she takes her first breath on earth or holds her breath, the sound of her voice and the movements and gestures of her body, can give us our first sense of the child's nature. This is a crowning cosmic moment when the forces of the stars and planets imprint themselves on the newborn child as her birth horoscope.

> After emerging from the birth canal, Jonathan lies with clenched hands held above his head, his body a dusky shade of blue, eyes open and holding his breath. There is a moment, before he takes his first breath, when he seems to be between two worlds; with clenched hands he holds on to the world from whence he came, with open eyes he looks out to the world that beckons towards him; then he draws his first breath and without a cry he quietly takes his place in the new order of his life.

Whoever has the good fortune to observe this momentous event, may experience in the instant of the first in-breath that a great transformation takes place in the newborn child. The first breath expands the lungs and initiates the breathing rhythm that will continue without interruption until life ends. But something else enters the body that was not there before; there is a new presence and awareness in the child: someone who can perceive her environment, who can sense and feel her body and who can make her presence felt in many different ways. Some children 'arrive' on the in-breath, others in the moment before breathing. Some are very vocal, others are quiet. As already mentioned the Greek word for breath – *psukhè* – is also the word for *psyche*; our ancient forefathers were aware of the connection between feeling, emotions and breathing; they knew that with the first breath of life the soul dives into the physical body.

The human being is born triumphantly into an earthly body. She enters the world of earthly matter as a citizen of the earth and can now cast off the outer protective sheath that sheltered her before she was ready to emerge – the placenta (the fused chorion and allantois) and amnion sheath (recognized by the waters which break during labour).

Birth Options

The newborn child's experience of birth will clearly depend on the type of birth the parents choose and how they wish to conduct the pregnancy and birth. A natural birth at home is a different experience for the newborn to one in the maternity home; a waterbirth is a different landing to a conventional 'earth' birth; and a Caesarean section, where the newborn baby leaves the mother's womb passively by surgical removal, has a very different impact on the child to one where she is actively involved in the process. The decision to deliver at home or in a maternity clinic may be clear from the outset or may be decided only in the final two to three months for medical or obstetrical reasons such as a narrow pelvis, multiple births, a baby lying awkwardly or maternal illnesses.

Natural Childbirth

As a birthing method, this refers to the practice in which medical interventions are minimal and the parents' prenatal preparation is encouraged. Most of the many natural childbirth programmes are based on the methods of Dick Read in England and Lamaze in France. Expectant mothers are encouraged to understand the birth process, learn specific exercises to relax, to breathe correctly and to control the muscles involved in childbirth. The consequent reduction in fear and tension reduces contraction in the muscles which in turn decreases birth pains. As a result, less or no medication is required and complications and the need for interventions can be minimized. Many studies claim that the birth process is shortened, less painful and more satisfying, less medication is needed, babies are healthier and babies and mothers bond better. Other studies dispute these findings. From the child's perspective however, a mother who is more relaxed and self-assured is a more supportive birth partner than one who is tense, frightened and medicated with painkillers.

Home Birth or Maternity Hospital

Virtually every mother who has had an uncomplicated natural birth at home will attest to the benefits for all involved: for the newborn child, herself, the father, and other members of the family. Giving birth in her familiar home environment will help the mother to relax in the best possible way and to offer her newborn child a warm, natural and personal welcome. The sanctity of this special event can more likely be found by the special personal touches that only the parents can provide. Furthermore, the child is welcomed into her new home by her new, chosen family. In developed countries and communities it is most likely that a midwife who has accompanied the pregnancy in part or whole will deliver the baby at home. The trust that develops between expectant mother and midwife undoubtedly improves the chances of a healthy delivery. In developing rural communities, babies are delivered by traditional birth attendants who make use of a wide range of medicinal plants and other procedures to bring on labour, ease labour difficulties, expel the placenta and stimulate the flow of breast milk. Nearly two-thirds of all babies born in the world are delivered in this manner. Where midwife expertise is not available however, risks to mother and child may of course exist.

Parents who wish to be fully involved in the birth process and who trust their attendant midwife will often favour a home birth over a hospital birth.

The socially and medically acceptable place for giving birth nowadays, in line with conventional medical attitudes regarding hygiene and centralized medical care, is the maternity hospital. Most expectant mothers in developed societies feel safer in this environment, and supported by their obstetricians who only deliver in clinical situations, they readily choose this option. The hospital environment undoubtedly offers greater facilities for dealing with complications but the newborn child will be exposed to harsher first impressions and other risks such as hospital infections and higher drug administration. Furthermore, state hospitals are not often able to provide the intimate and personal care which most enhances the birthing event. There are clinics in many countries that endeavour to meet the personal needs of parents, and actively involve the midwife in the birth process.

Water Birth

The proponents of this method believe that water is a more natural element for the baby's entry into life, allowing for a gentler transition from a maternal environment where she was suspended in fluid for many months to the new, solid earth environment. The mother gives birth in the comfort of a warm bath at home or in hospital. It is claimed that this provides many benefits for both mother and infant, including greater relaxation and less pain, and thus less chance of complications.[2]

Leboyer Method

F. Leboyer, a French obstetrician, was influenced by the idea that the birth process was traumatic for the child and could lead to later psycho-emotional problems in adult life.[3] He suggested a number of supportive measures that could reduce the stress on the newborn child:

- the birth room should be dimly lit
- noises should be restricted
- immediately after birth the baby with her attached umbilical cord should be placed gently on the mother's abdomen for some minutes, only after which the cord should be cut
- the baby should be gently bathed in warm water
- traditional plastic gloves should not be worn to offer natural tactile stimulation.

These methods have been criticized by other researchers who dispute the psychological benefits to the child and claim that the soft, supportive measures could place the baby at risk because:

- delay in cutting the cord could increase the chance of infection in mother or child
- the dim lighting could result in overlooking problems
- the cry of the newborn is necessary for stimulation of breathing.

Birth Interventions

Caesarean Section

Is the rising incidence of Caesarean section a cause for concern?[4]

There has been a progressive increase in the rate of Caesarean section (CS) deliveries worldwide in recent years. In the USA the overall rate increased from 5.5 percent in the 1970s to 30.2 percent in the year 2005; in the UK the incidence in 2004 was about 20 percent; in Brazil, the increase was from 30.3 percent to 50.8 percent, with the rate approaching 80 percent in private hospitals.[5] There is growing consensus that medical indications alone cannot explain these increases.[6] Based on the rates of CS with the lowest perinatal mortality, the ideal acceptable rate is widely regarded to be in the region of 15 percent, a figure endorsed by the World Health Organization. Currently, however, the rates vary greatly in different settings depending on a variety of factors. In all countries, CS rates in private hospitals are higher than in national health service hospitals. In South Africa the rate for the public sector is between 10 percent and 20 percent depending on the area; in the UK the average rate is 20 per cent, but varies between 13 and 30 percent from one centre to the next. However, in the private sector the rate is over 50 percent. This cannot be justified on clinical grounds alone. It is difficult to obtain precise information about the other non-clinical factors involved because all CS are ostensibly done for clinical reasons; the non-medical reasons are usually not stated. There are many obstetricians around the world who only deliver babies by CS, citing the safety of mother and child as the reason for this policy.

Faced with this striking increase in Caesarean deliveries, especially in the private sector, we need to consider what effect this might have on the child's overall health and indeed on the community. When there is an option to have a normal vaginal delivery, we have to ask whether this is not, in fact, in the child's best interests. Before seeking answers to these difficult questions, let us first try to understand the reasons for increased CS frequency.

Factors Influencing Rising Incidence

Maternal and perinatal risk factors have always been and will continue to be justifiable reasons for performing emergency or elective CS. There are definite medical indications for CS accepted worldwide, e.g. failure of labour to progress, foetal distress, and breech presentation – to mention a few. Advancing technology may give the clinician earlier warning of risk to mother or child and therefore increase the Caesarean rate. Yet these factors alone do not explain the increased prevalence. For instance, women with low income or socio-economic status are at higher obstetric risk, yet higher CS rates are associated with women of higher income and social class.

A host of other factors are associated with higher rates of Caesarean delivery.

- Socio-economic factors: high income/high level of maternal education/private insurance/urban residence.
- Demographic and reproductive factors: older maternal type/first pregnancy/previous miscarriage/previous stillbirth/low or high birthweight.
- Health service factors: private hospital/delivery in non-academic hospital/high number of prenatal visits/early initiation of prenatal care/recently graduated physician/male physician/individual obstetrician/solo practice setting/antenatal care under obstetrician working in the same hospital/request by patient or offer by obstetrician/delivery on Friday/medico-legal considerations.

If one searches among these factors for the underlying causes of the increase, two main reasons seem to stand out: *choice by the mother or pressure by the gynaecologist/obstetrician*.

Maternal choice appears to be influenced by intellectual sophistication and higher socio-economic status which permits greater health choices, i.e. private gynaecologist/private insurance/private hospital/more comprehensive antenatal care. These factors as mentioned above will increase the chances of having a Caesarean delivery.

The more informed the woman, the more likely she will know that normal vaginal delivery has a greater risk of incontinence in later life, and that Caesarean delivery may avoid complications for mother and child. The more sophisticated the woman, the more she may wish to preserve her figure and youthful appearance, and place a high value on suffering the least amount of inconvenience and discomfort when her baby is delivered.

The psycho-emotional status of the pregnant woman will also strongly influence the birth process and thus also the chance of delivery by CS. Most women choose the perceived safety of the controlled hospital environment. And many women will choose not to go through the natural birthing experience for fear of the physical and or emotional pain or discomfort of the birth.[7] Parents today have greater freedom to choose how they wish their babies to be born. Whatever their choice, which needs to be respected, they should always be as well informed as possible about all the factors involved, both the overt physical risks to mother and child and the psycho-emotional consequences.

Gynaecological pressure may influence the mother to choose Caesarean delivery, and is more frequent if the gynaecologist is male, recently graduated, in solo practice and if the due date is at a weekend. This is compounded by the ever-present threat of litigation for damage to mother or child incurred during normal delivery. In the UK, 70 percent of all litigation relates to obstetrical practice and therefore obstetricians pay more for medico-legal insurance than any other medical specialty. In the USA some cities have no private obstetricians as a result of the pervasive practice of litigation for the smallest damage to mother or child.

The Conventional Obstetrical Point of View

Apart from the few radical obstetricians who would deliver all babies by CS, most gynaecologists/obstetricians would agree that a normal vaginal birth would be the first prize.[8] This is because CS delivery is not without its complications, especially in developing countries or where medical facilities are lacking. It is well documented that there are more maternal deaths with CS (9/100,000) than with normal vaginal birth (2/100,000).[9] The overall complication rate for CS is between 11 and 14 percent, the most common complications being uterine lacerations, blood loss and infections. Elective Caesarean delivery has significantly less risk of complication. Recent research indicates that Caesarean delivery has been associated with unintended adverse maternal health outcomes.[10,11] Caesarean section will also impact on future pregnancies: such mothers will statistically have fewer children due to lessened desire for or reduced ability to have children, and the next pregnancy is more likely to be complicated through repeat CS or placental problems. There is also evidence that Caesarean mothers experience less immediate and long-term satisfaction with the birth, are less likely to breastfeed and have greater difficulty interacting with their babies after birth.[12,13] It has also been documented that lung function in the newborn baby is weaker when born by CS compared with normal delivery.[14,15] If there is any perceived risk to mother or child, most obstetricians would not hesitate to perform a CS and would prefer to do an elective rather than an emergency Caesarean delivery since the complication risk in the latter is higher. The worst scenario would be a bad vaginal birth with perineal tearing and foetal distress. Most gynaecologists believe that the increase in CS is associated with reduction in maternal and neonatal risk.[16] Obstetricians evidently differ in their use of Caesarean delivery, suggesting different practice guidelines and expectations for doing CS. This would suggest that other factors such as the risk of malpractice litigation, the emotional needs of the mother-to-be, convenience for both obstetrician and the pregnant woman, and financial considerations, may sometimes exert greater influence than the obstetrical indications to operate.

The Midwife's Point of View

Most private midwives are dismayed at the high incidence of Caesarean delivery in the private sector.[17,18] The rate of CS is much lower in women who are delivered by midwives. Why is this the case? Midwives can generally provide a variety of options and benefits to a pregnant woman that the gynaecologist cannot offer. They have the time and dedication to provide a warm and nurturing support system which engenders trust, less anxiety, and more insight and understanding for parents. Many midwives feel that gynaecologists are more focused on solving obstetrical problems than carrying out routine deliveries, have less time to support the individual psycho-emotional needs of their patients and are often not fully available for the mother in labour. It is probably this more personal relationship and relaxed environment that accounts for the much lower incidence of CS, perineal tears and the need for epidural anaesthesia.

In South Africa there are a number of ways in which a pregnant woman can work with a midwife. She may choose a private-practice midwife to accompany her through a part or all of the pregnancy and opt to have her baby at home, in a birth centre or in a hospital where the midwife may still be active in the birth process. Or she may choose to have an obstetrician deliver the baby or be on call for an emergency that the midwife cannot deal with. All midwives would certainly choose to have a good working relationship with an obstetrician as they see this as the optimal support for pregnancy and birth.

Effects of Caesarean Section on the Newborn Child

The process of being born into the physical world is the first major challenge that the child has to face in earthly life. It is a highly significant event and the way she experiences it will impact on her future life. It is a vastly different experience for a baby to be born naturally by her own labour through the birth canal than to be removed unnaturally from the mother's abdomen by surgical incision through the womb. Imagine and try to experience these two birthing experiences. Being pulled out from the warm, buoyant, enclosed space and thrust into the harsh glare of cold fluorescent light without preparation or participation is likely to have a very different impact on the child's sensibility and future life.

The Caesarian-born baby loses the intimate connection with her mother who is anaesthetized either fully through a general anaesthetic, or partially through spinal anaesthesia. She must then bear the shock of the surgical incision made in her mother's abdomen and uterus. Her first human contact is the obstetrician who pulls the baby sharply out of the womb, suctions her airways and forcefully stimulates her breathing because the amniotic fluid has not been squeezed out of the lungs as in a vaginal delivery. The umbilical cord is then cut and if the mother is anaesthetized, the baby is removed from her for some hours where she is washed and monitored by attendants who have no personal connection with her.

Many obstetrical units are more sensitive to the baby's inner needs and try to reduce her experience of separation and alienation: regional anaesthesia allows the mother to be awake during delivery and the presence of the father in the delivery room maintains the continuity of contact with the baby. More progressive approaches like those of Dr Robert Oliver advocate humanizing the Caesarian experience for all concerned, even in emergency circumstances.[19]

A number of authors have linked some of the personality traits of Caesarian-born individuals to their perinatal experience of missing the primal human experience of birthing naturally and having someone do the job for them:[20] they are described as having difficulty dealing with conflict, frustrations and obstacles to their goals, having a sense of entitlement and expecting and needing others to do things for them; because of this, they often are overstepping boundaries and getting themselves into difficult situations where they are hoping to be rescued or given clear direction. They are often highly sensitive especially around issues of separation, exclusion and abandonment and crave affection and acknowledgement. They are frequently looking to be born into something or to give birth to something. There is less flow-and-process, and more all-or-nothing in their lives.*

At the same time, they are described as being endowed with other positive attributes: such as enthusiasm, creativity, spontaneity, being spiritually open and having a pioneering spirit and leadership qualities. Macduff who was 'plucked untimely' from his mother's womb is the character that Shakespeare creates who has the power to defeat Macbeth. As so often happens, the child deprived becomes the child endowed.

There can be no doubt that Caesarian section plays an important role in modern child delivery, preventing a variety of maternal and neonatal complications. It therefore has to be seen as a necessary part of the destiny of many children. The question really is whether this procedure is avoidable or not and to what extent the child herself is

---

* These are the subjective observations of certain researchers, and may simply indicate a tendency in people born by Caesarian section; they should not be used to create a stereotype.

involved in the birthing process: is she simply a passive partner who merely responds to physiological changes or is she respected as an active partner in the birthing process? Does she actively participate in her own birth and does she have a right to some choice in the matter? Does she perhaps know better than anyone else when she is ready to be born? And what do we take away from the child by depriving her of the opportunity to be born in a natural way?

These questions cannot be answered intellectually, and no quantifiable research will provide clear-cut answers to the long-term impact that unnecessary Caesarean delivery will have on the life of the child. Nor will we gain insight in this way about the long-term effects on society of every second child being born by CS. My impression from speaking to insightful individuals born by Caesarean delivery is that they feel something remains unborn in their lives, that they continue to struggle existentially to go through the birthing process they missed.

I believe the only way to hear the answer to these questions for oneself is to enter into the experience of the unborn child and allow the question to resonate in our attentive inner experience. If we give the child the respect and reverence she deserves as a spiritual being, it is hard to imagine she is not actively involved as the central player in her own birthing process and birthing experience. And when we, as the parents, doctors and nurses involved in the destiny of the child, help the child to determine her own future, then we become the true midwives for this child's journey into life.

Birth by Forceps or Vacuum Extraction

These procedures have a very different effect. In Caesarian section the child is uninvolved and passive, simply lifted out, whereas here the child is actively helped or forced out by quite violent means: a hard instrument takes hold of the baby's head and pulls her rapidly and sometimes violently into the physical world. Imagine what it must be like for the baby to feel her tender, soft head suddenly in the grip of an iron vice or a powerful suction device that pulls her out into the world. These appliances can be life-saving and should, like Caesarean section, only be used for medical emergencies, and never for simply facilitating the birth or for the obstetrician's convenience.

A Family in Close-Up

Jonathan is the third child born in his parent's home by natural birth. He has an older brother Adam who is five and an older sister Maria who is three.

Surveying the period of childhood and adolescence on which this newborn child is about to embark, we can reflect on the forces that will shape her life and have a bearing on her future potential.

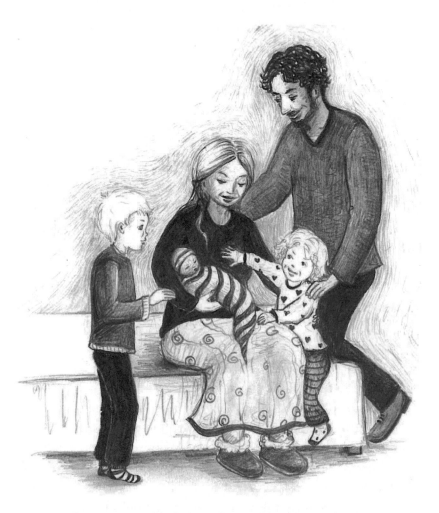

Adam, Maria and baby Jonathan with mother and father

- Firstly there is the stream of individuality that belongs uniquely to the child herself and, in our view, has an origin outside of the earthly dimension. This encompasses her I or higher self as the eternal core being of her existence that will invisibly guide and direct her onward journey. It also includes her soul that provides her with inner awareness and experience, enabling her to participate in this journey as a citizen of earth, as well as her life forces that endow her with all she needs for her growth, development and the maintenance of her bodily functions.
- Then there is the stream of inheritance handed down via the genetic material of fathers and mothers through the generations and bequeathed on her by the mother and father she has chosen. From them she receives her physical constitution and her gender; her life forces and temperament will also be influenced by this stream.
- Finally there is the stream of the environment which may significantly influence the physical nature and individuality of the child; unlike the first two streams, this comes to meet her from the outside world in which life and destiny place her.

The **gender** of a child and her **order of birth** in the family may also exert an important influence on her life and the extent to which she fulfils her potential.

Gender

The gender of the child is one of the first things that parents wish to know: *Is it a boy or girl?* To begin with male and female infants seem to be more alike than they are different, and apart from outer sexual characteristics, their sexual differences are not yet apparent. However, from the moment of birth, and even before, parents will often relate to a son differently from a daughter; this establishes a gender role from an early age that appears to have a strong determining influence on future behaviour.

We need to be aware that many gender stereotypes persist as a result of social and cultural attitudes. These preconceptions and expectations determine the way many parents rear their children and strongly affect the child's perception of (him- or) herself: for instance females are frequently regarded as good housekeepers, while males are more practical and technical; girls are more emotional, talkative and dependent, while boys are thought to be more logical and show higher achievement motivation. As a result of these attitudes, male infants tend to be handled more vigorously, female infants are cuddled more; fathers spend more time with infant sons and tend to be more aware of their adolescent son's concerns than of their daughter's anxieties; and boys are more likely to be disciplined physically. The child will frequently become what her parents want her to be, for instance the good-mannered, submissive type, thereby branding herself as a certain type of person that will determine her personality for years to come. Thus a child's gender influences parental attitudes in a variety of possible ways.

Gender identity and gender role develop from a wide range of factors including bio-physiological determinants (genetics, hormones), physical characteristics (physique, body shape, genitalia), social learning experiences with parents, siblings, teachers, friends, and cultural factors. There appears to be a sensitive period between 18 months and 3 years for the development of gender roles. Small children often imitate the toys and activities that are intended for girls or boys respectively, and copy what they see men and women doing around them: they may see women cooking and doing housework and men going to work and fixing things in the home (or vice versa!). Gender reinforcement also plays an important role, such as 'big boys like you don't cry', different kinds of dress and toys. A young boy will try to emulate his father who may encourage his son to behave in a typically 'masculine' manner. Outside of the home the peer group, school teachers, especially the nursery school teacher, and religious and cultural influences will put pressure on the child to experience him- or herself and behave according to a certain gender role. Boys who dress up as girls or play with dolls may be considered a little odd. Finally, storybooks, magazines and the media, especially television, frequently portray gender in a stereotypical way: men tend to be seen as active, dominant, innovative and independent, while women are passive, nurturing and dependent. TV commercials frequently use women to advertise household cleaning materials and men to advertise beer.

The Order of Siblings

The family constellation and the relationship of siblings to each other undoubtedly have a powerful influence on the development of personality and social behaviour. We can all give examples from our own family biography about how we were influenced by our siblings or they by us. A number of authors, including Karl König, have studied sibling order and tried to discover a common law that typifies these relationships.[21,22] We can all draw on our own personal experience or deepen our insights using the methodology of experience literacy described in Chapter two. While guarding against stereotyping children, we will find there does appear to be some law inherently determining certain general behaviour principles in the different birth order of children. Based on the dynamics found to exist within the family constellation, characterization of these broad traits in the first three children is given below. It is important to remember that there will be many exceptions to these general characteristics.

The First Child

The first child is usually met with the most wonder, joy, reverence, possessiveness, bewilderment, fear and uncertainty because she is the first. She is likely to be an only child for a certain period, during which time she enjoys the undivided and novel attention of her parents. This constant outpouring of love imprints itself into her being. If such undivided adult attention continues she may become precocious and prematurely adult, losing her easy connection with the world of children. Her closeness with her parents frequently induces her to take on the family mantle and assume natural responsibility and accountability for the family traditions. She tends to be conservative, conscientious, conscious of duty and oriented to the past. Traditionally in many cultures the first child takes over as the head of the family. The firstborn will therefore often assume a leadership role in life, becoming self-reliant, ambitious and defensive of her superior position. If her parents or another sibling are too strong for her, she may not be able to assume her rightful place and could suffer insecurity.

The Second Child

The second-born comes into the world knowing that someone has come before her. This often makes it easier for her because she has less responsibility: she is likely to carry fewer expectations. Her parents are more relaxed now, having done it all before. She generally accepts the importance of her older sibling's rank and will therefore be less bound to family traditions and less burdened by the past. She therefore tends to live more in the present, can be freer to explore her own nature and more open to the outer world than her older sibling. She is often relaxed, sociable, optimistic, content and seeks inner fulfilment; she is then the 'perfect sister'. But she may also challenge her older sibling, becoming stubborn, rebellious, difficult or frequently sick because she is up against the resistance of the ruling order.

The Third Child

The third-born accepts from the outset that there are two before her who may well have already teamed up, leaving her on the outside. Her parents have done this twice before and the glow of raising children may have worn a little thin. This may leave her with an innate sense of insecurity, inferiority and loneliness. She may feel different from others and somewhat marginalized, leading to a complex personality structure. On the other hand, being the youngest of three she is often pampered by the other people in her life, which may result in her taking less responsibility for herself. She may therefore find it difficult to engage her will fully, and may live in the future as an idealist, visionary and dreamer. But if she can overcome the inner obstacles of feeling victimized or entitled, the third child can be highly creative and perform major service for humanity. This is because she knows what it is like to be the underdog and has risen above it to be of help to others. In fairy tales the 'third son' is often a character with special powers of will who succeeds where others fail.

From the observations of researchers such as König[23] it appears that the further succession of siblings follows the tendencies of the first, second and third-born. Thus the fourth resembles the first, the fifth the second and the sixth the third, and so on.

It should be clear that what is indicated above are generalities that will be individually modified by the range of internal and external factors mentioned above. Specific family dynamics that also influence the personality include, of course, the parents' characters, the manner in which they rear their children, the number of siblings and the specific gender relationships.

The Effects of the Environment on the Newborn Child

Outside of the protective shelter of the maternal environment, the child is more exposed and therefore more vulnerable to external impressions. Her soul forces and life body have entered her physical constitution and therefore have begun to engage with the outer physical environment. The body of the child belongs to the material world of matter, providing the foundation through which her soul can work.

To understand the impact of the environment on the newborn child we shall need to expand our picture of the soul and its relationship to the body.

The Soul Body

To begin with, the unformed psyche of the newborn child creates wakefulness and awareness in contrast to her unconscious sleeping state when the psyche is not engaged in the physical body. What are the functions of this undeveloped part of the soul – which we can call the **soul body** or **sentient body**? These are the sense perceptions of the newborn child – for instance her sense of cold or warmth through the physical sense organs, and resulting sensations such as pain or pleasure, and the drives, impulses and desires, for instance, to still the pain of hunger or satisfy the need for comfort and security. In line with older literature it is also known as the **astral body**. This is a level of consciousness, possessed by the animal kingdom also, as the faculty to perceive and possess an inner awareness of pleasure and pain. The soul life here is primarily directed towards serving bodily functions that provide for the survival and preservation of the species. It sustains awareness only when the object of perception or sensation is present; when the object disappears, awareness vanishes.

How does the body transmit sense impressions from the outer world to the soul that perceives them? In this question lies the mystery of the body-soul connection.

The infant hears a loud sound and turns initially towards it; this sense impression enters through the sense organs of hearing and the child becomes aware of the sound. One observes by the way the child cries and turns away from the sound that she does not like it: perceiving leads to a bodily sensation which leads to feelings which lead to reactions. This interface where outer world becomes inner world lies in the soul body or astral body, a border between body and soul where impressions from the outer world resonate on the 'strings' of the soul body, creating the inner activity for sensation, feeling and reactivity. Steiner informs us that this soul body is the finer part of the life or etheric body which has been described above as 'a vibrating, resonating organized system of life forces'.[24] This is also the vehicle of our life memory, our immunological memory and our subconscious psycho-emotional memory where all impressions and experiences are stored. The implication of this is that every contact with the world has a resonating impact on the child's constitution.

The Impact of the Environment

We must realize therefore that the environment, both internal and external, will affect the child in a variety of ways.

* There will firstly be an impact on the physical body through food and drink that is ingested and assimilated, through gaseous substances that are inhaled and exhaled, through contact of substances with the semi-permeable barrier of the skin and

through the many sense organs that absorb a wide variety of sense impressions, including light and warmth. These physical and chemical gifts of nature are required to provide the building blocks for a body that can exist in the natural world; and a regular quantity and quality of these elements is needed for optimum health: for instance minerals such as calcium and magnesium, which are present in large quantities in dairy products, are needed for healthy bone structure. Lack of them can have long-term effects on the skeleton. But the impact of the environment does not stop here.

- The environment will also affect the child's vitality and functionality – an expression of her life forces. These impressions, whether physical, chemical or psychological – enter through the digestive system, breathing system, skin or sensory system and cause the energetic life matrix of the etheric body to resonate accordingly. Harsh impressions will impact more aggressively on the child's life forces. Many of these impressions will not become conscious but their specific resonances will be absorbed and imprinted indelibly into the resonating life body's 'memory bank'. They may well have a significant effect on the child's health, either immediately or later in life. The impressions that do come to sentient awareness (but not full consciousness) will be transmitted to the contiguous soul body and will be expressed positively or negatively in the child's behaviour. Thus the child's wellbeing may be significantly affected by environmental factors such as poor-quality food, sensory overload (TV, audio-visual stimuli), parental stress and premature burdening of the immune system by immunization and chemical medication. These factors can weaken vitality and cause a range of functional illnesses such as tiredness, tummy aches and recurrent illness.

- The outside world will further impact on the child's psychological nature or soul, encompassing all cognitive, sensory, emotional and volitional functions, out of which the personality emerges. These inner activities will also be affected by external sense impressions. For example, the newborn baby senses tension between her parents, feels the tension in her body; this constricts and cools down her body so that she develops tummy aches and begins to wake at night. But poor nutrition will also have the same effect on her behaviour. It is not difficult to imagine the profound effects the environment may have on the child's psyche. From inside herself she is sensitive to the impressions of her own body, from outside to impressions from nature, or the impact of another psyche in her environment. Every experience that impresses itself in the soft, receptive soul organization, is then sealed into the memory etheric life matrix. In this way all the faculties of sensing, thinking, feeling and will affect the growing child's potential of physical strength and energy for life.

- Finally, either directly or indirectly via the other three bodies, the I nature of the newborn child, which also interacts with body and soul, is likewise affected by the impact of the environment. Again, this impact can significantly affect a person's future potential. For instance, it is my impression that autistic children, who are especially sensitive to toxic environmental influences, make a choice at some point to withdraw from the world because they feel unable to face the rigours of a hostile environment. More will be said about autism in Part 2.

It will be clear from the above that the child's environment, and our affect on it as parents/carers, will impact on these four different aspects of the child's being, influencing her constitution in a positive or negative way.

Core Picture and Care for the Newborn Child

The newborn child comes into the world as a complete stranger, naked and vulnerable and needs the protection of those who will care for her. The kind of birth parents choose for themselves and their unborn child will have a profound effect on her birthing experience and future life. Whatever the birth option, the newborn child loses her highly protective maternal sheath and is immediately exposed to a radically different and potentially hazardous external environment. The newborn child places her fullest trust in her primary caregivers for her physical and psychological needs; her future custodians can come to meet this trust by trying to create the most healthy environment during and after birth.

Here we will only consider hazards that could be prevented by a more holistic perspective of birth, and not unforeseen medical complications that belong to obstetrical practice.

At the risk of sounding prescriptive, some suggestions can be given here for protecting and thereby enhancing the health of the newborn child.

Caring Measures During Birth

• Avoid or limit medication during labour.

Mothers who give birth in hospital are far more likely to receive medication to facilitate an easier birth. Currently this takes the form of morphine-type and other strong painkillers and spinal anaesthesia aimed at reducing or eliminating the pain of childbirth altogether. It is a symptom of our 'quick-fix' age that people wish to remove discomfort and suffering as swiftly as possible. Modern pharmaceutical drugs provide an easy way to do this. When in pain and feeling scared, it is very tempting for all involved to regard powerful drugs freely prescribed by a doctor as the normal and right course of action. One good reason not to take them however is the sedating effect these drugs have on the child, which may also impact on the natural timing of the birth. A second is the wish to remain conscious through a vitally important event in the life of a mother and her child. Another is the human value of dealing with pain and suffering and resisting the temptation to take the easy route. It is not a question of suffering like a martyr for the sake of suffering, but rather the empowering effect this can have for oneself, as well as the child on whose behalf one suffers. If it is possible to do without painkillers or at least to limit their quantity, the unborn child is protected from their powerful chemical effects; but more important, the mother gives a gift of full consciousness and endurance, an offering of her blood, tears and pain to accompany the child in her arrival on earth. The choice to suffer for the wellbeing of one's child and for the bond of love that protects the newborn in her

most vulnerable phase, may be of immense value for the future
life of mother and child. It is probably true that women in general
develop greater resilience than men precisely because they learn
through childbirth and child rearing to place their children before
themselves. The bio-psychological necessity innate in the intimate
bond between mother and child gives the mother a natural way of
practising selflessness, empathy and compassion.

Caring Measures After Birth

If birth attendants lack insight into the finer needs of the newborn child,
she might have to face a variety of 'safety and convenience procedures'
as well as a host of other unwelcoming environmental factors. There
are a number of important protective measures that can usually be
requested and implemented, and have a significant supporting effect
on the newborn baby's wellbeing in the first days of life.

- The umbilical cord should not be cut immediately after birth
  but only after it has stopped contracting. This will enable the
  child to receive that extra volume of blood which may reduce
  complications. The risks of infection are minimal in a clean
  environment.
- The child should not be separated from her mother but kept as
  close as possible, even sleeping in the same bed for the first days;
  alternatively she should be placed in a cot, cradle or crib that is
  as womb-like as possible, and placed next to the mother's bed.

  The newborn child is frequently removed from her mother
  to allow both to be cleaned up and to give the mother a chance
  to recover from her ordeal. Babies are frequently taken from the
  labour ward to the nursery some distance away where they are
  washed, examined and placed in an isolated cot alongside other
  babies. The mother usually fetches her baby when she needs to
  be fed, and the father may have access only in visiting hours.
  These 'practical arrangements' unwittingly hinder the mother's
  natural protection and nurturing. More enlightened maternity
  homes will allow the baby to stay close to the mother and the

father may have free access to mother and child, as is now often the case in the UK.

No mother who is connected with her true maternal feelings wishes to let her newborn child be taken away from her after giving birth.

- The baby should be allowed to latch onto the breast as soon after birth as possible, where she may drink her first earthly nourishment in the form of the all-important colostrum.

Colostrum is the pre-milk fluid produced by the mother's mammary glands at the beginning of lactation and is intended for ingestion by the newborn during the first hours of life.

It contains potent protein chemical substances (immune factors) that activate the baby's immune system to provide protection against a host of micro-organisms, as well as hormonal growth factors responsible for building and repairing tissue.

- The neuro-sensory system should not be overloaded by sense impressions that are too strong for highly sensitive sense organs: bright electric lights, cool temperatures or inadvertent cooling while bathing or changing, loud noises and synthetic garments. The newborn baby's thermostat function is not fully functional so that a constant warm temperature has to be maintained.
- The open fontanelles readily lose blood warmth and the head should therefore always be kept warm and covered in the first few months.
- Natural fibres like wool, cotton, silk or linen should always be used in preference to synthetics that may be harmful or irritating to delicate skin. Synthetic fibres are derived mainly from petrochemical products to which the human being has no natural relationship. Have you compared the different sensation on your own bare skin? Furthermore, synthetics are not able to retain warmth, and the skin tends to perspire more readily.
- The baby's eyes should be protected from bright light by hanging a combined light blue/rose pink-coloured double silk veil over the cradle. The mother may choose a different colour if she knows what feels right for her child. Most babies seem to be more content under these colours. Colours speak directly to young children's delicate senses and should be used consciously in the environment of the newborn child. The right colour may immediately soothe a fretful baby.

- The warmth-protective and nourishing vernix which covers the body of the newborn baby should not be washed off. The vernix caseosa is the natural cheesy, fatty substance that covers the newborn baby's skin; it lubricates the birth passage, insulates the body against fluctuations in temperature, moisturizes the skin against dehydration, nourishes it with fats, protein substances, vitamins and mineral salts and protects it against harmful bacteria and fungi.

  It is necessary only to clean the face and hands with a little warm oil. It is not advisable to bathe the baby or wash off the precious vernix in the first few days, since this deprives the baby of natural protection and valuable nutrients; the vernix will be absorbed naturally within this period.

  Babies able to receive the nutrients of their birthright – the warmth, the vernix and the colostrum – are less prone to neonatal jaundice.

- Individual decisions should be made about avoiding unnecessary exposure to chemical substances including immunization. Most babies delivered in South African hospitals are given their first immunization against polio and tuberculosis soon after birth. One should remember that breastfed babies are protected by the mother's natural immunity. Silver nitrate is an archaic routine measure that is still instilled into babies' eyes in some hospitals to prevent contracting sexually transmitted diseases, often causing eye irritation.

Natural Feeding Versus Bottle Feeding

It is widely believed that breast fed babies generally develop more harmoniously and with fewer problems.[25] This controversy has been raging for decades. Most serious researchers agree that breast milk remains the most ideal food for the baby. Yet many mothers choose not to breastfeed their babies or to feed only for a short period. The reasons are usually cultural, or for convenience. While these reasons are understandable, the reality is that the child is deprived of the ideal food, greater protection against infections, and the intimate bonding between mother and child that breastfeeding creates. Therefore every attempt should be made to breastfeed a child. There are many different points of view about how long one should breastfeed a baby, but there is general consensus that breast milk alone should usually extend only to the fifth or sixth month, approximately when the child is trying to sit up. The force of uprightness and individuality begins to make itself felt and the child will soon begin to crawl away from her mother; this is an opportune time also to begin to digest nutritive substances other than those that come from the mother. It is also possible to breastfeed too long. Certain schools of thought believe one should breastfeed as long as the child wishes. I know some mothers who have breastfed their children for four years! I personally do not think it is in the interests of the child to breastfeed longer than a year unless it is for nutritional purposes when food is scarce and the baby would otherwise be malnourished.

Cow's Milk

According to Steiner, donkey's milk is the best substitute for breast milk. Most paediatricians would however recommend cow's milk. Goat's milk does not contain sufficient protein. If donkey's milk or sheep's milk is not available and there is no surrogate milk from another lactating mother, my personal choice would be *fresh cow's milk* in preference to a formula feed. Unpasteurized milk contains far more life forces than pasteurized milk but must be obtained from a reliable source. Glöckler and Goebel in their highly recommended and comprehensive *Guide to Child Health*,[26] give practical guidance for early childhood feeding. One should be aware that cow's milk contains more than twice the amount of protein, but half the milk sugar content of breast milk. It also has a much greater mineral content, especially large amounts of calcium and phosphorus. Cow's milk-fed babies will usually have bigger muscles as a result, and more mineralized bodies.

Formula Milk

Although the most convenient baby food, containing the 'ideal' balance of nutrients, dried milk formulas are in my view the least suitable. They are often fortified with extra minerals and vitamins to counter their lack of natural vitality, and frequently lead to overfed and overweight babies; excessive minerals and vitamins such as vitamin D result in premature hardening of tissues. Excess weight and obesity in children have assumed epidemic proportions and are now a serious health risk factor. Because they are machine processed, these formula feeds contain very little in the way of life-sustaining forces. Life or etheric forces are present in the food we eat to the extent that these forces have not been leached out by refining methods. Have you tasted fresh, unpasteurized milk and compared it with longlife milk, or even ordinary pasteurized milk? Sensing the subtle qualities of the food we eat is another rich practice area for the experiential approach. What for instance is the gesture inherent in milk fresh from a cow compared to 'tired' milk that has been heat-treated and preserved?

The Diet of the Nursing Mother

Breastfeeding mothers should be aware that the outer environment as well as the mother's own inner environment will impact through the breast milk on their suckling child.

The food and drink the mother ingests can have a negative impact on the sensitive nature of the child, causing digestive disturbances (reflux, cramping, winds, diarrhoea) skin rashes or emotional distress. The nursing mother's diet should therefore be easily digestible, nutritionally balanced and free of fatty, rich, spicy and wind-producing foods (cabbage, onions, cauliflower, garlic), acidic fruit juices, excessive sugar products, wine and coffee. Many chemical medicines will also pass through the breast milk and their intake therefore needs to be carefully considered.

- The mother's emotional condition will likewise affect the child's wellbeing: for instance, mothers who suffer from postnatal depression tend to be more inconsistent with childcare; they generally have poorer coping strategies, feel more insecure and tend to avoid their babies, who are therefore less content than babies with happy mothers.

The newborn child has a right to expect a warm and caring reception. Just as she was given an unconditionally protected biological home, so she has the right to receive an equally nurturing and protective outer worldly environment. Can we be mindful of the earthly welcome that we ourselves would have hoped to receive?[27]

It is my will to enter this world, trusting fully in those who are there to receive me. In my naked innocence I open myself to this world and learn everything I can about it. In so doing I lay myself open to all its impressions, the good and the bad. I have no fear for the unknown around me; I do not doubt that what I meet is true and good. I accept myself unconditionally and because I trust myself, I also trust those who come to meet me. When I am met with harshness, resistance and uncertainty, I feel oppressed by cold and dark. When I am welcomed and received in love and openness, I feel bathed in warmth and joy.

CHAPTER 6

The Heavenly Years

Deep Devotion and Trust Enshrine and Empower my Early Years of Learning

The first three years of childhood touch us all in deep and mysterious ways: the otherworldly presence of the newborn child, whose unfocused gaze seems to rest on invisible, faraway places; the sheer joy of a young child standing up for the first time on his own two feet or courageously taking his first step; the total trust that children of this age give to us adults; or the helplessness of a toddler lost in a supermarket crying desperately for his mother. These and many other images call up powerful and deeply moving feelings.

This is a critical period of the child's life because it is the most impressionable time. What happens during these years will profoundly influence his physical and psycho-spiritual wellbeing. It is a time of innocence, absolute truthfulness and relative helplessness, with the child at the mercy of a potentially hostile environment. There is no period in life more trusting and accepting: the human being gives himself over in complete faith to the world that is given to him. The child may find himself in the most brutal, cruel and ugly world, but having no other to compare it with he accepts it without question. He may have the most uninterested, dysfunctional and cruel parents, yet remains loyal and devoted to them. Life is what it is: they cannot yet discern what is right or wrong, accepting what they are given without question.

In this chapter we will attempt to discover the grandeur of this period; in many ways it feels like entering a sacred temple where one does one's best to leave one's imperfections outside the portal before entering.

The Power of First Memories

We all have special memories and perhaps photographic images of children in this early phase of life. We may also have memories of our own early years. Can we recall the cot we slept in, some object like a blanket that we became attached to, a smell, a room, our house or garden, or some specific recollection of mother or father? What was your first memory in this life period? Most people can only remember pictures from around their third year of life, though some can certainly recall images from their second and even first year.

We have all been through this early period, largely unconsciously, and have stored our experiences deep in the innermost layers of our memory. As we saw in Chapter two, we can re-live our early experiences. We can call up feelings, bodily sensations and memory pictures. One way to consciously rediscover the experiences of early childhood is through psychotherapeutic counselling work. A short case history will illustrate how this can happen.

> The client wished to understand why she always felt shy and reserved in company. She remembered a recent incident when she had the feeling that she needed to withdraw from a group of people; she was asked to sense how this feeling affected her body and then to gesture how it felt. Her body gesture was one of contracting inwards and drawing herself away from something. When she detached herself from this position and looked at the after-image, she was deeply moved to see before her a small, highly sensitive, shy child, perhaps two years old, who was trying to hide away from people. She could describe exactly the white dress with lace around the sleeves and neckline. This memory picture opened up rich details of the early life of this child.

Anyone who has been able to relive these early years in this way will wake up to the nature of his early childhood, and will access some

conscious experience of what it is like to live in the world in the body
of such a child. This is how I experience it:

> I have left the haven of my universal home in search of something
> that I can only find on earth. I have acquired a body from my
> mother and father, and for a while this will become my new home;
> I know I must find the way to connect with it, but it is still new and
> unfamiliar and I do not yet fit properly into it. I am not yet part of
> this earthly world and still feel close to my true home. I completely
> trust in the powers that have guided me into this new life, that
> build up my body and enable me to function as a human being in
> this world. I surrender myself to the care and protection of my new
> caregivers to whom I entrust my life and my potential.

The Journey Begins

Let us join the newborn child as he sets off on his life journey.

This period begins when the physical body of the child is set free
from the sheaths created for his growth and protection within the
mother's womb. The physical environment can now work directly
on the child. He draws in his first breath of air – holds this cosmic
moment on the inbreath – and then presses out a cry as if in pain,
born of the feeling – *I have left something behind, something true and
precious.* One may often observe after this first breath a particular
kind of peace that descends on the child as if he were saying – *I will
strive to carry some of what I have left behind with me, at least for a
certain time, even though the earthly forces of gravity press down on me
and the light that shines on me is now the outer sun.*

The newborn child belongs to two worlds: that of earthly matter
and another more 'heavenly' world.

During these early years the child seems not fully of this world.
In the first weeks after birth, Jonathan hardly seems to be aware of
his surroundings: his soft blue eyes cannot yet fix on objects and
he seems to be connected much more deeply with another, unseen
dimension. If we pay close attention to the child's inner nature we
can sense this other reality. Young children experience the whole
world around them, including rocks, water, air and fire, as vibrant,
animated being. They are completely at home in a world where

every force is a living one, and therefore relate unquestioningly to nature spirits and angels. The child is present as much outside in his surroundings as inside himself and is therefore able to connect intensely with everything he perceives in both domains. When he plays with water he becomes one with the water, when he drinks milk he feels the very nature of the milk flowing through his body; his fingers and toes move in rhythm with the flow of milk.

The Roadmap of Early Childhood

As we saw in Chapter five, the young child's biographical journey unfolds according to an unalterable developmental plan. The neuro-sensory system grows at a much faster rate than the cardiovascular-respiratory system or the metabolic-motor system. The brain and sense organs are functionally well developed within the first year (whereas the digestive organs and the limbs, for example, remain relatively undeveloped). At birth the head is disproportionately large and the forehead and upper head are the parts that are most developed, in contrast to the little button nose and chin. In the first years of life the spherical tendency of the head predominates throughout the body because the dynamics of the neuro-sensory system are most active in this period. The tummy is round and protruding, the hands and feet mostly assume a curled shape. Young children love to move in circles, and early drawings always start from the sphere.

Because the body's rhythmic life is still relatively undeveloped, pulse and respiratory rate are rapid and irregular, and movements and metabolism are arrhythmic and spasmodic. A set rhythm of waking, sleeping, eating and moving will take some months to develop. The limbs and metabolic functions are still very unformed and immature. The lower limbs cannot initially support the weight of the body, and the digestive functions are still relatively underdeveloped and are therefore a vulnerable part of the infant's organism.

Yet it is in these biologically undeveloped limbs and metabolic organs that the life of the soul first awakens: very soon after birth the infant begins to move his limbs, kicking his legs, waving his hands, moving his eyes and constantly taking objects to the mouth to be tasted and swallowed. An infant who does not move in the first months is cause for concern, for the healthy child wakes up to the world through *movement*, which most visibly expresses the soul's will activity. We should be quite clear that feeling life is not yet properly developed in these early years: at this stage the feelings still function more in strong connection with organic functions. Thus an infant child will feel content when his bodily needs have been satisfied, and a toddler will quickly forget that his mother has left him if his physical needs are addressed by another caring person. Thinking at this age is likewise bound up with what is immediately present in the physical, sense-perceptible world. This is why you can easily distract an infant or toddler by turning his attention to some other immediate experience.

The young, awake child is unbridled activity, always busy doing, exploring and creating. Just observe a two-year-old in action!

Thus while the head and neuro-sensory system develop earliest through the activity of etheric life forces, will activity is the first faculty of soul to be born in the young child.

Neuro-Sensory System

If we wish to understand this early period of childhood, therefore, we need to have a clear picture both of the nature of the neuro-sensory system as it unfolds and predominates in this period, and of the nature of the will.

The sensory and cognitive activities of the soul require functional organ systems to transmit perceptual information from the outer world and process it cognitively. These systems comprise the sense organs, the nerves, spinal cord and brain. The sense organs are specifically designed to convey sense impressions derived from the outer or inner world via nerve pathways to organ centres – the spinal cord or brain – that can then utilize this information for the healthy functioning of the human organism.

The eye is constructed precisely for the purpose of recording and conveying visual impressions via nerve pathways to the central organ of the brain; the ear and auditory apparatus likewise is an organ perfected for transmitting auditory perceptions to the brain. It is not difficult to find comparisons between the sense organs and mechanical instruments: the eye with its aperture, lens, image formations and retinal film is very similar to the construction of a camera; the three tiny bones in the middle ear, the hammer, anvil and stirrup, operate like mechanical levers, and the fine hairs located in the inner ear resemble the strings of a piano. Likewise, the brain with its neural circuits is often likened to a vast computer that captures and stores data. The growth and formation of the brain in small children has been directly linked to the development of cognitive functions. It appears to act as a reflective organ that mirrors the outside world, enabling perceptive and cognitive functions to take place. Indeed, each hemisphere of the brain maps the whole body, and different portions of the brain are directly responsible for the movement and exchange of sensory and motor information in the rest of the body, such as touch sensitivity, cold, heat, pain, etc.

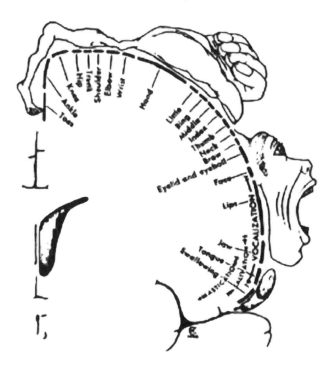

Image of brain homunculus: a miniature 'person' as symbolic representation on the brain surface of 'the body within the brain'.

This quasi-mechanical nature of the neuro-sensory system reflects the relatively lifeless nature of this system: nervous tissue does not regenerate easily and tissues involved in sensory and cognitive functions tend to have a poorer blood supply than metabolic-rich tissues; the lens and cornea have no blood supply at all. In addition, neuro-sensory organs tends to have a fixed, formed and finely differentiated nature and are largely symmetrical, as if they were constructed according to a well-organized mechanical design.

We should be clear that this mechanical construct pertains only to that part of the neuro-sensory system that serves the function of perception and cognition. For their healthy function these faculties require an organic structure and design that has an earthbound and quasi-mechanical nature.

We should also remember that as the cognitive functions develop in this period of life, some of the formative growth forces that build up the neuro-sensory tissue are diverted to support these cognitive functions. Therefore we should not be surprised to find relatively less etheric life force in this region and more material, earthly forces. However, this tissue is of course still alive and must therefore still be supported by other life processes such as nutrition, warmth, circulation and respiration.

The perception of sensory stimuli and their cognitive assimilation always requires a certain level of conscious awareness. It is the neuro-sensory system that allows us to be conscious and aware of external stimuli. The level of consciousness may range from the relatively unconscious sensitivity of the digestive system for the fat content of a meal, to the semi-unconscious awareness of some irritation on the skin, or to the conscious awareness of observing and naming an object.

In order for us to perceive something, we have to actively 'harness' it; this means that the living activity inherent in the object must be stilled, suppressed or even destroyed for the information to be 'captured' and used in specific ways. Life processes that come to rest 'cool down' and enter a devitalized state as a fundamental condition for consciousness; for as we have seen before, there is an inverse relationship between life and consciousness. When vegetative life predominates, as in lower forms of life, consciousness is dim; as consciousness increases in mammals and humans with the development of the nervous system, so burgeoning life diminishes. The reproductive forces that are so powerful in bacteria, amoeba, plant seeds and even the spawning of fish, become diminished as the reproductive capacity of the nervous system to reproduce mental images increases in higher forms of life. The same can be observed with respect to the growth forces: each part of an earthworm cut in two will replicate to form a complete earthworm, and a lizard that loses its tail will grow another tail; a frog that loses a limb will grow a stunted new limb, but a dog whose tail is amputated will never grow a new tail. The relatively new science of stem-cell research is based on this insight that primitive embryonic or adult stem cells have such an abundance of growth potential that they can differentiate into a diverse range of specialized cell types.

The neuro-sensory system thus captures and processes living realities by fixing, cooling, and converting them into dead images like photographs and computer data that can be used for cognitive activities.

Neuro-sensory activity is the easiest system to experience because its function corresponds to the sense-bound and cognitive mode of observation we use consciously during waking life. Think of a tree blowing in the wind. To absorb it fully we have to focus our attention on this object to the exclusion of all others, absorbing all the visual impressions – its shape, colour, and various parts; at the same time we notice its movement and hear the rustling of the leaves. But we cannot actually observe or experience what happens between our outward perception of the tree and our recognition of it as a tree. Neuro-physiology tells us that the eye harnesses the image, imprints it on the retina which then conveys a fixed, 'frozen' image of the tree along nerve pathways, to the ocular brain which consciously registers our perception of the tree. Likewise, the auditory apparatus conveys auditory perceptions via a complex system of vibrating membranes, oscillating bones and resonating hairs to nerve fibres which transmit them as recorded sound to the auditory brain. The conscious awareness that follows is only possible because the experience of an active, warm and living reality has been dampened down to a fixed immobile image or vibration of the tree.

Cognitive activity follows either subconsciously or consciously as we reflect on what we have perceived, naming the object *a tree moving in the wind*, reflecting on the nature of the wind that moves the tree and deciding perhaps that this tree is safe to climb. Earth-bound cognitive processes (see page 37) may initially fix the tree further by describing the details of the sense perceptible object, estranging it from its real nature. By enhancing thinking however, with life (experiencing it as a living, growing tree), soul (experiencing the inner effect it has on one), and spirit (discovering something about the tree that is common for every human being) as described in Chapter three, we can consciously reconstruct the object perceived into one that is again imbued with living reality.

The Will

The will is like a dynamo that energizes and activates all other functions. We can say that it is activity itself, a faculty of the soul that kindles our thinking, feeling, sensing and actions. We have little or no access to this part of the soul because will activities are either submerged in the body, in the organs of metabolism and the limbs, or live in our higher intuitions, awaiting discovery. We can say that we are asleep in our will, just as we dream in our feelings and sensing, and are awake in our thinking. Does this mean we have no way of understanding the nature of the will? Ordinary experience can give us a good starting point for exploring its nature.

Every day we convey ourselves inwardly or outwardly from point A to point B, doing so voluntarily or involuntarily. Either consciously or unconsciously we are constantly exercising our will in whatever we do, and could not exist without this capacity. It is an activity intrinsically bound up with who we are. The will must therefore exist in every part of our being, our body, soul and spirit. We also know what will power is, a force within us enabling us to overcome what may appear at first to be an insurmountable obstacle.

If we now attempt to empathically experience the nature of this will activity in the physical body, how will it express itself? If it lives in us, it must have some effect on the form and design of the body itself. A body shaped in a particular way will be designed to function in a certain way; the wisdom inherent in a young child's body will enable him to stand upright at the due time.

In a similar way we can try to enter the nature of the will as it works in the life body. How does it express itself through biological activities such as breathing or the absorption of nutrition? The function of breathing can only be maintained through the provision of air, that of nutrition through the provision of food. Here the will works in the drive for air, the drive for food. The basic drives are essential for the function of the life forces.

And what is the nature of the will as expressed through the soul body? The soul body enables us to sense and perceive the world. What happens in us as we sense something? First we become interested in it, we are curious about it. As the infant wakes into his sense life he becomes intensely interested in sensory objects and wants to grasp them. Here will expresses itself as desire.

The Sevenfold Will

Rudolf Steiner first systematically described the anatomy of the will in a course of lectures given to Waldorf teachers in 1919.[1] He indicated that the organ of the will has seven aspects, each of which is connected with a different level of the human constitution.

We can test this model as a working hypothesis and see whether it resonates with our own experiences and insights.

In this chapter we will be concerned chiefly with the three least conscious steps in the hierarchy of will activities.

- Instinct is seen as the most physical level of will life. It is powerfully present in the animal world, and the structural design of animals' physical bodies is a picture of this instinctive will. A honeybird has a long, curved beak which allows it to suck honey instinctively from flowers with deep tubular structures that are rich in nectar. All animals will manifest their instinctive character in their bodily form. The child too knows instinctively how to crawl, stand up and walk because of the will working through his physical body. His body is structured in a certain way to allow for these activities. No one needs to teach him to do this. It is a physically-based instinct that expresses the power of the will working through the physical body.

- Drive is regarded as a force of will working primarily in the life body. When the life forces meet instinct in the physical body, they change it into drive. The drives are powerful functional needs that are directed by the life processes in the physical body. The body requires food and water to operate all physiological functions. Powerful life forces working through the will, expressed as the drives of hunger and thirst, compel the infant to cry for attention to pacify his needs.

- Desire is said to arise when instinct or impulse become more conscious, that is to say, are taken up by the forces of the soul. Every desire is a will impulse created anew each time by the life of the soul or astral body. The toddler desires the colourful red sweets because he remembers the pleasure it gave him the first time.

The other four steps in the anatomy of will described by Steiner are: motivation, wish, intention and resolve.[2]

The will also drives the child's burgeoning sensory life: the sense organs, as we have seen, are an extension of the nervous system which is primarily developing at this period. It is therefore understandable that will forces naturally direct their activity through these specific organs. When the will directs its activity towards the outer world and comes to rest in these organs, perception arises at this boundary with perceptible objects.

The Child as Sense Organ

In his waking life the young child is fully absorbed in sensing the world with his whole being. He hears the dog barking and in this moment gives himself fully over to the sound. He becomes an ear with his whole organism and takes these sound impressions deep into his inner nature. So it is with all the senses that transmit impressions of the outer world into the inner world. The young child lives completely in his sensing life. This essential feature needs to be understood if we are to grasp the nature of the young child.

We are brought up to believe there are only five senses: hearing, sight, touch, taste and smell. This is a limited view of human sensitivity however, as we can experience at first hand. Dr A. Jean Ayres,[3] who studied children with sensory and motor problems, recognized four other senses.[4]

Before we proceed with a description of the different senses, stop reading for a moment and explore how many different senses you can discover in yourself. Begin by focusing on the sensing experience of the body at rest and in motion; then on the sensing experience in relation to the surrounding world; finally on the sensing experience in relation to another human being. Then try to enter the experience of the young child and discover what the senses convey to his awakening soul.

The Twelve Senses

Steiner described the human being as having twelve developed senses and three which are not yet developed but which can be developed through spiritual training.[5] We can take this description, once again, as a working hypothesis and see for ourselves if it concurs with our experience and understanding of the young child who is so intensely preoccupied with sensing the world.

When we turn our attention to the activity of sensing, we find that there are a wide range of sensory doorways through which we gain access to the internal and external world.[6]

1. Sense of touch

What do we discover about ourselves and the world through our sense of touch? Firstly we find that the touch-sensitive organs are located on the boundary of the body: on the skin and mucous membranes of the tongue, mouth, nasal passages, eyes and ears as well as the inner organs that open to the outside world, such as the pharynx and anal cavity. This sense brings us into direct contact with the outer world, informing us of its existence; but we can only be sure that it exists because at the same time it informs us of our own physical existence: here we are experiencing the world through direct contact with our physical body. It brings us close to something, but paradoxically in the act of touching we become aware of ourselves as separate from the world. Soesman refers to a quotation by Novalis who expresses the nature of touch exactly when he says: 'Touching is separation and connection both at once.'[7]

Through this boundary sense the child meets resistance and discovers the boundary of the physical world. He explores the outer nature of this world and wants to get to know what it is like; he senses whether it is hard or soft, rough or smooth and takes this experience into his inner, unconscious soul life.

The child senses the love and affection in the way his mother holds and caresses him; soft natural cotton fibre on his skin feels different from synthetic fabrics; a doll made from natural materials has an entirely different feel to a plastic doll. He must touch everything because this way he gets to know the world as well as his own body; he progressively will come to know the boundary between his own physicality and that of his physical environment and thereby learns to separate himself from the world. In this way he arrives at a consciousness of his self; he wakes up to himself.

Healthy tactile experiences create healthy boundaries for body and soul. They provide the foundation for a healthy feeling of identity, self-awareness, self-confidence and trust in life.

2. Sense of life

We perceive physical wellbeing in the broadest sense: at any moment we can sense how we feel in our body – comfortable or uncomfortable, tired or energized, tense or relaxed. This sense allows us to experience our independent physical existence. It also gives us warning signals when something is wrong, and thus the opportunity to correct the problem.

The physical organ system that mediates these sensations is the autonomic nervous system, a diffuse network of nervous tissue distributed throughout all the organs and tissues and comprising the sympathetic and parasympathetic nerve system. These organs have a great deal to do with the preservation of life; they sense conditions within the body and respond accordingly. For instance, when a toxic substance is present in the digestive system, the autonomic system will perceive the danger and take steps to expel it through parasympathetic nerve stimulation; this increases intestinal contraction which promotes peristalsis and intestinal secretions to eliminate the toxic substance. Here the life sense conveys the disturbed condition of the etheric life processes through feelings of nausea, cramps and pain.

This sense informs the child from the beginning of life whether his body is in harmony or not. Through it the child becomes aware of his hunger, thirst, digestive or emotional sensitivity and will cry to draw attention to his discomfort, and to ensure the problem is corrected or the discomfort is alleviated.

The environment will have a strong influence on the healthy development of the sense of life; for instance it will be enhanced by untainted mother's milk, health-giving food, adequate sleep, warmth, play and regular routines.

A healthy sense of life will develop an inner sense of harmony, a clear awareness of pain and discomfort, and the resilience to correct these imbalances.

3. *Sense of movement*

When I move my hand freely with eyes closed, I am aware that my hand is in movement and if I waggle my tongue I know it is moving. I know that it is moving because I also know when it is at rest. I move from one point to another; with few exceptions, I can only move certain parts of my body that are primarily those that I can perceive are moving; I cannot for instance move my heart at will and most of the time I cannot sense my heart. I am aware through this sense of movement that some part of me is active and in motion; I can also become aware of the movement of my thinking, feeling, sensing and impetus for action.

Through the sense of movement, the child perceives his own gross and fine movements. This sense grows as the child develops his musculo-skeletal system, moving his limbs, raising his head, crawling, standing up, walking, running and jumping. To begin with his movements are uncoordinated and uncontrolled. Through inner perception he gradually learns which movements are needed to perfect these bodily skills. He learns to conquer space and discovers his independence and self-control.

A child who is given the freedom to move will have the best opportunity to develop good motor coordination. In later life, an integrated sense of movement will lead to independence and an inner sense of freedom.

4. *Sense of balance*

When you move your head into different positions with eyes closed you will know where your head is in space; when you stand upright you will know the position and orientation of your body in space and whether it is steady and in equilibrium or not. Your body senses instinctively when it is in balance and is constantly correcting positions of imbalance. However, it can only do this in relation to the physical earth on which you stand; for the moment you float in water or in air, you will lose your sense of balance. You will need to exert a great deal of will power to maintain your balance within these elements. In fact one's sense of self, one's I, has a great deal to do with one's orientation in the world, location on the earth, and sense of balance.

The main organ of balance is located in the three semi-circular canals housed in the bony labyrinth of the inner ear. These three canals, each describing about two-thirds of a circle, are placed at right angles to one another and are filled with lymph fluid. They represent and detect the three planes of space. The inner lining of the three semi-circular ducts contains fine hair cells that connect with the vestibular nerve, and minute crystalline calcified bodies called otoliths which detect the dimensional changes made by the head.

By means of this sense, the child perceives his position in space in the three dimensions of above-below, left-right and forward-backward, and is able to adjust his position accordingly. His healthy motor development will depend on a healthy sense of balance working hand in hand with the sense of movement. When the child stands upright and finds his equilibrium in space for the first time, he discovers in this moment his sense of self. He comes to an awareness of himself as an I.

A child who develops a healthy sense of balance will acquire the foundations for a strong sense of self and a healthy orientation in the world.

These first four senses are predominantly connected with the physical **body** and the **will**, which are primarily developing during the first seven years of life. Healthy development of these senses is of utmost importance during this period. They allow the child to perceive the condition of his physical instrument. When nurtured in a healthy manner, the child will find a healthy relationship to his physical body and to his physical surroundings. These senses provide the foundation for trust, harmony, freedom and orientation in later life.

5. *Sense of taste*

Our sense of taste is a function of the taste buds in the mouth, mainly located on the tongue, but also on the palate and tonsils. For this sense to come into operation, we must open our mouths, place in it some substance and begin to dissolve it with the first digestive juice – the saliva. Tasting is the initial activity of 'digesting' the outer world. We begin inwardly to get to know the outer object. The taste buds are specialized cells at one end of which are taste hairs which protrude through a taste pore that opens into the mouth cavity. The taste cells connect with nerve fibres that convey sensation to the brain.

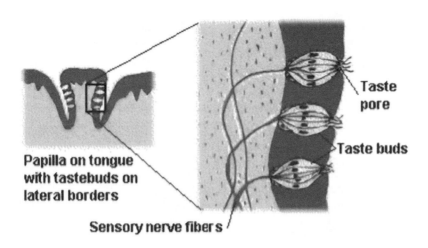

Papilla on tongue
with tastebuds on
lateral borders

Taste
pore

Taste buds

Sensory nerve fibers

We can detect four primary sensations of taste: *sour* – caused by acid substances; *salty* – due to ionized salts; *sweet* – caused by a wide range of chemicals including sugars, alcohols, amino acids and small proteins; *bitter* – due to mainly organic substances such as resins, tannins and alkaloids.

By constantly putting things into his mouth, the child inwardly learns to know about the world. He thereby forms a deep relationship with substance. He senses whether a substance is nutritious and wholesome for his body but also whether it is agreeable to his soul.

The development of a healthy sense of taste is the foundation for sensitivity, discernment and good 'taste' in later life.

6. *Sense of smell*

Whereas the sense of taste opens the soul to the world of solid and liquid substances and requires the digestive fluids to function, the sense of smell addresses the world of gaseous substances and is connected to the breathing system. Because we breathe continuously, we also smell continuously and therefore have little control over this sense. It takes us further into the outer world than the sense of taste.

The mucosal lining of the nasal cavity contains specialized olfactory cells that project into the mucus coating the inner surface of the nasal cavity. The other end of these cells is connected via nerve fibres directly to an outgrowth of the brain called the ophthalmic bulb. The sense of smell is thus very close to the brain itself.

We can easily discover that the sense of smell is much less conscious than the sense of taste: it is difficult to characterize an odour, and we usually ascribe it to some other quality we know such as camphoraceous, herby, fruity, or floral. Yet we know immediately whether an odour is pleasant and agreeable or unpleasant. The sense of smell is like a relic of the powerful instinct possessed by the animal world.

A healthy child will immediately sense the quality, scent, freshness and vitality of gaseous substances, and knows whether the smell is

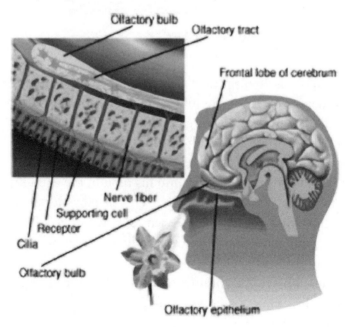

something good or bad. He intuitively knows this in the same way that he can sense or 'smell' another person's moral qualities.

A finely developed sense of smell paves the way later for good judgement and moral discernment.[8]

7. *Sense of sight*

Our eyesight is undoubtedly our most dominant sense. If you close your eyes for a moment and then open them, you can experience the far-reaching effects of vision. There is a world of difference in whether our eyes are open or closed. A glance will reveal more of the world to us than any other sense. Inwardly, it activates all the functions of the soul: thinking is stimulated by the wide range of impressions the eye is capable of picking up in an instant; our aesthetic sense is activated allowing us to appreciate beauty; our feelings and emotions are powerfully engaged and our will is mobilized to engage with what we see.

Soesman calls eyesight the 'all-encompassing sense' for it also contains all the other senses: our balance is physiologically connected to the muscles of the eye; our sense of movement is influenced by our vision; a repulsive scene will affect our sense of wellbeing and instinctively make us withdraw from it in the same way that a foul-smelling odour does; we 'touch' things, 'taste' things and even 'hear' things with our eyes because sight powerfully triggers our memory and earlier experience of the object: the sight of a lemon can evoke a sense of its leathery surface, its sour taste or the sound of squeezing out the juice; and we speak about warm and cold colours.

This all-embracing nature of the visual sense becomes understandable when we realize that the eye – which is placed in the most strategic position for facing the world that lies before us – is actually an extension of the brain that opens out into the world: embryologically it develops as a protrusion of the primitive brain; when one examines the eye medically, one is looking directly at the layers of the brain and the optic nerve that transmits visual information to the brain. There is no other nerve that can be perceived so directly and no other sense that opens to us so much of the world. This sense perceives light and dark, and thus enables us to discern objects, but it also creates a world of colour to the extent that an object allows light to shine through it. The rose only allows red light to shine through it, and this in itself conveys something about the quality of a rose. The world of colour enriches and beautifies the world.

From the second or third month the child begins to discover the world actively through his visual sense and this continues throughout life as an essential organ for learning about the world. A rich sense of sight will strengthen the child's ability to observe accurately – a necessary step towards deeper 'insight' into life; it will also enhance an aesthetic appreciation of the world.

8. Sense of warmth

We have a sense that allows us to become aware of our own bodily warmth and through it the warmth of the environment. We do not have to touch an object to sense its degree of warmth. However, there does need to be a difference in temperature, or a flow of warmth or cold between myself and the surrounding temperature for me to experience my state of warmth. The various gradations of warmth are experienced quite differently both physically and psychologically. A cold object which doesn't allow warmth to flow through it has a very different nature to a hot object which freely permits warmth to permeate it. You may notice how the cold freezes, constricts and slows down the body and closes one down emotionally. On the other hand, warmth frees up, stimulates and expands the body, and opens up one's feelings. When cold and heat reach a certain extreme temperature, they are both experienced exactly the same – as pain.

The cold and warmth receptors are unspecialized nerve fibres located immediately under the skin; they transmit warmth sensations via the spinal cord to particular areas in the brain. These nerve receptors, which lie close to capillary blood vessels, are able to detect temperature changes caused by warmth that is either withdrawn by the capillaries or given up by them.

It is thought that thermal detection results not from the direct physical effects of heat or cold on the nerve endings, but from changes in their metabolic rates, which lead to intracellular chemical changes. This finding is important because it connects the changes in warmth to metabolic changes that are always connected with the soul's will activites.

Steiner suggested that the sense of warmth is the archetypal sense out of which all the other senses developed. It is a sense that is spread out over the whole body, has a continuous subliminal interest in the outer and inner world, and produces continuous metabolic reactions that physiologically mirror the activity of the will. This in essence is the nature of the senses: to carry will or interest towards the outer world.

This sense connects the child even more deeply with his immediate surroundings. Through it he has an instinctive awareness of his own inner warmth; he knows what level of warmth is right for him and can therefore relate intimately to heat and cold in his external environment. Warmth or lack of it informs the child about the inner nature of things. It also enables him to relate with warmth to the outer world.

In the second seven-year cycle, the child opens his soul to the world through his feeling life while he strives to establish a balance in his rhythmic life (all the rhythmic activities including circulation). These four senses require special attention during this period of the child's life. They convey to the **soul** an inner experience of the outer world that lies in close proximity to our sense-perceiving organism. Through embracing the polarities of light and darkness, cold and warmth, as well as the wide spectrum of odours and tastes, the child explores his soul life through the fine shades of feeling called up by these senses. The groundwork for future emotional intelligence is laid down through these senses, as well as the gifts of discernment, morality, sensitivity, aesthetics, insight and inner warmth.

9. *Sense of hearing*

When listening to the sounds that our hearing perceives, it is interesting to discover that we can experience them in various parts of the body, although they are initially perceived by the auditory apparatus: the grating of teeth, a trumpet call, a violin played beautifully or discordantly, a deep sounding bell or the beating of a drum, all appear to resonate in different parts of the body. This becomes comprehensible when one realizes that the main function of the auditory apparatus is to translate sound vibrations that are transmitted by the air into resonating vibrations conveyed

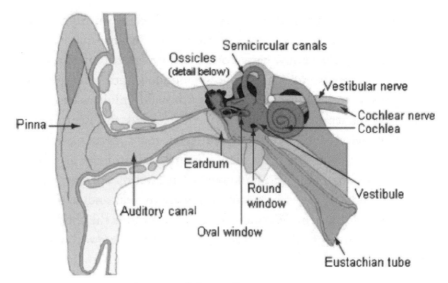

Diagram of the auditory apparatus

as impulses to the brain. The etheric body, as we have seen, is a resonating sound body, and it is therefore readily understandable that it will carry these inner vibrations thoughout the organism.

Let us try to follow the transformation of sound from a resonating object like a bell to the internalized experience of a child who hears this sound. The bell resonates when it is struck by another object; it resonates in a very different way from a solid rock because it has been lifted out of the earthly into the airy realm. These sound vibrations, which can be exactly measured and mathematically numbered, are mediated via the air and received by the outer ear where they strike the eardrum. In the middle ear they are transformed into the mechanical vibrations of three bony ear ossicles – the hammer, anvil and stirrup – that function together as mechanical levers. These vibrations in turn impinge via a second vibrating window upon the lymph fluid-filled space of the inner ear, which is housed in the temple bone of the skull, one of the hardest bones of the skeleton; here they are carried by the fine ripples of fluid resonance to the end point of the hearing organ where they pass through a spiral shaped cochlea. Fine hair cells located on the inner lining of the cochlea are stimulated by the resonating fluid and generate the nerve impulses that are conveyed to the brain. One may well ask why the cochlea has a spiral shape. Imagine you become sound vibrations that are sucked

– like water into a vortex – into the funnel-shaped opening of the spiral cochlea, driven ever deeper and compressed ever more as the space narrows down towards the apex. What happens at this point? One arrives, as it were, at the 'eye of the needle', at the point where, in the digestive system for instance, food is completely broken down in the great spiral of the intestines and where something entirely new can come into being, because the old has been completely erased.

From the above description it would appear that the ear is able to take in sound vibrating in air, pass it through fluid and solid matter and transform it into pure sound experience that is freed from earthly influences. It receives sound waves that can be physically measured, passes them through mechanical bony levers and through a labyrinthine bony structure housed deep in a cave of the hardest bone, and offers it up to the human organism in a completely new form. It can now be experienced by the whole body through the resonating etheric system of the organism.

The auditory organ is obviously closely connected to the organ of balance; it internalizes the three-dimensional earthly world that the organ of balance opens to us, in the way described above, revealing a creative world of soul and spirit.

Through this internalizing process, the child acquires even more intimate knowledge of the outer world than through the sense of warmth. Whereas heat is evenly distributed through an object, sound may cause a part of the object to vibrate, informing us about the resonating quality of that particular part. The sound may also originate from an object far away, enabling us to discover much about the object before it meets the eye.

Through his sense of hearing, enhanced by his sense of balance, the child acquires an inner depth of soul and a deep empathy for his environment. The sounds of nature, the way his parents speak, live or recorded music, will all have an influence on the child's healthy development.

10. Sense of speech, word or tone

When we listen to someone speaking we hear the sound qualities of the words; but we can go further and also understand the meaning behind the words. Specific words convey specific meanings and each language will offer a slightly different meaning for the same object. A sense other than hearing is needed to detect the meaning within a word, tone or sequence of speech. We have to listen more with our hearts than with our heads and we can discover that this sense is closely connected with the power of empathy. Through this sense we hear something about the person behind the sound or word. In listening to the meaning behind the words, it is as if we move towards the person speaking, and meet their individual qualities.

Indeed, this sense appears to be intimately connected with movement: we shall see later in this chapter that speaking is a natural developmental progression of movement in the young child, who learns to speak and understand words only after he learns to stand and walk. Furthermore, the centres for speech and motor function of the dominant side of the body are located in the same part of the brain; thus right-sided individuals have the speech and motor centres in the left cerebral cortex and left-sided people have these centres in the right cerebral cortex. This centre also represents all the muscles of the mouth and voice box that are needed to move and shape speech. It is well known that the vocal cords of the larynx move as they shape each vowel or consonant. Kinesics, the study of body movements and gestures, has shown by fine film and soundtrack analysis of someone speaking, that every word or letter is associated with quite specific movements of the body. It has further been shown that the listener also moves his body in sympathetic synchronicity to the articulated structure of the speaker's words. The inference is that every language will create a different movement in the speaker and the listener, and a different nuance of feeling and meaning for the same word spoken in different languages. Thus the sequence of letters in the word 'tree' or *Baum* (German) will be experienced very differently.

A child who lives in natural sympathy with the world will therefore enter into the meaning behind words and the particular inflections of the voice, and will instinctively imitate what he senses. The creative power of the Word can become a source of creative expression when language is conveyed to the child in a wholesome manner.

11. *Sense of thought*

We all have had the experience of unconsciously sensing what someone thinks. We listen to someone speaking or read what someone writes and we can grasp the idea behind the words. We can observe a child's frightened movements or gestures and perceive the thought that stands behind the movement –'I am scared'. This ability to sense another person's thoughts, concepts or mental pictures requires one to put aside even more of oneself than the sense of speech. For even the word or the gesture must be dissolved if one is to sense the idea behind the outer expression. One then enters a world that is universally human, where ideas and concepts live.

When we develop this sense more consciously, it permits us to sense another person's thoughts underlying their spoken or written words, or their actions. This rests on a healthy development of the sense of life, which, like the life forces, are transformed into forces for thinking.

Children intuitively use this sense to pick up what lives in others' thoughts. It enables them to grasp concepts behind words and actions. An environment that reflects wholesome concepts will have a health-giving influence on their growth and development.

12. *Sense of I*

When we meet another human being, we can sense a uniquely individual I living in him. We perceive this through any form of expression he manifests: his words, gaze, handshake, handwriting, gait or gestures. We know intuitively whether someone is standing with his whole being behind what he says. We can sense when someone is being authentic, honest, truthful or the opposite. We can do this because we have a sense for another person's I. But how do we do this? We have to look past what we hear in the words of a particular language; we have to ignore the meaning of the words and even the ideas. Then only do we arrive through deep empathy at the individuality of the human being. Steiner suggests that this sense is an unconscious organ of knowing, spread out over the whole human being.[9]

Children instinctively sense the I-nature of those with whom they live. They will feel others' intentions and morality, and this will impact positively or negatively on their health. This sense, which builds on the sense of touch, will enable the child in later life to recognize other human beings' true nature. As we saw above, the sense of touch helps the child to wake up to a sense of his own self, which is the first step towards recognizing the self of the other.

These four senses are connected with the **spirit** nature of the human being. In the third seven-year cycle, the adolescent experiences the world actively with his thinking and it is these higher senses that need to be consciously nurtured. The adolescent can thereby discover a healthy relationship to his own spiritual life as well as to the life of society around him. The foundation for clarity of thinking as well as self-awareness, inner depth of soul, deep empathy, intuition, open-mindedness and creative expression are provided by the development of these senses.

The Twelve Senses in Summary

These twelve senses inform the child about the world in which he lives: the four lower bodily senses tell him about his physical instrument; his four middle soul senses inform him about his immediate sense-perceptible environment; his four higher senses provide him with information about a more refined supersensible reality.

4 Lower senses:	Touch, life, movement, balance	Body-based senses	Inform about body
4 Middle senses:	Warmth, sight, taste, smell	Soul-based senses	Inform about sense-perceptible world
4 Higher senses:	Hearing, word, thought, I	Spirit-based senses	Inform about supersensible world

Immediately after birth the soul body of the child becomes highly active, working primarily with those senses closest to his physical being. Through his sense of touch, life and warmth, he learns to appreciate the sensory impressions that feel good and nurturing for him: for instance, the tactile sensation of the nipple that carries the warm flowing milk gives him evident pleasure and sense of wellbeing.

He develops awareness and an inner mental picture of the stance and location of his whole body and its parts through his sense of movement, balance and sight. He learns to find the optimum position of his body in space to satisfy his needs. Through trying out new positions and discovering his body, he learns to pass objects from one hand to the other (bilateral integration), develops left or right handedness (laterality), improves his postural responses and thereby learns to raise his head, crawl, stand and walk.

His other organs of hearing, smell and taste also evolve as he experiences new sensations. As these senses become more organized, integrated and functional he can extend his sentient activity towards the surrounding world. He can now direct more energy to his other senses, his auditory, visual, speech, thought and I sense.

Imagine for a moment you were able to surrender your whole being to the taste impression of, say, chocolate, without forming any judgments or thoughts like 'this is delicious' or 'I shouldn't really be having this'. You are fully present in tasting the chocolate with your whole organism, letting its nature enter and make an impression on your body. And now you try to express what it does to your body through some gesture or movement. If you accurately observe the sensations and feelings that chocolate creates in you, you will be able to discover the nature of chocolate as it affects your body.[10]

This is exactly how the young child explores and discovers his environment. He surrenders himself completely through his sense perceptions to the objects of the outer world, allows these impressions to resonate within and then gestures or **imitates** them outwardly.

Imitation

This is the basis for all learning in early childhood, without which one cannot understand the young child. It is a natural faculty with which all small children are endowed, making learning for developmentally healthy children easy and automatic. Everyone who lives or works with children will appreciate their natural talent for absorbing and then imitating what they perceive around them. If you build up blocks with a child in a certain way the child will copy this, if you hammer he will hammer in like manner. He observes his mother standing upright and when his body is sturdy enough, he will want to stand up; he hears words being spoken and he speaks these words; he sees his mother or father kneading the dough and he too wants to knead.

Because the child does not yet have a strongly individuated sense of self, he does not feel separated from the surrounding world and is therefore able to live actively and fully present in this world, experiencing outer objects as if he were inside them. Thus when he sees a tree, one can imagine he becomes one with the tree, when he hears a bird call he inwardly resonates with the sound, and intuitively experiences the nature of the bird.

Experience imaginatively what it is like to lose your sense of a personal self separating you from everyone else; imagine losing your finite boundaries and sense of self and notice how much more connected you feel to everything outside you – less conscious and more dreamy. Feel how open you become and how much easier it is to absorb sense impressions; you connect with these impressions, identify with them and then express them outwardly through some action; you may find how easy it is to imitate these perceptions.

How does the child turn sense impressions into actions? How is he able to copy something immediately after perceiving it? With the awakening of the soul, outer world becomes inner experience for the child. The life body, as we have seen, activates all living processes in the physical body such as growth, digestion, respiration, etc. The finer part of this life body is the soul body, that organization of awareness that mediates, among other things, the life of sensation. The sensory impressions that enter through the twelve senses cause the vibrating nature of the life forces to reverberate as resonating impulses, much as a particular gust of wind ripples the water surface in a specific way. The life body as the organ of memory absorbs and copies these sensory impressions just as the soft sand beneath the water surface allows the movement of the water to imprint and hold its form within it. Outer impressions are thereby transcribed into inner experience.

For instance a child observes the way his mother or father irons a garment. These impressions are taken in by the soul body and cause the life body to reverberate accordingly. In this moment the learning process begins; the memory of ironing is stored inside. Now when he wishes to iron his doll's clothes and takes up his play iron he knows exactly how to do it; his physical body merely carries out what his life body has internalized.

In this way the child learns to know things from the inside without having to study them like an adult; he does things quite naturally because he has a genuine master imitator in his etheric body.

If this picture has reality, it has obvious implications for the health of young children since all environmental impressions – health-giving or harmful – penetrate directly into the child's organism through etheric transcription. For instance, loud sounds create a stronger and harsher etheric resonance compared to soft melodious sounds, and over time will impact negatively on the young and impressionable body. Thus the quality of the sense impressions in the early years of childhood will have a deep effect on the overall functioning of the life forces, determining the foundation of health far into the future.

Three Human Capacities: Standing/Walking – Speaking – Thinking

Among all the things a child must learn during this early period, there are three human capacities that are fundamental for the child's future life: his **upright posture** and ability to **walk**, his ability to speak and his ability to **think**.

These three human functions are not given to the child in the way that species of the animal kingdom are instinctively and quickly endowed from earliest life with specific abilities; for instance a baby chick can walk, scratch in the soil and feed itself soon after emerging from the egg. The child has to acquire these capacities through his own will, sense perception, imitation and actions.

The first year is concerned with learning to move the body, stand and walk; the second year is the period when speech develops; and the third year is characterized by the development of conscious thinking.

The developmental sequence is never absolutely fixed and linear, and there is unquestionably an overlap between different functions. Nevertheless, as we have seen in our study of embryology and developmental morphology, and as we will see throughout our exploration of the child's biography, there are definite, discernable developmental tendencies and predominant activities which occur at predictable times. These point to an underlying biographical law which allows developmental psychologists to speak unanimously about developmental periods and developmental milestones. We have identified these developmental laws and milestones as intrinsic to the biography of the universal child.

From this point of view, and knowing that the growing science of developmental psychology is highly controversial and in constant flux, we can propose the idea that each landmark achievement appears to prepare the way for the development of the following one: out of movement, standing and walking emerges speaking, and out of speaking, thinking proceeds.

Standing/Walking

The ability to walk is the culmination of intense activity in learning to orientate and move in space that begins soon after birth and continues through the first year of life. The child shows a great deal of mobility immediately after birth: watch the reflex muscular actions in a screaming child, or the fine movements of the mouth, lips and tongue as he sucks at the breast. The little hands and toes are very mobile as he experiences the milk flowing through his body. These movements are uncoordinated, to begin with. As his sense perception awakens the child begins, from his horizontal position, to be more aware of his environment.

In the first month his vision becomes more focused, his hearing more directed. We observe spontaneous, uncontrolled and seemingly purposeless movements of legs and arms. He begins to explore his world with a sense of touch that is distributed over the whole surface of his body: his hands probe surfaces and objects, his limbs become more active, he discovers parts of his own body, his hands, fingers, feet and toes. Then he wants to see further: how many times must he raise and drop his heavy head before he develops the strength to keep it aloft?

In the third month he has it finally under control: the head is the first part of the body to be properly mastered. Then he begins to move his body by rocking sideways, squirming forwards and backwards, rolling over. He raises his chest by pushing upwards with his arms.

By five to six months he is sitting upright, surveying his world with delight at his achievement. He now has firm control over his chest and arms.

At about six months one can sense the child's urge actively to explore his environment. He starts by shifting around from the sitting position, then begins to push or pull himself around.

By seven to eight months he is crawling on all fours. He is still confined to the horizontal plane. Joan Salter describes how the infant recapitulates in his early movements and gestures all the earlier evolutionary stages, passing through fish, frog, reptilian, bird and mammalian phases of movement.[11] Then comes the triumphant moment between nine to twelve months when he raises himself into the truly human position, standing freely on his own two feet, his spine vertical, overcoming the forces of gravity and thereby creating the first real separation between himself and the world. To observe this moment is to catch one of the great moments of childhood – one can sense the child's joy in this freedom.

> I have arrived at my humanity, I have found my position in space; my head looks out freely into the world, my voice can now receive the gift of speech and my hands are free for creative deeds.

He stands up and falls down many times before he stands firmly and securely. He gains control over his legs.

And then between twelve and sixteen months, he takes his first step into the world: a further step towards freedom.

Thus, through his own efforts, the child overcomes gravity and acquires mastery in orientating and stabilizing himself in space, working once again from the head down through the chest to the feet. The head has attained a position of rest which allows him to perceive the world calmly; his arms are free to explore the world, his legs have the mobility to carry him through the world.

It is essential that we allow the child to learn these body skills himself in his own good time and in his own unique way and resist the urge to help him along in this process. The innate intelligence of a developmentally healthy child is far wiser than our desire for a milestone to be reached at a particular time. At the same time we should be aware of obvious developmental delays: an infant who scarcely moves, who cannot sit by nine months, stand by fifteen months or walk by eighteen months needs to be seen by a paediatrician or other child health specialist.

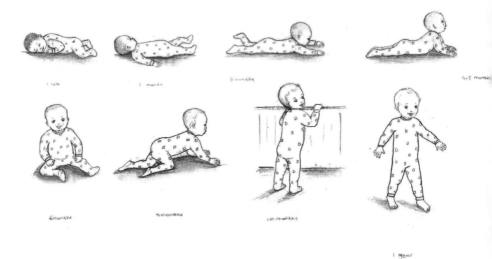

Speaking

Before a child can speak we have to try and interpret from his body language and his bodily sounds what he is experiencing and what he needs. So often we stand in front of a young child totally perplexed, wondering what is going on in his soul, and wishing that he could express himself through words. This is because speech is our accustomed means of communication. What a relief it is then to hear the first words of a child and to be able to relate to him increasingly through a common language. This will take place in the second year of life.

Just as walking comes about through progressive development of bodily movements, so speech develops through the movement and elaboration of sound in the body. This begins with the child's first cry after birth, and for the first three months crying and cooing are the means by which the child communicates his inner experiences to the world.

By the third month babbling has begun, consisting of random combinations of vowels and consonants as the infant begins to exercise the various organs and muscles of the speech apparatus: the larynx (voice box), the parts of the mouth – tongue, lips, teeth, palate, cheeks – and the nasal cavity and sinuses as resonator. Through interaction of these organs of speech and the air present in these spaces, the sounds of speech are produced.[12] These sounds combine to form syllables which make up the unique baby talk common to all babies from different cultures and are the building blocks for the future 'mother tongue'. Children born deaf babble in the same way as those who can hear, indicating the reflexive nature of babbling as the child discovers his organs of speech.

At the beginning of the second year the first true expressions of speech as such begin, as syllables learned through babbling are connected with the unfolding of new inner experiences: for instance the child has learnt to sound the syllable 'ma' and hears the word 'mama'; with reinforcement and feedback, he gradually associates this word with the presence of his mother and the inner feelings of comfort that she calls up in him. When one tries to enter the child's inner sense for the tone or word, one is left with the impression that the single words conjure up in him a complete inner experience: the child appears to live actively in the experience underlying a word. He expresses his inner experience through it. Thus *moo-cow* expresses the child's full engagement with what he experiences when he sees the cow.

Between the twelfth and fourteenth month, the child realizes that objects can be named. He discovers that he has the power through speech to give the things in his world a name. He may borrow the names through imitation or he may invent his own name for things on the basis of his experience. These protonames may be entirely different from one child to the next and often very different from our preconceived concepts. Thus a dog may be called *ha* (one that often pants), *woo* or *ti* (short for Rusty).

His first words are usually object-related – cat, ball, hat – but later they become action-related, i.e. verbs which indicate the moving and doing realm in which the child is so much at home. As he learns to recognize and name objects, he is learning at the same time to separate himself slowly from a world with which he originally felt completely united. Through words connected with the material world he is learning to find his relationship to space; through words related to action he is coming into a more objective relationship to time.

During the next months the child grows his vocabulary and starts to string words together with huge delight in his new-found creative power.

By the end of the second year, sentence construction gradually emerges through the blending of nouns, adjectives and verbs, and in the third year the mother tongue begins to fully emerge.

Through standing and walking, the child has learnt to conquer space and move freely in the world. By naming his world he starts inwardly to take ownership of this world as if it was his own creation and to bring order and meaning into the overwhelming diversity of his experience. And through talking he enters into a community of language that opens the door to social experience.

Speech and Movement

It is well known that the speech centre in the brain – the so-called *Broca's area* – is located in the same section of the frontal brain as the motor centre for the dominant side of the body. In other words the left side of the frontal brain represents the centre both for moving the right side of the body and the muscles needed for speech – the muscles of the mouth, larynx and respiratory system.

By the time the child has learnt to stand on his own, a great deal of motor development has taken place in all regions of the body, including the organs of speech. This has developed the motor area of the brain, where the speech centre is located. One may infer from this that the development of speaking is a natural progression of the bodily movements which culminate in the child learning to stand upright and to walk.

It is widely accepted that movement precedes and influences speech: The first words are spoken between the tenth and fourteenth month, almost always after the child has learnt to stand upright and has acquired his orientation in space. Both low and high muscular tone will influence the development of speech. For instance flaccid children with low muscle tone cannot develop the respiratory and interoral pressure needed for plosive (b, d, g, k) sounds; likewise spastic children cannot move their tongues freely and therefore cannot articulate clearly.

It follows that the healthy development of movement in an infant will have a bearing on subsequent speech. Allowing the child freedom of movement and providing an environment where the child can imitate clearly articulated language, will give the child the best opportunity to master speech.

One often hears a baby being spoken to in baby talk that is very different to a person's accustomed manner of speaking. While there is evidence that raising the pitch of the voice, slowing the rate of speaking and simplifying the language structure and concepts, can enhance learning to speak, it is important to articulate clearly and to steer the child gently and progressively to the customary way of speaking, as his verbal abilities develop. Thus the *woo* will change to *woof woof*, then to *doggy*, and finally to *dog* as the child hears this concept articulated in different ways. Because the child absorbs and imitates everything that he perceives, and because the brain and other organs will be physically influenced by these sense impressions, we will need to take care of the way we speak to children.

Thinking

Thinking appears to awaken as a conscious mental activity in the third year of life once certain basic structures and activities are in place. Cognitive activity before this time is limited to sensory-motor reflexive behaviour of varying complexity. Actions and behaviour will be largely determined by internal bodily or external sensory stimulation. On this foundation he will build the whole edifice of his thinking life. An infant cannot yet direct his life through conscious thought processes. He experiences his hunger and need for nourishment and cries to be fed; his bodily needs determine his action. Or he perceives his mother or recognizes the nipple and cries to be fed: an association between his sensory experience and his bodily needs leads to a very definite response. This is conditioned reflex at the level of the will. Later it is desire coupled with perceptions that lead to actions. These are also still conditioned reflexes that lead to purposeful action, though more complex.

Let us examine the conditions that need to be in place before the first level of independent thinking can take place, acknowledging König, Piaget and others for their comprehensive research in this field.[13]

Memory

This first prerequisite is the mental ability to store information at a subconscious level for later use and its retrieval for conscious experience. The child perceives an object for the first time, say a bird. This image is pressed into his memory body – his etheric body – as we explored in Chapter two. When he sees the bird again, it triggers the memory image and he recognizes it as a known object. Much recent research on memory claims that children can remember more and earlier than was previously thought.[14] But what kind of memory is the child exhibiting?

In the first year the child remembers past objects and events by perceiving these again in the present. A newborn baby recognizes his mother through visual, auditory and even olfactory stimuli that awaken his memory of being fed or needing comfort. The one-year-old child recognizes the furry cat and wants to grasp hold again of the soft, warm fur. Each time Daniel came into my consulting room he would search among all the toys for the tiny yellow porcelain bee ornament that he had played with on his first visit. This is how memory operates chiefly during the first year of life, based on recognition of the same perceptions. These then activate bodily processes such as the digestive system or the motor system, leading to the conditioned reflexes mentioned above.

Steiner informs us that our ancient forefathers possessed this localized memory which led them to erect memorials, signs or landmarks of different kinds to mark important events and to enable them to relive these again at a later time.[15] These monuments can be found today all over the world – the stone formations of the Celts in Brittany or Stonehenge in England, the Matopa ruins in Zimbabwe, the giant rocks of Easter Island. These point to a consciousness that today is present in the child when the memory is still strongly bound to the will and limbs, and can only be awoken by images of the sense world in which the child is living so strongly during this time.

Towards the end of the first year, the child realizes that an object exists even when it is out of sight, and will search for an object in the place he remembers having seen it. This is called object permanence, and this stage is still dependent on localized memory.

During the second year, the child develops a second kind of memory alongside localized memory. This is memory based on repetition, whereby something is imprinted into the life memory matrix by repeated activities of one kind or another; for instance the child will practise walking until it becomes an automatic activity, he will repeat words over and over, and wants to hear certain stories or rhymes repeatedly. He experiences great joy in this rhythmic repetition and never seems to tire of it: he is engaging in the life of rhythm, an activity underlying all life processes. This is the basis of the child's early learning: he learns by imitation and repetition, imprinting into the body a memory that will direct his basic bodily functions for life, skills that we all take completely for granted. Our automatic pilot runs our body without our conscious engagement, and is a function of this early, inbuilt memory which Steiner calls rhythmic memory.

Our forefathers needed to imprint their life experiences into their bodies through rhythmic activities such as singing, dancing, reciting, drumming, etc. In such activity these rhythmic movements which are associated with particular feelings are carried into the bodily will functions. Memories can be invoked again by re-awakening the same rhythmic repetition. This allows small children to retain memory of things which before required the object to be present in their direct field of perception. The topic of rhythm will be dealt with more fully in the next chapter.

Gradually, during the latter part of the second and the third year, certain events or objects that made a strong impression on the child can be recalled without being present again, or invoked through repetition. This mental representation is the forerunner of independent cognitive memory. The mental picture is now strong enough to exist as an independent picture memory. This becomes possible only when the child has separated himself to some extent from his surrounding world; he begins to experience himself as a separate part of the world and starts in a dim way to become aware of time. He is no longer living completely in the present moment. In his mental life he can recall things that happened in the past and can bring them back into the present. These inner experiences are no longer the real living world but an internalized image of this world. He has also named many things that he now can retrieve from his memory.

These three forms of memory are linked once again to the threefold nature of the developing child:

Localized memory	metabolic-limb system and the will
Rhythmic memory	rhythmic system and feeling life
Picture memory	neuro-sensory system and thinking life

We can wonder here whether the child develops a concept by first perceiving the parts of an object – for instance do the trunk, branches and leaves of many such objects lead him eventually to the concept and the naming of such an object 'tree' – or does he have a concept of the whole tree from the start and later becomes aware of the individual parts?[16] We shall leave this question for a later chapter.

The Relationship Between Thinking and Speech

It also seems that the development of speech is necessary for the development of independent thinking. That language and thought are closely connected cannot be disputed; how often do you find yourself saying out loud what you are thinking? The nature of the relationship however, is highly controversial. The idea that language is a necessary condition for thinking is as old as Aristotle, who believed that language was essential to instruction. We have seen that children typically learn the foundations of speech in the second year before they develop picture memory. The child plays with the different parts of language and thereby connects increasingly with the outside world: for instance nouns are the object things that he recognizes and names – cat, table, tree; verbs are the active, doing things in the world – meeouw, stand, grow ; while the adjectives and adverbs define and describe the things of the world – furry, gently, strong. All aspects of the language – declensions of the nouns, conjugations of the verbs, pronouns, singular, plural, past, present and future – define, differentiate and enlarge the child's world, empowering him with a tool for creating and defining his own world. One may say that the world is reflected in the child's soul through the fine differentiation of language. But for the child at this stage speaking is not thinking. He is able to speak the word 'doggy' before he has an independent mental picture of a dog.

Can we try to experience where in the psyche speaking arises? We have seen that it develops from primal sounds that ultimately become formed and differentiated into speech. It appears to be a will-based activity that is more conscious than feeling but not as conscious as thinking – seemingly somewhere in between. Of course speaking may be an expression of one's thinking, but most of the time speaking does not rely on us first thinking what we express in words. Speech unfolds and expresses itself through us and only afterwards can we reflect on what we have said, sometimes with huge surprise. *Where did that come from?*

When our ancient forefathers first developed language, words expressed what was for them a living reality. Take the words *headstrong, lion-hearted, encourage, handy*. By penetrating a word actively with the modes of experience we have been developing here – for instance visualizing, sensing, feeling and gesturing a *headstrong* person – we can access the power of language and the realities underlying it.

Children create words out of the innate plasticity of language and their deep perceptive powers. Thus the words *riverfall* and *rainbrella* tell us more about the *waterfall* and *umbrella* than these words themselves. These examples show how, through language, children take part in a universal process that prepares them for the inner structuring that is later needed for thinking as reasoning individuals. In other words, one can say that language possesses its own intelligence that begins to inform the way children think as they imitate it.

With due respect to the controversy surrounding this subject, many phenomena seem to indicate that conscious thinking begins *after* the child begins to speak and that thinking develops with and through speech. Speech thus appears to be an important building block for thinking. The way in which the mother tongue is articulated, the words and images used and the grammar and syntax chosen, seem to significantly affect the development of the thinking process in these early years. The environment of language in which the child learns to speak, and which he therefore imitates, is thus of utmost importance during this early phase of childhood. In children who die before they have learnt to speak, the surface of the brain responsible for speech has a smooth and even appearance; as the child learns to speak this becomes progressively more convoluted and differentiated. As the child learns to move his organs of speech, he simultaneously begins to mould and form his brain just as a sculptor carves a form out of clay. Steiner claims that the contours of the brain surface are formed differently by the formative effects of different languages.[17]

Play and Imagination

A third condition for conscious thinking is the activity of **imagination** and its outward expression in children's play.

Where does the child draw his faculty of imagination from? This creative power can turn stones into shining diamonds, mud cakes into delicious puddings and sticks into farm animals. At a deep, unconscious level, the child seems to have access to a fountainhead of universal life that bubbles up in his imagination, and incorporates everything around him – material objects, activities or ideas. Watch how happy and content the small child is when engrossed in his fantasy world. He is still in close connection and great sympathy with an invisible world of creative activity. Play brings the content of this invisible world into his daily earthly life. Here he can create the world just as he wishes it, like a master puppeteer creating the personalities of his choice. It helps us to understand the world of childhood when we realize that the young child is in touch with the world of archetypes; he knows the ideal reality of mother, father and child and can create a story line where these ideal realities manifest for instance in the form of sticks and stones. In play he can bring this universal world of creative existence into relationship with everything that he has perceived and imitated.

These preconditions of memory, speech and imagination appear to be the three cardinal soul activities needed before thinking can develop as a new and delicate human faculty.

At the same time, these activities are also at work in moulding the brain to become the instrument of thinking. We have seen that at birth the convolutions of the brain have a comparatively smooth surface; as the child awakens in his soul and engages with the world, his brain becomes more defined and differentiated over the following two to three years. And as it thus matures, the brain and especially the forebrain becomes a more efficient instrument for the I to use for conscious thinking and thus for self-awareness.

Neuroplasticity is a well-researched field,[18] which examines how environmental influences change or modify the brain. A baby is born with all the brain cells it will need for the rest of his life. These neuronal cells will grow significantly in size during the first year. In the following years up to the change of teeth, neurons connect progressively with each other by means of synapses to reach a peak at about the age of three-and-a-half. Life experiences have been shown to stimulate the formation of these synapses and their connection with the higher senses, leading to significant shaping and reorganizing of the immature brain in the first two to three years. Young children have more neurons and synapses than older children; as the child develops they reduce in number through a process referred to as neural pruning, whereby the brain loses its capacity to adapt as effectively to change. This process will be determined to a great extent by environmental influences, so that neuronal networks not sufficiently used are eliminated while those frequently used expand and become more interconnected.[19]

It is evident that neuroplasticity early in life is greatest because new connecting pathways are being constantly established and because synapses and neurons have not yet been significantly pruned.

While it is well-established that life experience will have an actual structural and functional effect on the brain, what is not so easy to establish scientifically is the particular effects of certain kinds of environmental impression. What for example is the specific effect of TV on the unformed brain of an infant child? Although no exact data are available, the American Academy of Paediatrics recommends that children under the age of two years should not watch TV because it 'can negatively affect early brain development'. The works by Martin Large – *Set Free Childhood* and Keith Buzell – *The Children of Cyclops*, describe cogently the influence of television viewing on the developing brain.[20] In

Part 2, the harmful effects of audio-visual and electronic media on the developing child will be presented. There can be no doubt that environmental impressions significantly shape the developing brain. We therefore all have a moral duty to use our common sense and healthy judgement to create an optimal environment for young children.

Self-discovery

In his third year the toddler starts to express himself as an individual personality able to make rational statements and to take purposeful action; his cognitive processes are now less directed by his bodily and emotional activities.

> Jonathan wanted to retrieve his ball from the chest of drawers; he tried to reach for the ball and realized he was too small; he remembered the last time he ran to call his mother to fetch it for him; he pondered the situation for a moment, then ran to the kitchen to fetch a chair and with great satisfaction reached over for the ball. Excitedly, he rushed to tell his mother – 'Mummy, I fetched the ball myself!'

For the first time Jonathan had named himself here not as *me* or *Johnny* but I. He has discovered his own I nature; he himself was able to fetch his ball and he was conscious of this act! He could carry out this action because he could see himself as smaller in relation to the table, because he could remember it happened before, because he could imagine what he would have to do to retrieve the ball – to find something to make him taller – and because he had the physical power and skill to perform the task.

He has therefore found a relationship to his own body, to time and space and to cause and effect, seeing himself for the first time as a separate personality. And thinking has become the faculty that makes this new awareness possible. Thinking becomes the new power through which he can master his world, giving guidance and direction to his power of movement and of speaking that he already possessed.

Upright Posture, Speaking and Thinking

These three cardinal human functions provide the foundation for all future human action. Where do the wisdom and power implicit in the unfolding of these three essential functions come from? Certainly not from the world of physical matter, nor from the etheric body's realm of life forces, that only provide the blueprint for the growth and development of the physical body. The forces working through these activities are not bodily functions. The soul realm, likewise, is itself involved in a dynamic process of development and cannot provide the impetus for the awakening of these activities.

The I has only just become aware of itself: for instance at the moment when Jonathan named himself 'I'. Although still very much hidden, it is the main actor in the drama. Is it the I that writes the child's early script and instructs him so well to stand, speak and think or is the I empowered by something else to discover these capacities? As we have seen through accompanying the child in this process, the first year is chiefly concerned with learning to move the body, standing and walking; the second year is the period when speech develops; the third year is characterized by the development of thinking. Each landmark achievement appears to prepare the way for the development of the following one: out of movement, standing and walking, speaking emerges; out of speaking, thinking proceeds. When one opens oneself in reverence to the young child's nature and tries to stand imaginatively in his experience of learning to walk, to speak and to think, one may have a sense of something that goes beyond the child himself: a sense of the higher wisdom and power working through the child's I deeply into his bodily nature – into his limbs, his larynx and his brain – and providing the driving force that brings into being these three fundamental human characteristics.

Thus, during the first three years of life, these three essential instruments develop that the child's self requires for his journey in the physical world. Only once these functions are in place can the child's I take proper possession of his body. This happens in the third year in that glorious moment when the child discovers that he is separate from the world around him and addresses himself as 'I' for the first time. It is a rare gift to witness such a moment. This is usually the point in time to which the continuity of our memory can return.

Core Picture and Care in Early Childhood

- During the first three years the child is a citizen of two worlds. He is still faithfully connected with the unseen world whence he came, and he bears this devotion, trust and sense of rightness and goodness into the earthly world.
- He surrenders himself with complete trust, loyalty and unquestioning acceptance to the care and protection of his caregivers and to the sense impressions of the outer world. He places his life and potential in the hands of his caregivers and in the world of earthly matter.
- He learns everything through his surrender to sensing and his natural capacity to imitate.
- Through imitation and the power of a higher wisdom working through him, he acquires the three fundamental human characteristics of: upright posture, speaking and thinking. These abilities develop sequentially as a preparation for the child's I to enter and take hold of his body in a new way.
- The will and the sensing functions are the first organs of the soul to awaken, propelling the child into the world of the senses and making it a priority that the head and neuro-sensory system grow first and fastest.
- The child is highly impressionable, nakedly innocent and relatively helpless and this is a time more than any other when we need to be the child's advocate and protector.

The more we can live into the sensitive and impressionable life of the young child and empathize with his trusting nature, the more readily we can realize that this vital period of childhood is today threatened and compromised in countless ways. Parents, educators, healthcare practitioners and all those who love children, need to recognize the vital importance of these years for later life and to protect the child against the potential hazards of an ever-increasing materialistic and technological age. We can best do this when we learn to respect the world of early childhood and to value its gift for every individual and for humanity as a whole.[21]

Risks and Threats

Calm and Consistency

Our modern life so often imposes on the child's secure state by taking him into situations that are harmful to his sensitive constitution. While only a child living in the country can perhaps avoid this completely, we should do our utmost to avoid carrying him around in fast-moving vehicles through busy traffic, into sensory-overloaded supermarkets and shopping malls, to large gatherings of people, and to events at night when he should be asleep. The young child does not thrive on over-stimulation of this kind and it is easy to see how he is thrown out of his restful equilibrium. Frequent air travel and moving home is also injurious to his health. This is because young children need stability and constancy above all: a settled, calm environment.

Vaccinations

If parents accept without question this now established approach to the prevention of certain illnesses, the young child will receive some thirty foreign-protein inoculations in the first two years of his life, with a wide range of potential side-effects. These vaccinations are aimed at preventing dangerous illnesses but these include some childhood infectious conditions that have benefits for healthy development. Parents need to be informed and to be discerning about the immunizations they should subject their children to.[22]

Childhood Illnesses

Fevers occur most frequently in the first seven years. They may be a natural response to inner or outer stress and an important part of the body's immune and defence system. Or they may occur without obvious external cause, signalling the dynamic engagement of the child's higher self in biological processes. As we have seen, warmth is the medium through which the I engages in the body. Adequate warmth is essential for the child to connect properly with his body and when this is not happening sufficiently, enhanced warmth, namely fever, will be the result. The current medical doctrine of suppressing every fever as a matter of course, as well as administering many other chemical medicines for trivial ailments, should be reassessed in the interests of child health.[23] In illness the healing process can be supported with natural medicines and therapies. Childhood illnesses can be regarded as a normo-regulative activity of balancing out inner weaknesses and disturbances and will be dealt with in great detail in Part 2.

Nutrition

This plays a vital role in the healthy development of the young child's biological systems. Young children should ideally receive a balanced and life-rich nutrition including, where possible, unprocessed and organic foods. There are many schools of nutrition, a wide range of different diets that come and go according to current fashion and hundreds of different claims, both scientific and non-scientific that propound the virtues and vices of all kinds of foods, nutrients and food supplements. It is important that parents can find their way through the hype of controversy and contradiction, fads and fashions and come to a sensible and rational approach to providing their children with healthy food. In addition, the nutritional quality of food and drink available today is steadily being eroded, either because the soil is increasingly depleted of essential minerals or because the refining process impoverishes the food. Processed foods have far less biological value than unprocessed foods. A good knowledge of the nutritional needs of the child will be therefore be helpful.[24] A guide to children's nutrition will be given in Part 3, where it will be shown that a natural correspondence exists between the child's constitution and the natural world (the source of all our natural food). This will enable parents to work creatively to provide a wholesome and balanced nutrition using the nutritional discipline of their choice for each and every child, as well as for each stage of the child's development.

Environmental Impressions

Because the child is living so actively in his sensory world, he is highly vulnerable to these impressions. Through imitation he faithfully imitates everything he perceives. Unlike an adult the young child's protective power of thinking has not yet developed. Very strong environmental impressions, such as harsh sounds, audio-visual and electronic stimulation, violence and other immoral social behaviour, especially when they are recurrent or persistent, will imprint into the life matrix of the child as a subconscious memory. These may manifest in childhood as minor health, personality or developmental problems, or in well-known disorders such as allergies, immune disorders, attention deficit disorders, autism, phobias, or panic attacks. Alternatively, these may be triggered later in life by exposure to similar sensory or psycho-emotional associations, causing illnesses of all kinds and dysfunctional psychosocial patterns.

In Summary

A Health-Giving Environment

We therefore need to create an environment that offers the child the most health-giving sense impressions.

- The adults living and working with children are their role models and teachers. What one says is not as important as what one is. How one speaks, stands, walks, feels, thinks and acts will enter the child's soul and will shape his personality. Speaking in baby talk does not give the child a good example of how he should speak. Uncontrolled emotions and negative thoughts have a constricting and cooling effect on the child's psyche.
- Over-stimulation of the senses, especially excess audio-visual stimulation from TV and computers create an unbalanced and unnaturally stimulated soul experience.
- Live music resonates more harmoniously in the child's soul than recorded music.

- The natural environment is supportive to healthy growth and development and provides health-giving sense impressions; the young child should therefore as far as possible be surrounded with natural objects rather than synthetic materials.

- The young child should be provided at all times with adequate warmth. This is essential because the thermo-regulatory mechanisms are immature in neonates and young infants. They only mature toward the end of the first year of life and remain labile for the first two or three years of life. The sweat glands develop and start functioning only by 6–8 months of age. As a result the young child has no way of informing himself of his state of warmth. It is also important to know that the body temperature in children tends to be higher than in adults. A decrease toward adult levels begins at age 1, and slowly declines to normal body temperature through puberty, stabilizing at 13–14 in girls and 17–18 years in boys. Thus all parts of the body should be kept at even warmth at all times. The head, which radiates the blood warmth of the brain through the open fontanelles, should always be covered for the first year by a light cotton or woollen bonnet depending on the outside temperature. As we shall see in the further course of this book, warmth is the driving force of the metabolism and the power underlying the child's will life. A lack of warmth in the early years of life may predispose the individual to a range of sclerotic-type illnesses in later life.

- The child's bedroom should ideally be airy, light, warm and quiet. There should not be too much clutter in the room. Colours of the walls, ceiling and furniture should be consciously chosen. The cradle, cot or bed should be placed as far away as possible from electrical wall points because of the electro-magnetic radiations that are emitted there. It is worth turning off all appliances at the wall plug at night, and removing plugs from sockets.

Movement, Play and Self-expression

We have seen the immensely powerful drive of the will to enter the world, to imitate and thus absorb the environment and to know what is living there. This is the same will activity that initiates and drives the child's whole development, brings him into the typically upright human posture, guides him to communicate by speech, and mirrors his world of perceptions through thought images. This will is the energy dynamo driving the child, and the power behind all creativity and all natural self-healing. We need to nurture this power carefully as it expresses itself through the child's movement and creativity.

- The child should be allowed to express himself in free movement and free speech under the ever-watchful guiding caregiver. It is not good to continually 'correct' or control a child's activity or self-expression.
- Free play should be encouraged, avoiding toys that limit free movement and free expression; for example dolls with fixed facial expressions that perform certain fixed functions may limit the child's free play and imagination.
- Fantasy, free imagination and creativity should be fostered through imaginative games and stories.
- While freedom should be encouraged, healthy boundaries also need to be created, not only for the obvious protection of the child and his environment, but also to support the individual nature of the child: thus quieter, less creative children should be given more rein and be encouraged to be more expressive, while more boisterous and overactive children should be held back and given firmer boundaries.

Rhythms and Routines

All biological processes function in a rhythmic way, and arrhythmic functioning is unhealthy. When we help the child to live rhythmically, and to establish a pattern of rhythm in his life, we are strengthening these life rhythms. At the same time we strengthen the child's inner feeling life which is intrinsically connected with biological and rhythmic activities. We can do this in a number of ways.

- Healthy routines of eating, sleeping, playing and interacting with other children and adults should be provided.

- Regular experience of rhythmic activities such as hearing live music and song, storytelling, nursery rhymes and rhythmic games.[25]

I carry the forces that can help rejuvenate humanity and I help you to participate in this rejuvenation when you connect yourself with my inner life. Observe my nature with the reverence it deserves and it will reveal great wonders: impulses for true fraternity, love, peace and goodwill on earth, for these are my natural virtues. There is a higher wisdom that guides early childhood and even the wisest may learn from my nature. You can imaginatively revisit your own inner child, tapping back in to the original power that was living in you as a small child, that lives in me. Here you may find the power of the higher self which is the source of your creativity, your knowing, your healing, your joy, fun and laughter, your love, and peace of heart. In reclaiming your own inner child you can find fulfilment in your life.

CHAPTER 7

The Golden Years

My Will Activity and Vibrant Life of Sensing Create My New Body

These years span the journey between birth and the change of teeth, a phase that covers approximately seven years. We have already experienced the first three years – like an exquisite, untarnished jewel that radiates its power and light through the rest of the child's biography. We have welcomed the child as a newborn baby into an unfamiliar world that, step by step, she learns to make her own. We have travelled with her, exploring and remembering a world of great vibrancy and power, a world we have largely lost touch with, and which some of us perhaps are striving to recover. This incomparable time of purity and trust in the world needed to be characterized on its own, and experienced in its own special way. At the same time these heavenly years also belong dynamically, as we shall see, to the whole of the first seven-year period. In this chapter, recalling our experience of the child in the first three years, we will now move forward with her until the change of teeth at the age of seven.

This is the primary formative period of the child's life during which the essential structure and function of all the organ systems are established: the substructure as well as the 'service utilities' of the house she will live in for the rest of her life are being constructed.

Certain systems will need to be completed first; for instance, the neuro-sensory system is virtually fully formed and functional by the change of teeth, and the immune system will be well developed by this time. We observe tremendous growth and development taking place in the body and we sense that the child herself is actively engaged in transforming the body she inherited from her parents into the individual substance of a new body.

At the same time we notice the child beginning to express herself in certain ways, creating her first configuration of soul and personality. This will have a strong bearing on the development of her future psychological make-up. From an early age Adam was a very sensitive, shy child; his younger brother Jonathan in contrast was far more robust and extrovert.

During this epoch the child will learn more about the world and about her own body than at any other period; she develops her basic life skills: she learns to walk, speak, think and socialize; she attains her first level of independence in movement, play, feeling and thinking.

Recalling the First Seven Years

What can you remember about your first seven years of life?

Those who cared for you were the principal human beings with whom you spent the greatest part of your waking life. Imbued with prebirth archetypes of father and mother, you instinctively accorded them a position and a role that was impossible for them to fulfil, since people are not, after all, perfect. It will take some while before the child awakens to the reality of an imperfect and limited world.

Can you remember your bedroom and the toys you played with? A tricycle perhaps with a certain shape and colour, a tree in the garden, a secret place where you always liked to go? Do you remember other members of your family – sisters, brothers, aunts and uncles, grandmothers and grandfathers; or a carer who was your special friend, who carried you around and perhaps made you food? Then there was the time when you left the safe place of home to attend school; was it exciting, gratifying or terrifying? How was it to meet your first teacher in nursery school and a group of other small children? There are so many things to do and so much to play with. And then that big day, your first day in junior school. What pictures and feelings about it touch your body and fill your soul? Can you *re-member* with the vividness of the present how you are, where you are, what you are you doing and what is going on there? There is much that can be remembered and recovered by entering into childhood memories in this way because the complete experience of childhood is always present in the life-body's memory.[1]

Three Phases

The first seven years of a child's life can be divided into three periods which naturally and gradually flow into each other.

Infancy	from birth to approximately 2⅓ years
Toddler phase	from 2⅓ years to 4⅔ years
Preschool phase	from 4⅔ years to approximately 7 years

This first, three-phase epoch is a reflection of the whole of child-hood on a smaller scale. The growth process in the first seven years mirrors what happens in the wider span of twenty-one years: for instance, in infancy Adam's metabolism and limbs are still weak and undeveloped, but by the seventh year they have attained a degree of sturdiness that reflects the future completion of his limb growth by the twenty-first year; likewise, the awakening of his picture thinking and abstract memory at the change of teeth is a harbinger of the intellectual thinking that matures at the end of his third seven-year cycle. Every aspect of the first seven-year period is an anticipation of what comes to completion at a later time.

We have already highlighted the universal principle (Chapter 4) whereby the whole is always reflected in the parts. The microcosm is a reflection of the macrocosm. We saw this manifesting spatially in the morphological realm, where the threefold structure of the human being is reflected in the cell, an organ, a body part, the face, a limb and the whole body. Here we see it again expressing itself in a time-sequential way in the developmental realm.

In the first three years we can also discover a preparation for and reflection of the first seven years: thus, by the third year the child's limbs are strong enough to carry her on her journey, and her thinking has attained a level of independence that can allow her to live as a more independent person. The first three years are a miniature representation of what takes place in the first seven years, which in turn reflect on a smaller scale what happens during the first twenty-one years. This law of correspondences is a fundamental law of growth and development that will help us to understand children rightly and meet their needs in the most fruitful way.

Physical Growth

This first period of seven years is characterized by the growth and development of the physical body by virtue of the unseen formative life forces active within it. We have seen that at this period these forces work most forcefully within the head region – what we have designated the neuro-sensory system. These formative powers give structure and form to substance. This system manifests its character through the dynamic forces of the sphere and directs its activity centripetally from outside inwards, bringing substance into compact form, and steering the child down into the earthly realm.

As part of the developing nervous system, the sense organs are also developing. The senses allow the child to perceive her surrounding world, thereby bringing her into contact with this outer world which includes her own bodily nature. Working through her sense perceptions, her will can now engage actively with this world. It is her will that impelled her into life and that drives her now to meet the world with such great enthusiasm and zest for life; it directs her sense perceptions and drives her continual activity, her imitative nature and need for repetition. In the infant, everything assumes the character of will.

My first task is to construct my physical body so that it may carry me through this earthly life. I shall need first to create a nervous system and sense organs to inform me about the world and to guide my limbs on my chosen path.

Observe how the young child experiences the world through will activities; and how her whole nature is still very much bound up with her physical body: her activities of will, and her sensory life are strongly connected to her physical body. She is also forming concepts and developing feelings which, though less visible, are still closely linked to her bodily and will nature. It is important to realize that in the first seven years all these activities are still intimately connected with the physical body, growing and maturing within the respective 'embryonic' sheaths of the life and soul bodies.

As we accompany the young child through her first seven years of life, let us, to begin with, trace the transformations of the physical body up to the change of teeth.

The Physical Roadmap

If we observe Adam, Jonathan's older brother, as an infant we may be struck by his relatively large round head, which is about a quarter of his total body length. The skull and upper part of his face are also more prominent than the rest of his face, giving it a distinctly spherical form; his soft round eyes, his button-shaped nose and his frequently pouting or sucking mouth are striking features.

The lower half of his face in contrast is underdeveloped, with the lower jaw small and receding. His head is as large as his chest and does not appear separate from the chest because a fully formed neck has not yet developed. There is also no separation between chest and abdomen, and his round belly is also typical of infancy. His arms and legs are relatively short – babies cannot touch their fingertips with outstretched arms above their heads – and his legs are only one-and-a-half times longer than his head.

These features begin to change in the middle of Adam's third year, as the 'toddler' emerges. His body has begun to grow more quickly than his head, and a ratio of about 1:5 is established during the toddler phase. His forehead is still quite prominent and his chin starts to emerge. The neck begins to show itself. The increased growth is usually more in the chest and abdomen than the legs. There is still no clear separation between chest and abdomen and his tummy still protrudes. His legs look sturdier but his limbs are still chubby from the underlying subcutaneous fat. His limbs often appear to move in a circular and spherical fashion. He loves to walk in circles and gesticulates with spherical movements.

Adam's preschool phase (up to the age of 6)[2] is characterized by dramatic growth in his limbs so that by the age of seven his head-to-body ratio has changed to 1:6. His head grows little in this phase, his forehead gradually becomes less prominent, his nose becomes more defined and his mouth and chin assume a character of their own. His neck likewise becomes a separate feature.

As the trunk region becomes slimmer, a clear demarcation between chest and abdomen emerges and the tummy flattens out. His limbs, especially his legs, stretch to become longer, more slender and contoured so that muscles, joints and bony parts become visible. By the time Adam is ready for school at the age of six he has lost the soft features of early childhood, and his chubby, rounded form. His appearance is more graceful and his movements have become more coordinated and purposeful.

He loses his first teeth, signalling the birth of the etheric body and the liberation of a portion of these life forces for cognitive activities that will be required for school learning. One does encounter individual variations in the age of loss of the first teeth, signifying presumably an individual pace in the rate at which the new body is constructed. His nervous system is almost completely developed and, together with his body, which has attained a certain degree of solidity, it can now support his new-found independence.

This transformation of form is a striking phenomenon of child development and is more evident when we stand apart from this growing process and see the child at intervals of several months.

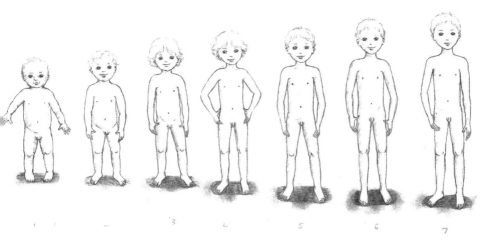

Adam's physical transformation through the first seven years

Let us be clear that the physical body is a complex combination of mineral substances that, on its own, cannot grow and develop in the manner described above. The awe-inspiring transformation that takes place in each and every child in this universal fashion is the result of the unfolding dynamic activity of the etheric body, working first to bring the neuro-sensory system to maturity, then the rhythmic system and finally the metabolic limb system.

We shall now trace in greater detail the nature of the life body, which has everything to do with developmental processes, morphology and physiology in the human being.

The Life/Etheric Roadmap

We have described the etheric body as a self-contained and autonomously resonating organized body of life forces. This dynamic force system, working through every cell of the physical body, transforms lifeless mineral substance into living substance, giving it form and shape. We may therefore also call these life forces, *formative forces*. They have everything to do with the form of the body, its tissues and its organs, as well as their functions. What is the nature of these forces and where do they come from?

The Opposite of Gravity

We know that gravity works from the centre of the earth, drawing matter back towards the earth; the plant root grows downwards into the earth because it is under the influence of earthly, physical forces. However, the plant stem grows upwards towards the sun because of the forces of light and warmth streaming downwards towards it. These downward streaming forces have the effect of drawing matter upwards towards the source where it originates.

This force is so powerful that it can draw thousands of tons of tree sap through the finest capillaries of the tallest trees. With the help of light, the material substance and form of these huge trees come into being; photosynthesis, the process in which the energy of sunlight is used by plants to synthesize carbohydrates, means 'construction through light'.

These are forces that clearly work in a contrary direction to those of the physical world; we can characterize these as etheric forces which act from the peripheral cosmos towards the earth; they create levity and buoyancy whereas the earthly forces of gravity create heaviness. Thus, as mineral substance is drawn into the force field of the etheric stream, it loses its physical nature and assumes a different character, one that is imbued with life and form. When the life forces are no longer present, matter falls back into the lifeless realm of the physical forces and begins to disintegrate. The human body without an etheric body becomes a dead corpse and immediately begins to break down.

Sun, Moon and Planets

The plant knows where to find its source of life, for it grows upwards towards the sun, the source of our light and warmth. Life of course would be unthinkable without the sun, which is certainly the source of all life on earth. But the other planets also have an effect.

The moon has well-known effects on the ocean tides, on the sap of plants, and on the reproductive life of plants and animals; and the moon's orbital cycle of approximately 29 days is the average duration of the female menstrual cycle.

Less well known are the subtler effects on life processes of the other primary planets, Venus, Mercury, Mars, Jupiter and Saturn. From ancient times these seven primary planets have been known to influence life on earth in various ways.

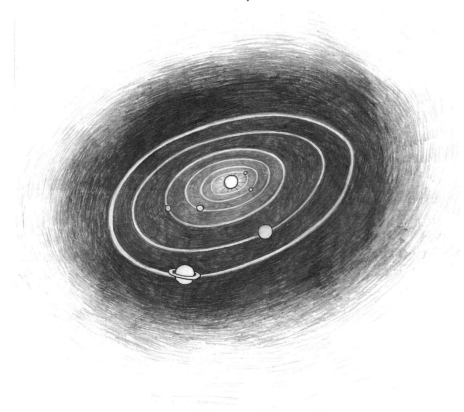

Diagram of our solar system

We have to imagine the etheric organization in the human being as a delicate body of forces that works down essentially from the broad expanse of the universe but in an individualized and organized form. Just as every child has an individualized physical body with its organs and tissues, so she also has her own particular etheric body. However, while the parts of the physical body may be seen as separate, the etheric body is in constant streaming, interweaving motion, connecting all parts of a whole organism.

The Cosmos Within

If the law of correspondences is true and the macrocosm is present within the microcosm, then the external universe with its stars and planets must also be present within the human being. We can therefore imagine the forces of the sun and planetary bodies as being present in an individualized way in the human etheric body. Paracelsus, a physician and alchemist living in the fifteenth century, spoke about the inner sun and the inner planets within the human being.

Light brings the form of things into existence. We see nothing in the dark; but switch on the light and objects become visible. The light of the sun working with a gas – carbon dioxide and water – brings about the substance and forms of plants. The plant forms in nature are infinitely variable, as are, likewise, the organs and tissues of the human body: the finely structured nervous system is very different from the round soft forms of the liver. The various tissues and organs of the human body also exhibit varying degrees of vitality, which can be seen, for example, in the physiological balance created between cell generation and cell destruction.

There are tissues belonging to the sense organs that are almost as lifeless as a physical apparatus: we have mentioned for instance the lens of the eye which functions like a glass prism and has very little vital or regenerative function. The central nervous tissue is not quite as lifeless but does not grow new cells and has a very limited capacity to regenerate when injured.

In contrast, metabolic organs such as the digestive system and the liver are very vital organs with a high rate of cell turnover. Yet even these organs have mechanisms which destroy cells and limit cell growth. The reproductive organs and the bone marrow have the highest capacity of cell vitality: here new cells are in continuous production and very little cell degradation takes place.

What is it that determines the differentiated forms and life potential in the tissues and organs of the human body? We know that the sun is the source of life, and have seen that light helps to create or synthesize form. But what is it that modifies sunlight to bring about such variation in the form and vitality both of nature and the human being? Steiner informs us that the life forces radiating from the sun are influenced by the six primary planetary bodies and the orbits they traverse in our solar system.[3] Let us imagine that through prenatal microcosmic interiorization, both before and during the embryonic stage, these seven planetary forces have become active in the human body, bringing about certain effects in seven main regions. Steiner describes, as did the alchemists before him, the correspondence between these planets and human physiological functions: Saturn weakens the life forces in the organs of the senses so that virtually no life exists there but consciousness can prevail instead. Jupiter creates the finely formed, contracted life of the nerve tissue that facilitates reflected awareness.[4] Mars is the force that influences the life of respiration. The sun builds up and stimulates the life of the circulation; Mercury is the power behind the life of metabolism. Venus activates and determines the life of movement and the moon determines reproductive life.[5]

Neuro-sensory system	Sensory life	Saturn
	Nervous life	Jupiter
Rhythmic system	Breathing life	Mars
	Circulatory life	Sun
Metabolic-limb system	Metabolic life	Mercury
	Movement life	Venus
	Reproductive life	Moon

These planetary forces will be described in greater detail in Chapter nine.

Experiencing the Etheric

Can we, without higher perceptive faculties,[6] experience the reality of these etheric forces that clearly have everything to do with the growth and development of the child?

We have seen that in contrast to our sense perception, our capacity of thinking brings us into a completely different relationship with the world.

Observing a child at different stages of development, we can note the different features first at the infant stage, later at the toddler stage. If we do not reflect about what we observe and stay only in our sensing of all the observable features – for instance the size, shape and roundness of the upper head, and the lower part of the face – we will be directing our full attention to each separate feature, going from one to the next; there is no distinction or connection between any of these features, nor can these features have much further significance. My perception will depend on a number of factors concerned with who and where I am, for instance the nature of my sensory apparatus, which may be different to yours, and the position from which I am looking at the child. I can never know exactly how you, as distinct from me, perceive a particular child. My feelings while observing a child are likewise my own personal experience and may be totally different from your feelings. Thus our sense perceptions and our feelings are subjective experiences, separating us from the objective world as self-contained, individual people; there is little agreement or certainty and little communication between us.

However, the moment we apply our thinking to our observations of the child, the picture changes radically.

Let us try to penetrate the act of thinking in greater depth.

The Nature of Thinking

We look at the features of an infant's head – eyes, nose, ears, etc. Long ago, as children, we found the concepts for these features and named them accordingly. We have also at some early stage connected all these concepts together, realizing that there is some relationship between them, and have thereby created a broader concept called 'head' that incorporates all the smaller features.

We have likewise discovered the concepts of 'size', 'shape', 'roundness' and can identify the feature of the upper head being 'round'. The feature of the lower head is 'less round'. The forming of concepts and the connecting of concepts can only come about through thinking.

We likewise discover through our thinking the idea of 'comparison', namely that we can relate the 'shape' of one perception with the 'shape' of another. We can come to the conclusion that the upper head is 'rounder' than the lower.

In the same way we can compare the roundness of the head in infancy with that of the toddler and can conclude that the overriding shape of the younger child's head is 'rounder' than the older child. We can all agree on this conclusion simply on the basis of a commonality inherent in everyone's thinking. Our thinking evidently has the ability to connect us with a universal truth that allows us to feel united with all things and all people. We can liken thinking to a universal force, similar to the way etheric forces are drawn in from the universal circumference.

Our sensory life compels us to see the terrestrial character of separate objects, and our life of feeling has a uniquely personal and individualizing character. The activity of thinking on the other hand has a universal nature. In this quality it shares a common nature with the etheric forces.

The Etheric and Thinking

We will recall that with the birth of the etheric body at the change of teeth, a portion of these same forces that were engaged in organic growth and transformation is freed to become the forces that create the basis for ordinary thinking. We must therefore regard thinking as a pure etheric activity, but one that is not bound organically to the physical body.

By investigating our activity of thinking, we can find that thinking has four principle characteristic qualities.

• Its universal character brings together and connects separate sense impressions to form new observable phenomena through the creation of new concepts that we name accordingly; in the example above, the concept of 'head' arises by connecting the perceptions: round, eyes, nose, etc. We feel satisfied when we have given things a name; we feel united with the world and with one another because we can agree that the upper part of the head is rounder than the lower. We are then able to communicate with one another. We can call this integrated thinking that unifies the world.

- Thinking also has the character of organizing the world, breaking it down in an analytical manner or building it up synthetically: we can break the concept 'head' down into many different concepts and build it up again; we can 'grow' the idea of a plant from a seed form and let it develop in our thought life to form a seedling, a sprouting plant, a plant that flowers, fruits and goes to seed again. It is only in our mobile fluid thinking that we can imagine the unfolding plant in its complete transformation. This is fluid thinking that organizes the world.

- Thinking also illuminates the world for us. It is through thinking that we acquire knowledge of life. Without thinking we would observe thousands of sense impressions all separate and without any real distinctions between them. Everything would be a grey sameness. 'Round' and 'angular' would not exist, since they depend on conceptual distinctions. Thinking creates the awareness of difference, waking one up to the reality of the world; it is like shining a light on the world to create a rich tapestry of colour, textures, shapes and differences. This is light thinking that illumines the world.

- Finally, thinking has the capacity to set things in motion, to generate activity and to create new worlds. We may become aware of the round, dome-shaped head of a baby, and that it elicits a warm feeling: How beautiful! We wish to stroke it tenderly. Thinking sets in motion feelings and actions. The idea that there is a growth force that works downwards from the head to the limbs may kindle in us warmth, enthusiasm and the will to search and understand this law further. This is warmth thinking that creates the world.

I am aware that other authors have examined the relationship between thinking and the etheric forces and have found other functional qualities that characterize thinking. For instance, Glöckler[7] describes the digestive and assimilative nature of thinking which analyzes thoughts critically and then builds them up synthetically. Close scrutiny will show that these activities, and others such as those of growth, reproduction, regeneration, maintenance and protection, as well as the rhythmic functions of respiration and circulation, belong to one of the four primary qualities described above.

Locating Etheric Activity

If thinking is an etheric activity with four essential characteristic elements, it begs the question whether these four etheric qualities can be found in the *organic* domain of the growing child. Where are these etheric forces at work?

The **unifying quality** is connected with that essential vitalizing force that unites and integrates parts of a whole, providing the blueprint that allows restoration and healing to take place in the organism when there is deformation or injury; it creates and maintains forms and shapes and provides the means by which all cells and tissues can communicate with each other. We find here the life processes involved in maintenance and regeneration.

The **organizing quality** may be discerned in the aspect of the life body that breaks down and builds up substance, divides cells but builds them into tissues; that forms the different qualities, shapes, parts and organs; that regulates the variety of processes, functions and phases in the body of the growing child, orders chemical reactions and governs the specific frequencies of matter. Here we see the life functions of digestion, secretion and metabolism.

The **illuminating quality** of the light-active life forces allows matter to unfold in space with a specific size, volume and expansiveness. This is a characteristic of light which, as we have seen, helps engender form and substance. Once physically manifest in bringing matter into form, it can be perceived in all its differentiation. Here we find the forces that have to do with the growth of the child.

The **generating quality** may be experienced in the aspect of the life force that activates all life processes, setting them in motion, creating all sequential phases of the child's developmental cycles and bringing them to ripeness and maturity. Warmth, reproduction and development are functions of this life quality.

We thus discover a singular relationship between thinking and the human etheric or life forces. Let us recall our imaginative prenatal picture of the human etheric body drawn together shortly before conception out of universal life forces; they find their way via the amniotic embryonic sheath into the body of the child where they begin to unfold their life and growth-creating functions.

Steiner describes the universal etheric forces that stream down towards the earth as being constituted of four distinct ether qualities. He names these four ethers as follows: life ether, chemical or sound ether, light ether and warmth ether – but says relatively little about their specific characteristics. He leaves it up to us to attempt to discover their intrinsic nature.[8] By investigating and experiencing the differentiated nature of thinking, we may be able to come to an inner experience of the differentiated nature of the etheric body. Such an exploration can connect us directly with the living organic forces that underlie child development.

Life ether	unifying quality	wholeness, healing, form, communication
Chemical/tone ether	organizing quality	chemistry, frequency, membering, order
Light ether	illuminating quality	growth, size, expansion, volume
Warmth ether	generating quality	creation, activation, time, age, maturity

These qualities work together to bring about all aspects relating to the development of the physical body in childhood and adolescence. Thus the interaction of life and chemical ether enable the separate parts of an organ to be united in an integrated whole: for instance, all the various parts of a cell are organized as individual parts (chemical ether) but also function as a whole (life ether); the co-operation of light and warmth ether manifests as growth of the child in time: the child grows through the force of the light ether and matures through the power of the warmth ether; the working together of chemical ether and sound ether results in the growth of specific parts such as the limbs.[9]

Heredity and Individuality

It will be useful at this stage to look at the struggle between heredity and individuality, in the course of which the child creates a physical body she can call her own.

As we have seen, the body into which the child is born is an inherited body that her parents and forefathers have helped to build.

During this first cycle of seven years, the child's own formative life forces take hold of the raw inherited material of this 'model body', expanding, shaping and replacing it until by the change of teeth it has been thoroughly transformed by the child's own individual powers.[10] This can be likened to a sculptor working on a clay model, wrestling with it to shape it in his own likeness. An unseen struggle takes place here between the resistance of the clay and the will and forming power of the sculptor. We see the outcome of this struggle in the growth of the child; some children bear a strong resemblance to one or other parent or relative, others bear very little resemblance to anyone. Much will depend on the individual forces in their confrontation with the inherited form. The childhood illnesses that occur in these early years are symptomatic of this encounter between the inherited substance and the individual identity of the child, a subject that will be dealt with in Part 2.

We should remember that while this is all happening, the life forces are still in gestation, developing and maturing within the inherited model on which they are working. These forces of growth are embedded in the protective etheric sheath of the mother, just as the body of the embryo and foetus grows and develops within the protective sheaths of the mother's physical womb. This means that the child will experience the world partially through the life of the mother, sharing in her biological and emotional experiences. Just as the physical growth of the child in the womb is strongly influenced by her surrounding environment – both that of the womb and beyond – so is etheric development – and hence its effect on the physical organs – strongly influenced by the living environment in which the child finds herself. As we saw in the previous chapter, the child faithfully and innocently absorbs this environment directly into her life organization through the sense impressions that flood in through the twelve senses. The life forces repeatedly imprint the pliable physical material, shaping it into organ systems that become permanent for life. It is essential that the physical organs are formed in as healthy a way as is possible during this life period, because all future development is based on the growth processes that take place here:

'We can never repair what we have neglected as educators in the first seven years'.[11]

From this we can see that the awakening soul life impacts on the developing physical body. But how does the soul itself awaken in this first seven-year cycle? For as the life body is unfolding and developing its forces within the material substrate of the inherited body and within the etheric sheath of mother and father, the soul body is likewise involved in a synchronous process of development.

The Soul Roadmap

The will is the first faculty of the soul to awaken in infancy. It is this power that drives the young child to connect with the surrounding physical world using her limbs, her twelve senses and her natural ability to imitate – to take the world into her inner life. Thus movement, sense perception and imitation are the early manifestations of the soul through which young children relate to their environment.

Let us follow this process in more detail: we have seen that movement first expresses the soul's will activity. In the first few weeks, the undeveloped will of the child in the form of basic drives is directed towards sleep and nourishment, where the metabolism is highly mobile, and actively absorbs, assimilates and eliminates material substances. Jonathan, the newborn child whose development we are following, does very little other than sleep and drink, with short periods of wakefulness. Through sound and body movement, he will make known his needs. In his waking hours, his hands and feet soon become more active, grasping and kicking in an uncoordinated manner. His eyes are mobile but cannot yet focus properly. A smile may sometimes appear fleetingly on his face but as yet there is no conscious recognition of people around him.

In the second month he begins to spend more time awake, recognizes those close to him and smiles purposefully. He has become aware of his environment and from this point onwards it is as if an unstoppable force has been released within his soul, intent on absorbing the world into itself. He becomes a mobile, multifaceted sense organ driven by his desire to discover the world. He learns everything by perceiving the world in a completely open way and imitating what he has perceived.

> Imagine an insatiable drive within you to discover everything about a new place: you give yourself over completely to learning all you can about your new environment; you absorb thousands of sense impressions, imprint them dynamically into your life body and then, like a natural actor, you confirm and express through your body what you know in your body, through the dramatic art of imitation.[12]

By three months, Jonathan's movements are more directed: for instance his hand can take objects to his mouth. Now the task of finding a new spatial relationship to the body begins. He lifts his head, then learns to sit up.

At about six months, he moves away from his mother in his first show of independence and begins to crawl; he is standing at approximately nine months; he takes his first step at about one year.

The manner in which each child goes through these phases of finding her walking feet will give many pointers to her future potential. Some children need more or less time to develop healthy functions. We discovered in the previous chapter how she finds this new orientation. With unfettered hands and mobile legs, the child is now free to explore her world; she gradually learns to take hold of and control her limbs so that she becomes more co-ordinated, dexterous and agile.

> Bulani at eighteen months can run stiffly, pile three cubes and feed himself.
> Maria at two years walks up and down stairs with support, builds six cubes and can help to undress herself.
> Rajan at three years can ride a tricycle, build a tower of nine cubes, helps in undressing, can roughly copy a circle and can play simple games and puzzles.
> Thandi at four years hops on one foot, climbs well, can use a pair of scissors for simple cutouts and can interact socially with several children.

Adam at five years is learning to hop-skip, dress and undress and take part in domestic activities.

Saskia at six years can count comfortably up to ten, draw a human figure and house with features, ride a bicycle and play with planning and purpose.

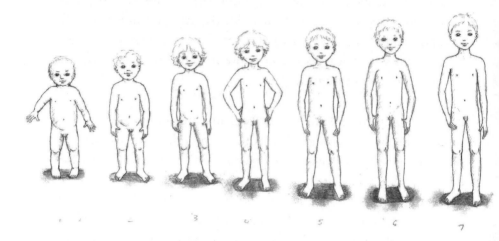

From Movement to Speech

Once the will has facilitated free and independent movement, it can turn its attention to the activity of speaking; Jonathan begins to babble, then he speaks his first words, repeating them over and over, getting to know the sounds and the speaking apparatus that forms them. To begin with these are words heard and imitated and have no meaning for the child; gradually however, in the second year, he begins to name the objects he has perceived. In the third year he begins to put words together to form phrases and sentences. Through speaking, he has discovered a new world and in the next few years he takes great pleasure in practising this new skill. His insatiable curiosity about anything and everything call forth endless questions that do not expect logical answers. In his sixth year Jonathan wants to know: 'Where do I come from?' Without waiting for the answer he responds himself: 'From the stars!'

The individual way a child learns to speak will say much about her individual nature: From the age of one Thandi was babbling incessantly; she would take hold of anything that looked like a telephone and speak into it. By two she was highly verbal, an indication of her later headstrong nature. Bulani on the other hand spoke no words until he was two; but he listened to everything intently, indicative of someone who in later life would be sensitive and receptive.

The Development of Feeling Through Rhythm

As movement consolidates and speaking evolves, so feeling life unfolds.

In her infancy Maria's feelings are completely dependent on the organic functions of her body; she is happy when her body tells her she is content, and unhappy when her bodily needs are not met. These needs have a cyclical and rhythmical nature: for instance, her digestive system needs nourishment on a regular basis, her waking and sleeping life gradually settles into a stable rhythm. Later the outside world will increasingly impact on Maria's emotional life: she feels angry and upset when her older brother stops her from taking his toys. Her drives and desires control her behaviour and also her emotional life. Her desire to have the toy arises from a soul life that is still closely connected with the body; and when her will is blocked this triggers her emotions.

Maria is exploring her relationship to space: in her second year she can move through the world and interact with the objects in the world. She is also discovering the world of sounds and speech and begins to name the things around her. She starts to experience the power of repetition and rhythm in moving, speaking, drawing and playing; she practises all kinds of movements, going round in circles, and learning to hop, run and jump; she repeats words that she hears, and invents some; she wants to hear the same story repeatedly, and asks continual questions; she builds things up and breaks them down, plays for hours in the sandpit making endless sand cakes.

All these activities are establishing the bodily foundation for the life of feeling. This faculty is sustained by the rhythmic activities of bodily functions. By her third year, Maria has found names for many objects in her world, and in this process she has become more distinct and detached from it; she becomes aware that she likes some things and dislikes others, and that liking something is very different from disliking it; she learns that she can become personally involved in what she likes and dislikes; she also discovers that she can assert herself by saying 'no' to what she doesn't like.

In this defiance and stubbornness she experiences herself more strongly. She starts to become aware of herself as a self-contained individual, and the glorious moment arrives when, for the first time, she discovers that the simple word 'I' is the only word of her new-found language that truly expresses her identity. This awakened consciousness of self also leads to a change in her feeling life when she starts to experience feelings within herself that are not simply reactions to her own body or her outer environment. Lievegoed describes this moment as 'the birth of feelings'.[13] Now the inner imagination burgeons forth in contrast to the immutable reality of the outside, objective world. This new faculty announces itself strikingly in the way in which the child's play changes.

Play

For the young child, life on earth is a natural playground where she can discover herself through playing with the world. Within the first few months of his life, Jonathan begins to explore his immediate environment; he begins to play with his body, his hands and toes and then with a play object like a rattle. For the first two years he can only play with what he has in front of him, forgetting entirely what is outside his perception. This will naturally cause a great deal of sibling friction because Jonathan wants to play with and imitate whatever he sees around him. He loves to construct things and then pull them down again, expressing in his behaviour what is happening in the organic world of synthesizing and assimilating matter and then breaking it down again. It is in his fourth year of life that Jonathan has separated his consciousness sufficiently to withdraw in play to some degree from his environment. Where does he then go? He enters the living and creative world of his own fantasy and imagination. We caught a glimpse of this magical world in the previous chapter. He breathes himself heart and soul into this dreamlike, imaginative world. Now his world of play becomes richer and vaster. Play with a four- or five-year-old whose imagination has not been suppressed by modern media images, and you can experience an enchanted world of kings and queens, castles and dungeons. Jonathan is fully in this world, completely involved in all the characters he creates. And in this real world of imagination, the child experiences the first surges of her real feeling life; she starts to experience the ebb and flow of feelings through the different characters that she herself creates and acts out. She becomes the good, wise king or queen and experiences the feeling of firmness, strength and power; she lives into the warm, loving mother and feels her warm, heart-felt nature; she enters the evil soul life of the wicked witch and experiences hate and anger; she experiences the fear and doubt of the helpless child locked in a dark dungeon. Through her playful imagination and imaginative play she comes gently into contact with the material world, encounters and acts out manifold personality types, faces obstacles and challenges, and discovers innovative and creative ways of dealing with these realities. She is rehearsing for life ahead. But until a certain stage is reached she cannot distinguish her imaginative life from reality.

Toys

It follows from this that the toys with which she plays should allow for an experience of this inner fantasy and free movement. Sophisticated toys that can do everything, such as dolls that function like small children, and even 'speak' mechanically, or electronic cars that open and shut, prevent the child from exploring this hidden kingdom that helps to develop feeling life.

Stories

The fabulous world of stories is soul food for the young child. Just as food ingested and enjoyed appeases hunger, children find sustenance in books and stories told or read to them. Stories and storybooks activate and invigorate the imagination, which as we have seen is a necessary precondition for conscious thinking. Many adults set great store by the stories they first heard when young, and that accompanied them like friends as they grew. Do you recall the picture books and stories that made an impression on your growing soul?

Already in their first year, infants are drawn to simple picture books portraying objects and scenes from life. They become part of the landscape of new or familiar impressions that come to meet the desire to learn about the world. They also offer a microcosmic image of the world where concepts and language can be nurtured by their first tutors, their primary caregivers. (*This is a cat; and this is a cow.*)

The illustrations offered to small children should be simple, clear and true to life, allowing the eye to explore the image in comfort and freedom. Pictures that are too busy or active may make it difficult for the child to enter into them easily.

The toddler will soon become ready for storybooks portraying basic daily activities that he experiences around him, such as a mother ironing clothes or a father fixing a gate. A nursery-rhyme picture book, artistically illustrated, can soon become a daily necessity: the young child delights in endless repetitions of the same verses. Simple nature stories about trees and animals, insects and worms will enchant the young child, who still feels part of the natural world. This is why the world of nature spirits, fairies and gnomes is so familiar and completely natural to preschool children. They are still close to what we have conceived to be their original, invisible home. Is this why they are so easily comforted and reassured by stories about heaven and angels? The stories accompanying the festivals of all religions fill the young child, who seems to be innately religious, with a deep sense of satisfaction.

When the child begins to express her imagination actively in play, the fairytales that were created out of the same imaginative dimension that she now experiences naturally can be introduced.

Our early ancestors experienced life in a simpler, more open and childlike manner than we do today; we can still find remnants of this mystical or magical consciousness in indigenous tribal folk who have not encountered Western civilization. These ancestors lived in a world rich with soul-spiritual reality; what we speak about abstractly today was real and visible to them: for instance, someone who expressed hate and selfishness might well be perceived to assume the form of a witch, whereas a wise and benevolent person could be experienced as looking regal, or king-like. For people of earlier cultures the great mythological figures of folklore were profoundly real. Gradually humanity began to lose its natural connection with nature and spirits, and stories relating to these realities were created to preserve this memory. The oral traditions found in all older cultures, were later written down by people such as the Grimm brothers in Germany, and survive today as fairytales, fables, myths and legends.[14, 15, 16]

There are many developmental phenomena that appear to validate the view that the child's soul development recapitulates the soul-spiritual journey of mankind. The imaginative picture consciousness of preschool children and their natural sense of affinity with the content of fairy tales, support this idea. The universal child unfolding through childhood and adolescence gives us a true picture of humanity's long evolution.

The idea that the development of the child proceeds in an ordered and predictable way, and that it is a recapitulation of the development of humanity in general, has profound educational and therapeutic implications. *It means that the child is critically ready at every stage of her development to absorb specific learning experiences.* We can either use or neglect these opportunities for optimum learning. Thus the child will only be open to the gift of fairytales for a few critical years, after which she will be ready for other things because her soul life is now different. This is a cardinal principle of the Waldorf method of education, which will be discussed in the following chapter.

In a rhythmic fashion, episodes of imaginative play will abruptly end; Jonathan will breathe himself back into the ordinary sense-perceptive world, where the table that had become an underground cave is now used for eating.

He will continue to play in this creative way until roughly the change of teeth, concerned only with creative activity and not with any specific outcomes. He will repeat the same play over and over because, as we mentioned above, he has entered the period in his development when the activity of rhythm – characteristic of those organs that underlie the life of feeling, the heart and lungs – has begun to unfold. This is an activity that comes to completion in the second seven-year period. With the change of teeth, the nature of children's play moves away from being completely open-ended towards more goal-oriented activity.

From Feeling to Thinking

On the foundation laid down by movement, speaking and feeling can unfold. And as these capacities take root in the child's life, they create the soul space for the will to grow active in the development of thinking.

In the previous chapter we examined in some depth the complex soul preparation that needs to be in place before thinking can unfold. We saw that thinking in Adam's infant phase is conditioned reflex at the level of the will, first directed by the biological drives of his bodily needs, later by his soul desires that become more and more powerful. 'I want' becomes a powerful thought process that characterized his 'terrible twos' and that was able to tyrannize his family because they were not finding ways to manage it. These conditioned reflexes lead to the formation of habits, and a 'good upbringing' ensures that the child learns good habits. Thus Adam is trained to use the potty, learns to wash his hands when they are dirty and brushes his teeth before going to sleep. These habits are the automatic imprinting of the memory body, bringing about the reflex actions which bypass conscious thinking. With further development, memory, speech and imagination find their rightful place and the brain attains a level of mature formation enabling it to become the instrument for the activity of conscious thinking for the rest of life.

At the right moment Adam names himself I, and the birth of a new way of thinking takes place. Now his conceptual thinking process can begin in earnest. He begins to form his own mental pictures which may contradict what habit formation has instilled in him. For instance Adam sees the dog doing a wee in the garden. He memorizes this image and the next time he feels the urge, this image comes to mind; he decides not to use the potty but goes outside and does it on the lawn.

Over the next few years, Adam's life will be directed on the one hand by a habitual kind of thinking, determined by biological and psychological impulses; but more and more he will discover his own independent picture thinking and picture memory as a certain part of his life forces are liberated from organic functions for the activity of thinking.

We discovered that this birth of thinking is at the same time the birth of the etheric body that takes place with the loss of the milk teeth.

Daycare, Play Groups and Nursery School

In the first three years the child generally prefers to play alone with her own toys, inside her own imagination, and does not readily join groups of other children. During this time it is generally preferable for her to stay at home, exercizing her will and absorbing, through her active sense life an environment that ideally offers her the most protection. Removing the infant from her home and placing her in daycare with a large group of young children is often the beginning of problems. I frequently find that many crèche children are often sick and 'pick up every virus'. It is likely that their inner feelings of insecurity and lack of protection predispose them to recurrent illnesses. If treated with chemical medication – antibiotics, decongestants and antipyretics – this is likely to have a weakening effect on their health in the long run.

There is divided opinion among researchers about the value of play groups and nursery school at various ages. Sally Goddard Blythe reviews this debate in her book *What Babies and Children Really Need*.[17] A number of studies show that before the age of two, large non-maternal daycare groups can be detrimental to some aspects of emotional and social development. A meta-analysis of peer-reviewed studies over some forty years indicated clear evidence of adverse outcomes which included attachment insecurities, socio-emotional dysfunctional development (anger and anxiety in boys, over-dependency, anxiety, depression in girls) and behavioural problems (hyperactivity, aggression and non-compliance).[18] These studies opposed the view that high quality daycare is an acceptable substitute for parental care.[19] However, by three years of age, studies indicate that children benefit educationally *and* emotionally from some time spent in daycare. On the other hand, children who had three years or more preschool experience showed a greater degree of anti-social behaviour. Other research has found that daycare children exhibited higher levels of cortisol than children cared for in their own homes. Since cortisol is a hormone that responds to conditions of stress, it would appear to indicate that children attending daycare in general experience more stress than those in their natural home environment. This accords with common sense that tells us that very young children feel most relaxed in their own homes and generally do not thrive on group experiences.

If the parents have to go to work it is far healthier for very young children to be cared for by grandparents, relatives or other child minders in a familiar environment. This is usually possible where there is access to an extended family. When this is not possible the next best alternative is the small playgroup currently in vogue in many parts of the world. Here a mother, often with her own small children, will make her home available to a small group of other children, providing home activities, healthy routines and free play. This may also have other advantages both for mother and child: it may give the mother time out for herself, allows her to meet other parents with young children, to discuss, compare, question and help each other with the myriad issues concerning child rearing. The child observes other children her own age which may stimulate her development, and finds playmates that may foster play visits which are desirable at this age.

From three years of age, the child is ready for group play but many children are only mature enough for nursery school from the age of four. The decision as to whether or when to send the child to nursery school is an individual one, and should be based on the home environment, the availability of suitable home care and the individual nature of the child. Organized preschool groups are a comparatively recent social phenomenon, associated with the growth of industrialized society. A child who grows up in a rural environment or in a home with a garden, who is well looked after by a parent or close relative and has other children to play with, does not need to go to nursery school.

However, when home conditions are not ideal, a nursery school can be considered from the fourth year. Ideally, the nursery school should be designed to resemble a home as far as possible and, within safe boundaries, should offer the child freedom of movement, free play, stimulation of the imagination and routine home activities such as sweeping, washing up, digging, planting, kneading dough, etc. In this safe and protected environment, the preschool child can engage in a range of activities that may not be available at home and that encourage her free movement and artistic expression: artistic activities such as painting and modelling, rhythmical movements such as dancing and eurythmy,* singing, story-telling and play-acting. The nursery school should be a natural continuation of the home environment; whatever happens here should be carried back into home life, and what happens at home should be brought back into the nursery school. This gives a young child the sense of continuity and wholeness which she needs as the foundation of her sense of security.

It should be noted that the preschool programmes that are currently being designed in many countries to 'kick-start education', especially those that utilize computerized technology, are in my view harmful to the healthy development of the child in this phase of her life.

Repetition and Rhythm

We saw that repetition and rhythm are essential elements in the life of a toddler. She loves to have the same story told to her repeatedly, sing the same nursery rhyme and play the same games, testing the patience of all parents and child carers. Repetition allows the child to methodically exercise her will. Repetition imprints imitation into memory. Her will is now not merely

---

* A form of movement developed by Rudolf Steiner that expresses speech and sound through the instrument of the body

under the control of her drives and desires, but instead a more purposeful focus for her actions and activities develops. Her own creative imagination and the feelings that arise guide her in self-directed play. The preschooler begins to set goals for herself; this means she can think beyond the present moment into future time – e.g. 'I also want to go to big school' – and in her play she seeks to achieve certain goals – for instance she plays being at big school. The birth of her conscious will has taken place at a time when her life forces are completing their work on the neuro-sensory system, and some of these forces are freeing themselves for the activity of abstract thinking.

The child now also realizes that she needs the help of more experienced people to help her achieve her goals. She learns to respect the superior strength and expertise of her seniors and is not shy about asking for help. Imitation transforms into respect for authority and now the child is ready for school. We will see in Chapter eight, though, that imitation remains active in the first two years of school, and is still a resource in the child on which the teacher can draw.

Synchronization of Etheric and Soul Streams

The child's 'I' has arrived on earth and is intent on gradually penetrating her earthly body. At the same time there are two other geniuses at work, two other streams of formative creative forces that have also entered earthly existence. The **life stream** working downwards in time from head through chest to the limbs; and the **soul stream** working 'upwards' through the will into feeling and then thinking. A picture emerges of two synchronous streams of transformation. (See diagram on page 93.)

The brain and sense organs are developed at an early stage in order that the activity of perception can awaken and connect the child to the world of senses; the will, working through imitation, movement and speech, requires the child to develop limbs and muscles sufficiently to support her upright position, and to develop the larynx for discovery of her mother tongue.

When the brain and nervous system are sufficiently mature to carry mental picturing and conscious thinking, the first self-aware experiences can take place; then, as feeling life prepares for its first independent activity, the rhythmic organs are stimulated in their growth; only when the etheric forces have completed their work on the brain and senses, and the limbs and metabolism have been sufficiently strengthened for appropriate will activities, can forces be freed for goal-directed thinking and memory.

This close correspondence between biological and psychological functions and development is fundamental to understanding the development of childhood and adolescence and has major implications for the wellbeing and future health of the growing child. What is stated above, in a very compressed and summarized fashion, will be explored and elucidated in greater detail in the following chapters.

Physical Constitution

Before we leave this phase of child development, it will be helpful to understand what may be called the *physical constitution* of the child. We use this term to differentiate it from the *human constitution*, which is the term used to embrace the whole human being – body soul and spirit, his fourfold nature of physical body, etheric body, soul and spirit. The child's physical appearance tells us already at a very early age a great deal about her nature. My first impression of Adam as a baby was his small head, his thin legs, his fine features and his extreme alertness. In contrast, Bulani distinguished himself by the prominence of his head, his large and protuberant abdomen, coarser features and his love of food.

The constitution in this context will be used to refer to the morphological appearance of the physical body, with a bearing also on function and behaviour. It is strongly determined by heredity and has a powerful influence on the development of the child in the first seven years. It can be of diagnostic and therapeutic value throughout childhood and adolescence. One can distinguish three main types of physical constitution that correspond to the threefold nature of the human being.

The Head Type

Here the characteristics of the neuro-sensory system penetrate the whole constitution too vigorously, making it more difficult for metabolic activities to permeate the body. This child is usually pale and small-headed with a firm body, dry skin and thin limbs. She will tend to lose her childhood softness quite early. She cannot concentrate well, is restless and easily distracted, and lacks creative fantasy. One notices already in preschool that her drawings and paintings are unimaginative and lack artistic feeling. Later she excels in the more cognitive subjects such as arithmetic, reading and spelling but does poorly in creative subjects like writing, story-telling and artistic subjects. Steiner characteristically named this child the *small-headed child* and, in her more one-sided nature, the *earthly child*. I have found this type to have two subdivisions.

- *The cerebral type* tends to be more introvert and brooding and is the typical precocious child who behaves like a small adult. Adam looks older than his age and has woken intellectually too quickly; this is because his soul and I forces engage his central nervous system too early at the expense of his organic growth and metabolic system. This type often exhibits digestive disturbances of various kinds.
- *The sensory type* tends to be more extrovert and over-active. Saskia is a highly sensitive child who lives too strongly in her sensory life. She tends to lose herself in her environment and therefore experiences life very intensely. There may be heightened sensitivity in any of the twelve senses. This type often has digestive sensitivities, liver or kidney weaknesses.

Anthroposophical physicians and Waldorf teachers have found the suggestions given by Steiner for these children to be very helpful in balancing out one-sided constitutional tendencies. These children do well with more sweet food, such as dried fruits, dates and honey, a warm compress on the tummy at night and the use of silver remedies to encourage warmth and fluid metabolism in organic processes.

The Metabolic Type

These are children whose metabolic processes predominate and whose neuro-sensory organization is not vigorous enough. Such a child has a large or domed head with a child-like, roundish face, soft warm body and weak legs. She generally has a warm pleasant disposition, an active imagination, leading to dreaming and fanciful ideas; she generally concentrates well, experiences the world more in pictures and is therefore a good artist but weak in analytical activities such as arithmetic and grammar. Steiner called this type of child the *large-headed child*, and in her more exaggerated form the *cosmic child*. I have likewise found that this group may be divided into two subgroups.

- *The digestive type* tends to be quite placid, dreamy and inactive in nature. Bulani can lose himself in his own world; he loves his food and his basic comforts. He tends to have glandular and congestive mucous problems.
- *The muscular/limb type* is characterized by a strong physique, powerful limbs and a strong will. Jonathan has little inclination for learning and loves any kind of physical activities. His predisposition is towards inflammations such as tonsillitis, bronchitis and ear infections.

The constitution of these children can be balanced by giving them more salt in their diet, and root vegetables, by washing the head with cold water in the morning and using natural remedies such as lead in homeopathic doses to strengthen the neuro-sensory dynamic in the constitution.

The Chest Type

This is the most harmonious of the three types, in whom neither the neuro-sensory nor the metabolic-limb systems predominate. The chest regions tends to be prominent, either being very long and flat, too hollow or too protuberant. This child displays a powerful feeling life, and can swing from introversion to extroversion very quickly. She has an artistic but also an analytical sense.

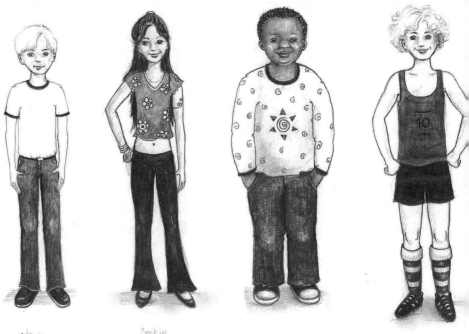

From left to right: Adam (cerebral), Saskia (sensory), Bulani (metabolic), Jonathan (muscular).

There also appear to be two types in this group.

- The respiratory type tends to be more anxious in her feelings and therefore more reactive in her behaviour; as an introvert, she can either withdraw too much, in which case her chest is more hollow in shape; or she pushes herself outward and develops a more extrovert nature. Thandi's wilful nature expresses itself in her prominent chest. These children often have a bronchitic or asthmatic tendency.
- The cardiac type is often a sensitive, caring child, and may tend to be too open to the environment. Maria has a long and delicately shaped chest; she is a shallow breather and her heart rate is slightly raised. These children are often allergic to environmental agents, being unable to fully protect themselves.

Children of this constitutional type need close monitoring of their feeling life; those who are more anxious need constant support and encouragement, while those who are too open need to learn to acquire firmer boundaries.

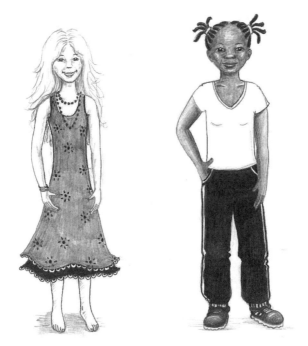

From left to right: Maria (cardiac), Thandi (respiratory).

Core Picture and Care of the Young Child

- During this first period of seven years, the etheric formative forces are dedicated to the growth and development of the physical body, as well as to the active transformation of the inherited body into the individual substance of a new body.

- The formation of all the organ systems develops simultaneously with the primary configuration of soul life and personality; this enables the child to discover the world, attain her first level of independence in movement, feeling and thinking, and learn life's basic skills.

- The formative forces are incipient in the growth of the musculo-skeletal system, enabling the will to work through sense perception, imitation and movement.

- The formative forces are most active within the neuro-sensory system, developing functional sense organs for the activity of perception; with further maturation, the brain can become the instrument for thinking; thinking in the form of picture thinking and memory can only emerge as transformed formative forces that have completed their primary shaping and modelling function of the brain.

- This signals, together with the change of teeth, the birth of the etheric body.

An understanding of these developmental principles offers a clear and rational approach for supporting the healthy development of the young child. These principles build further on those which underlie care for the first three years of life, and naturally also apply to the child up to the change of teeth.

- The greatest care should be taken that the organs of the physical body be allowed to develop in as healthy a way as possible. This is only possible if the etheric formative forces are supported and not hindered in their organic constructive functions:
  - Healthy food and drink, optimum light and warmth, adequate sleep, healthy routines and frequent access to nature
  - Intellectual demands on the young child's thinking before the change of teeth draw formative forces away from their organic tasks; therefore one should forgo the temptation to teach her to read and write, or to answer her questions intellectually. As far as possible, drawing on the faculty of imagination, one should give pictures rather than abstract, cause-effect answers, and avoid treating the child like a little adult
  - For the same reasons the child should not be schooled too early and should be carefully assessed for school readiness
  - Other factors that hinder healthy development of the body include indiscriminate inoculations, chemical medication, suppression of fever and injurious sense impressions.

Organs that are structurally or functionally weak predispose to both physical and psychological illness in later life. In Chapter ten we will explore the intimate continuum between the body and the soul in greater depth.

- The child should be allowed to unfold her soul life in the most health-giving way possible:
  - She should be allowed to express her will in an unrestricted manner through free movement and free creativity. Naturally this is within reasonable boundaries since the will is also educated by meeting appropriate resistance. To tell a child all the time not to touch is very obstructive and debilitating for her. I have found that small children, for instance, who are not given freedom to move and whose first efforts at walking are over-controlled by adults, will be prone to metabolic illnesses in later life
  - Since the child opens her body and soul through her sentient functions, the health of her physical, etheric and soul life will be strongly influenced by her surrounding sense impressions. Everything that the child perceives through her senses must be regarded as her environment. This includes not only the material and physical objects that surround her, the air she breathes and the food she eats, but also the aesthetic and moral environment in which she lives: sound, colour and harmonious forms as well as the thoughts, moods, speech and moral behaviour of the adults around her, will all impact on her
  - The natural faculty of imitation represents an enormous responsibility and challenge for us to provide a worthy environment in which the child can grow up
  - The feeling life of the child should be encouraged and never suppressed: 'Big boys don't cry' and 'It's not really so bad' are sentiments that can restrict a child's personality for life. Children who grow up in an environment of fear or excessive control develop anxious and nervous dispositions
  - The healthy unfolding of thinking can be supported through avoiding the intellectual approach mentioned above and through appropriate mental stimulation: encourage fantasy, free imagination and creativity through imaginative games and stories appropriate for each age. Inappropriate stimulation through TV, cinema, computer games and so-called educational computerized material for preschool children should be emphatically avoided.

Out of a vibrantly real spiritual life, the young child carries high ideals into the earthly world. She brings them as a gift to humanity. If we are open and respectful they can enrich our life. In her natural innocence the child expects the world to be good, and feels she has a right to be nurtured and protected. Can we live up to the innocent expectations of early childhood and offer her a good home in the broadest sense?

CHAPTER 8

The Beautiful, Healthy Years

Intense Feelings Shape My Soul Through the Rhythms of Breathing

The years between seven and fourteen are generally the healthiest years of the child's life. The most accident-prone years have passed and a certain level of immunity has been achieved, making this a time of relatively few illnesses and injuries. Indeed the mortality rate during these years is far lower than in the previous seven-year period (17 per 100,000 compared to 32 per 100,000).

This is a time when the child lives strongly in the pulse and breath of *rhythmical activities* – in free rhythmical movement, in singing, skipping, jumping and dancing. It is a time when the heart and lungs, whose health-giving rhythmical functions never tire, are supported and built up by the child's life activities. We will see that the healthy condition of this stage has much to do with the vibrant nature of the rhythmic life processes in the body.

Although many phases of childhood can be described as beautiful, this phase exhibits a special beauty as the child begins to unfold harmonious body proportions and graceful movements, like a young sapling moving in the wind.

Maria has thrown off the puppy fat of early childhood, and for the next five to seven years her sleek, lithe body, innocent and unpretentious, exudes the beauty and grace of a young Greek goddess. Rajan at nine or ten reminded me of the handsome statue of Michelangelo's David.

These are the years when the life of feeling awakens from its unconscious working in the bodily realm to become active as an independent and free soul activity. At the same time, an unbounded curiosity and thirst for knowledge takes over from a natural and self-evident trusting acceptance of the world; now the child experiences the world outside himself in a new way and he wants to get to know it consciously.

> My body has become distinct from the world, but in my feelings I still feel part of the world: here I am in the world; I feel the sun, the clouds, the rain, the trees, the birds – they speak to my heart. I long to learn everything about the world; the adults know so much about so many things and I too wish to know these things.

Most of us can remember these years well. We stepped out into the world, into a new community of many children and new caregivers. The school environment was very different from home life. For some hours every weekday, you left the safe protection of home and parents. How did you experience this? You were no longer the prime focus of attention, and had to learn instead to be part of a whole class of children, forming new relationships with teachers and classmates. Many things happened in the course of each day. After school there was life at home but the very familiar people – mother, father and siblings – began to look and feel different. You looked at them freshly as though seeing them for the first time – yet they remained your trustworthy anchors. Brothers and sisters became less important than new friends. There were weekends, holidays, birthdays and celebrations, new interests, hobbies, pets, and always exciting things to look forward to.

What lives imprinted in your memory of this time? How does it still affect your life now? Certain events may rise up as a clear memory picture often associated with certain feelings. It is often the unpleasant memories that come into consciousness out of the distant, dreamlike awareness of this time. Because all the experiences of our childhood are embedded in our memory, they are always accessible to our awareness.[1]

The Heart of Childhood

This is the middle period of childhood that spans the time between the change of teeth and puberty. Like the first period of seven years, this middle period mirrors the whole of childhood, except that here the *feeling life* is the dominant characteristic, rather than the will. This period can also be divided for the purpose of clarity into three divisions that flow one into the other with no fixed boundaries. The first third corresponds to the first seven years where, as we have seen, the life of will is dominant. Here we can observe how the will lives strongly through pictorial thinking and the impetuous unfolding of feelings. The second third reflects this second period of seven years itself, and is the very heart and centre of the phase when the feeling life awakens. The third phase that sees a blossoming of thinking activities corresponds, as we shall see, to the awakening of intellectual thinking in the third period of seven years.

Early school phase	Change of teeth to 9th year	**Will phase** (preponderance of will)
Heart of childhood	9th–12th year	**Feeling phase** (feeling and imagination dominate)
Pubescence	12th year – puberty	**Thinking phase** (more conscious thinking dominates)

Physical Transformation

We saw in Chapter four that the change of teeth signifies the beginning of a new way of being for the child. It is a striking picture of the birth of the etheric body, with significant implications for the future development of the child. Life forces that up to this point were completely directed towards the growth and development of the body, now become free to serve the activity of thinking.

We must assume that this transformation happens gradually over several years since the loss of the milk teeth takes the best part of seven years to complete. Contrary to common beliefs, the first permanent tooth is usually a molar tooth that appears behind the two milk molars before the first milk teeth are shed. This is the first sign that the child is ready for school since he now has at his disposal the faculties he will need for intellectual memory and thinking.

The first teeth lost are usually in the order in which they first arrived, commonly incisors first, bottom and top, and then the canines. Between ten and twelve years, the milk molars are lost and the second permanent molar appears behind the first one. By twelve years the canines have been replaced, and by puberty the full set of permanent teeth is present.

The bursting forth of new teeth accompanies the growth of the physical body. As we travel alongside the child we should be aware that all the physical changes we witness are an outer expression of the corresponding activity of life forces weaving and working through the body, growing and shaping its organs.

When Thandi was assessed for school readiness, she had her first permanent molar tooth and had shed her first lower milk incisor; she had lost the round chubby features of early childhood and had a slender body form. Her neck, chest and abdomen were clearly demarcated and her tummy was relatively flat. Her arms were long enough for the fingers of one hand to reach over her head and touch the opposite ear.

The growth rate in the middle period of childhood is slower in comparison with the earlier pre-school period and the subsequent adolescent period. The average annual increase in height and weight is approximately 6 cm and 2 kg respectively.

By her ninth and tenth year, Thandi's body has filled out largely through growth of the chest, trunk and limbs which have lengthened and are broader. In the prepuberty years there is a sudden growth surge, similar to the pre-school phase, primarily in the arms and legs. *How you have grown!* people often say. Thandi was quite pleased when people frequently called her big and strong; but Maria, who was much more sensitive, was embarrassed and irritated to be reminded constantly of her growing body, especially when it had become particularly skinny and awkward. Teenagers may suddenly need a complete change of clothes, girls at an earlier age (10 to 11) – than boys (12–13). As growth of the extremities of the limbs and lower jaw accelerates, the fine, childlike features of the middle phase give way to the somewhat lopsided look of puberty: the jaw becomes more defined, the face less refined, the limbs clumsy and gangly, the hands and legs top heavy. Indeed a self-conscious teenager can be an uncomfortable spectacle to witness.

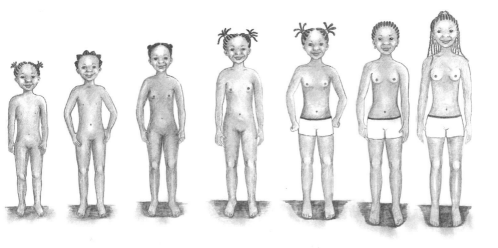

In the course of middle childhood the brain reaches its adult size and weight, and the neuro-sensory functions attain their full maturity. Most of the work on these organs has already taken place during the previous seven years.

Now it is the *respiratory* and *circulatory systems* that are preferentially subject to the developmental process; the heart and lungs increase in weight and size and a strengthening and consolidation of the rhythms of breathing and circulation take place. In the first years the pulse and respiratory rate compared to later years is rapid, often irregular, and easily affected by factors such as movement, metabolic activity and emotional changes. As can be seen in the table below, the pulse and breathing rates gradually settle down to attain by the 14th year a relatively steady rhythm, fairly close to the adult rate.

Average pulse and respiratory rates

	Pulse rate	Respiratory rate
Newborn	125	30
2 years	110	28
4 years	100	25
6 years	100	23
8 years	90	22
10 years	90	20
12 years	88	19
14 years	85	18
16 years	77	18
18 years	72	18

It is important to recognize that the transformation and consolidation of **rhythmic processes** is taking place at this time. The rhythms of the heart and lungs, and their interplay, are two of the most striking rhythmic activities we can become conscious of.

Simply turn your attention to your breathing and observe its rhythm. We breathe air containing mainly oxygen and nitrogen into our lungs, the breathing pauses for a moment and then we breathe out air containing mainly carbon dioxide into the atmosphere; again there is a slight pause before we breathe in again. The rhythm of our breathing determines the exchange and flow of oxygen into the blood stream and thence into every bodily cell, as well as the elimination of carbon dioxide, an end product of cell metabolism, from the body.

Once we know where to find the pulse at the wrist we can tune in to our circulatory rhythm. We feel the pulse surge as the heart contracts in systole; there is a momentary pause before the pulse subsides as the heart relaxes in diastole, followed by another pause before the next contraction. The rhythm of our pulse will influence the manner in which fluids, nutrients, blood cells and all bodily substances such as hormones, chemical transmitters, antibodies, etc. circulate throughout the body.

It follows that these two rhythmic processes will to a great extent determine the physiology of breathing and circulation. And so it is with all the other physiological processes. According to Steiner there are seven primary life processes that constitute the functioning activity of the life body, all of which are regulated by rhythmic activity inherent to them.[2] The rhythmic activities of all life processes undergo a strengthening and consolidation during this seven-year period.

Since the rhythmic life is an essential feature of this developmental epoch, we need to explore the nature of rhythm more deeply.

Rhythm

The nature of rhythm has been extensively investigated both from the scientific and the spiritual-scientific point of view.[3] Let us focus on the breathing rhythm because it is so close to the inner core of our being and so easily accessible.

As we breathe in and out we notice we are moving the breath in two opposite directions: inwards and outwards towards two extreme points at maximal inhalation and maximal exhalation. These are the two points furthest apart in the cycle of one breath; they both lead to a rest phase, a pause in breathing; they are also turning points and the point of greatest tension where we cannot go further but must instead go back in the opposite direction. Tension builds up towards the extremes, and at the 'turn' of the breath the tension is released and balanced. As Hoerner describes it, 'each breath is a polar event between two turning points'.

Breathing is not only a polar event in terms of its direction, but also in its whole dynamic. Inhalation is an active process in which the lungs, diaphragm, chest cage, ribs and intercostal muscles stretch and expand; in contrast, normal exhalation is a passive process in which lungs recoil elastically and the rest of the breathing apparatus relaxes with little apparent effort. We also experience the distinct polarity between movement of the breathing and the resting pause. Thus each breath consists of two one-sided and opposite components that are continuously balanced out by something that happens at the turning points between the two polarities. In fact, it is the very nature of rhythm to balance two extreme polarities that on their own would be destructive; if the breathing became fixed in either inhalation or exhalation, the excess of the one and lack of the other would quickly kill us. This breakdown in rhythm is essentially the basis of all pathology and is a subject we shall explore in greater detail in Part 2.

This dual event is one continuously repeated: one breath followed by the next. But in fact no breath is ever exactly the same as the previous one. Exact repetition can only be produced by robot-like machines designed specifically to reproduce commodities which are exactly alike. A time-piece must provide us with accurate, reproducible time; a factory making cars must have equipment that reproduces identical engine parts.

The sphere of life never functions in such a mechanical way: every leaf on an oak tree is slightly different from the next; no cloud or wave, or day or summer, is the same as the one before or after it. Therefore every breath may appear very similar, but is never exactly the same. Hoerner describes this process as a *renewal* of the previous event, or constant renewal. A metronome is designed to give a steady beat, with consistently identical repetition of two extremes: beat and no beat; the heart however cannot be said to beat, and least of all to pump, because its rhythm is continuously modifying the preceding rhythmic event. The metronome may well be more exact and predictable, but by its nature is unalterable, rigid and unsuited for the living world. The heart in contrast is adaptable and flexible and is constantly open and responding to new possibilities.

We can easily experience the different quality of something mechanical or life-endowed by comparing how tired one becomes when observing a mechanical activity (such as a traffic light going from green to red to green to red); and how, in contrast, one is enlivened by watching the ebb and flow of waves at the sea shore.

Next we can observe how our breathing rhythm is affected by movement or exertion. Simply by pushing your hands together you will notice how the breath changes and then settles down when the exertion ceases. The breathing rhythm is able to adapt constantly to inner and outer changes. Hoerner calls this 'elastic adaptability'. It is the means by which harmony is achieved.

Finally we must acknowledge that our breathing takes place in the course of time. It is not a spatial event but a temporal one which unfolds in specific sequential periods.

Our breathing rhythm is thus characterized by these five essential features:

- Polarity and balance
- Constant renewal
- Elastic adaptability
- Related to life
- Periodicity based on time.

All life processes in the universe and the human being are carried out in a temporal sequence by rhythms that balance polarities, are constantly renewing preceding events and are able to adapt elastically to changing circumstances.

Here, once more, we encounter the body of forces in the human being that encompasses and sustains life processes: the life or etheric body. This time we meet it in the element of rhythm, which is found only in the sphere of the living.

It is not easy to grasp the nature of rhythm. Where is it to be found? If we observe our breathing, where do we experience it? It is an invisible mediating element, living somewhere between the tangible aspects of inhalation and exhalation and the intangible realm of the soul and spirit. The life body is a mercurial reality that provides the mediating activity for the incarnating soul and spirit to enter the earthly material world. And rhythm is the activity of the etheric body enabling this interaction to take place.

Dynamic Transformation

This life body is not a body that exists in space. The physical body occupies space and can be weighed and measured as can a stone; but the human physical body of a child grows and develops in the course of **time.** It can do this because it is sustained by a life body that unfolds in rhythmic, living processes, one of which is growth and development. The etheric body is a time organism and unfolds its activity in rhythmic cycles.

The development of the child from conception to adulthood takes place in time and is carried and regulated by many different rhythms. The etheric body is the conductor holding together this symphony of rhythm in masterful harmony. There are many rhythms taking place over seconds, minutes, hours, days, weeks, months and years and they are influenced and invisibly bound up with universal cosmic rhythms.

Steiner frequently alluded to the relationship between the breathing rhythm, the human lifespan and the Platonic year. The average adult resting breathing rate is 18 breaths per minute, or 25,920 in 24 hours. This is the same number of days that a human being will live in an average life of 72 years. This means that we sleep and wake in an average lifetime the same number of times that we breathe in and out in the course of one day. And if we take one human life of 72 years and regard it as one day in a cosmic year of 360 days, we find it takes the same number of years for the sun to travel through the zodiac and arrive again exactly at the same point, namely 25, 920 years.[4] A cosmic or Platonic year – one could also say a solar year of the sun, the source of our life on earth – thus encompasses approximately the same number of years as the number of breaths in the course of 24 hours and the same number of waking-sleeping cycles in the course of an average human life.

The menstrual cycle of 28 days is a monthly rhythm connected with the moon cycle, which we know is related to reproductive life. This human life rhythm has become emancipated from the cosmic lunar rhythm, although some women still have their periods at full moon.

A larger rhythm, the seven-year cycle that governs the developmental process in childhood and adolescence, as well as the further life phases of the human being, is an expression of the unfolding panoramic activity of the etheric body.

We can catch a glimpse of the etheric body's nature in the act of remembering. We saw previously that memory resides in the resonating activity of the life body and that thinking is an etheric activity. Whenever we call up a mental picture out of our memory we are tapping into the pictorial life matrix of the etheric forces. Even the mental pictures of ordinary consciousness, that are dreamlike and shadowy compared with our sensory experience of the physical world, proceed from the life body.

This ordinary thinking, however, can be strengthened through specific thinking exercises. For instance, summon a simple mental picture in your mind such as a pin or pencil, and concentrate with all your power of thinking on this mental object to the exclusion of all other thoughts. Through repeating such exercises many times, thinking can be strengthened to the point at which the etheric body becomes direct experience.[5] Even before this stage is reached one can already enhance mental imagery by this and similar means to the point where it becomes more vivid and vibrant.

By focusing awareness on a specific memory picture, it is possible as we have seen to go back in time to any period in one's biography and re-experience as an intense reality, say, one's seventh or ninth year of life.

In the psychophonetics counselling process described earlier, images of periods and events in the client's life arise as a normal part of a session through gesturing and observing the bodily form that has been created through the gesture.

A client who had a fear of being attacked by a dog every time she went out jogging, gestured how she felt when she was anxious; when she looked at the form she had created as an after-image, she was astonished to see herself as a four-year-old child being beaten by her father.

This biographical picture is recalled or re-invoked by the gesture that the adult client gives to the anxiety she feels inside her. It is the same anxiety and gesture that the life memory has been carrying since four years of age. Through the power of visualization, the drama of that time opens up before her mind's eye. She is now able consciously to come to the child's help, deal with the hurt and fear in a way she could not previously and thereby resolve her current fear of dogs.

The whole etheric body is in dynamic activity through time and contains, in a compressed seed form, a person's whole

biography. This is why violent shocks or near-death experiences
that momentarily separate the life body from the physical body,
frequently result in a person seeing his whole life unfolding
panoramically in reverse order, or in flashbacks to specific life
events. Repressed or forgotten memories of past traumas – e.g.
concentration camp syndrome (a post-traumatic stress disorder in
clients who had repressed the traumatic ordeals they had experienced
in some kind of harsh internment) – may be powerfully re-evoked.
Indeed all post-traumatic stress disorders may be regarded as the
persistent recall of a traumatic event that reverberates continuously
through the etheric body.

Rhythm as an essential activity of the etheric forces, balances
extremes and sustains life. An experience I had some years ago will
illustrate this phenomenon.

As a young doctor I was fortunate enough to spend some time
at the WALA plant laboratory in Eckwälden, Germany, learning
to manufacture plant remedies without the use of alcohol as a
preservative. It is well known that when one adds organic material
to water, it will begin to smell and ferment within a few days, and
after a week will show signs of fungal growth. I was somewhat
incredulous to learn that all the rhythmically produced WALA
remedies were preserved by rhythm alone. This I had to see for
myself!

So we harvested the plant, chopped up the material finely,
mixed it with spring water and then placed the mixture for the rest
of the day in a dark chamber warmed to 37 degrees Celsius for an
hour around sunset and sunrise; the mixture was brought into the
light and kept cold with ice at 4 degrees Celsius; thereafter it was
returned to the warmth and darkness. This process was continued
for seven or fourteen days, during which I noticed the fragrance
and colour improving by the day. Within a week a murky opaque
liquid can become a clear extract, violet-coloured and sweet
smelling. To my amazement, the preparation stabilized after this
period and would no longer ferment, even after years. I still have
in my possession a rose tincture that I prepared in 1980 using this
method, and to this day it has not lost its freshness and fragrance.

The seven-day rhythmic activity of exposing the plant substances
to *dark – light/warmth – cold,* creates in the tincture sufficient power

of life to counteract the forces of breakdown and destruction by fungi and bacteria. Steiner indicated that the morning and evening cosmic forces around sunrise and sunset are times when the earth is exposed to the most powerful life impulses.

We have all experienced the vitality and exhilaration present in nature during these times: the birds sing in a more intense way and nature's creatures all become more active. Based on these suggestions, Rudolf Hauschka developed the WALA plant remedies whose name derives from the rhythmic activity of *Wärme Ansatz/Licht Ansatz* – meaning warmth preparation/light preparation.

Rhythms in Homeopathy

All mineral, plant and animal substances can be processed further according to the homeopathic principle of potentization and rhythmic succussion developed by Samuel Hahnemann. The new plant tincture that I helped to harvest for instance can be diluted to one part in ten or one part in a hundred, and shaken rhythmically in a certain way, for a certain time. The result is a first-level potentized remedy (D1 or 1× or CH1) whereby the latent life force present in the plant substance is released by the rhythmic process into the fluid medium. This process can be continued sequentially by dilution and rhythmic potentizing to produce a sequence of potentized remedies of increasing potency. The manufacture of homeopathic and anthroposophical remedies is based on these principles.

Here we see once again how the activity of rhythm can release the life potential latent in all living substance.

Rhythm and Life

Rhythm is a basic condition of life. Loss of rhythm leads to loss of life function and ultimately death; arrhythmic physiological functions lead to illness, and all illnesses can be looked at from the angle of rhythm disturbance: for instance the heart rate may become irregular, can accelerate or slow down, can be stimulated by amphetamines to race so fast that it contracts violently and comes to a standstill. Sleep disturbances, constipation, hay fever, asthma are likewise a result of disturbance in rhythm. Most of us lead an arrhythmic life, some more than others: too much food, too little sleep, too much work, too little exercise, etc. Yet we are constantly able to balance out the excesses or deficiencies through our rhythmic self-regulating or *life-maintaining processes*.

This healing capacity of rhythmical activities in an epoch when these life processes are being consolidated, will explain why this period is the most healthy time of life.

Rhythmic System

Having laid a foundation for an understanding of rhythm, we can now gain an understanding of the *rhythmic system* which is undergoing consolidation from the seventh to fourteenth years.

From birth to the seventh year, the physical body and nerve-sense system were primarily being developed. The life body was fully engaged at this organic level. With the change of teeth, some of these forces became free to serve the functions of thinking and memory. The other etheric forces begin to work more in the realm of soul and spirit and now become engaged in the consolidation of the highly complex organization of rhythmic processes that we may call the rhythmic system.

Wherever life processes are present, from the countless invisible biochemical activities of all cells and tissues to the visible physiological functions of organs such as the heart and lungs, rhythmic processes are continually balancing out polarities in sequential cycles. The rhythmic system comprises the integrated totality of all rhythmic activities in the human organism. Like rhythm itself, at work in every rhythmic process, it mediates between two extremes which, at the broad level of the human organization, we have called the neuro-sensory system and the metabolic-limb system.

In previous chapters we saw how these two systems operate in diametric opposition to each other: the neuro-sensory system is like a self-centred egotist trying to draw the world in towards itself, with the brain acting as the information-receiving centre, and the senses transporting the world content from outside towards the inside. The metabolic limb system is quite the opposite; it is an altruist wishing to give everything away: metabolic generation and transformation, transportation of substances, energy production, movement and activity.

The neuro-sensory system is the resting pole that draws the world inwards towards its resting centre: the metabolic-limb system is the moving pole that drives the world of matter outwards towards the circumference in constant motion. The rhythmic system is tirelessly working like a wise and caring healer to mediate between these extremes and to balance out their polar activities.

Can you imagine what would happen to the egotist were he only to take from the world and give nothing of himself to it? He would be completely focused on satisfying his own needs. If one tries to feel into this experience and to give expression to it physically, one may discover a cold, thin, dry and shrivelled-up individual whose body and soul become hard and contracted; and one could imagine he might succumb to some kind of hardening or sclerotic illness, such as arthritis, hardening of the arteries or blood thrombosis.

What would happen to the altruist who created and produced continuously for others, keeping nothing for himself? If one inwardly experiences this type, one may notice that one becomes too warm, congested and puffed up. Body and soul become too soft and expansive, and he may tend to inflammatory illnesses, like pneumonia, softening of the bones or blood haemorrhage.

One can view pathology as originating in a predominance either of the neuro-sensory system leading to sclerotic illnesses, or of the metabolic limb system leading to inflammatory illnesses.

Sclerotic illnesses generally create a preponderance of mineral deposition, conditions that can be characterized as *earthly*; inflammatory illnesses manifest the opposite tendency, where excessive demineralization and the breakdown of mineral substance into fluidic, gaseous, warmth and light dominates: such conditions may be characterized as *cosmic*. This polarity will be explored in greater detail in Part 2.

It is the presence of rhythm working through every rhythmic process within the rhythmic system that maintains the healthy state of the body. An invisible genius is at work somewhere in the interval between the two balancing pans of the scale, constantly sensing how much of the one, how much of the other is needed at every moment to maintain healthy balance.

How can we gain a tangible experience of the rhythmic system? It certainly cannot be discovered in the sense-bound cognitive mode of experience that we make use of in visualizing, reflecting on or describing the rhythmic system. This cognitive mode is appropriate for the neuro-sensory system. Nor however can it be found by directly engaging in rhythmic activity, for such direct engagement belongs to the metabolic-limb system. We can only experience the rhythmic system in the ever-present movement between two extremes of rest and activity, which is that of *feeling* life. While sensing and reflecting lead us to an experience of the neuro-sensory system, and will activity bring us to an experience of the metabolic limb system, only the experience of feeling enables us to enter the nature of the rhythmic system.

Mercury is the name given by the ancients to the power that rules in this twilight zone, mediating between the earthly and cosmic powers. They saw him as bringing messages of the heavenly realms down to earth, and carrying back the fruits of the earth to realms of spirit. As a solid-liquid metallic substance, mercury has the ability to unite two opposing tendencies: cohesion into matter, dispersion into spirit. Observe the way in which droplets of mercury coalesce but then as easily split apart again into tiny droplets. By bringing them to rest in a container the finely dispersed droplets coalesce into one compact, united droplet – metaphorically into a more earthly material form; by shaking the cohesive mercury onto an open tray, it can again be dispersed into many finer droplets, into a more immaterial form.

There is a bronze statue by the Renaissance sculptor Giovani da Bologna of the three-winged Mercury, clothed only in a winged helmet, with wings on his ankles. With his left hand, he holds a winged staff thrice wound round by two snakes: this, the caduceus, is the magic wand given to him by Apollo to balance polarities; with his right hand he points backwards to the spirit world from where he came. To this day, Mercury is the symbol of the healing art of medicine. Many medical institutions and associations use the staff of Mercury to symbolize the healing power of the dynamic space between two extremes.

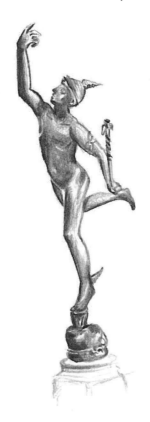

Breathing

There is an ancient saying that the secret of all healing lies in the breathing. Among the many interesting features of the statue above is the picture of Mercury poised in flight on the breath emanating from the upturned face of Neolus, the wind god. This cosmic breath appears like a flame or fountainhead of power through which Mercury, the paragon of healing, can carry out his healing tasks. This ancient dictum, embodied in this striking statue of Mercury, suggests that if we can comprehend the nature of the breath we may understand the healing forces in the human being's breathing system. It will also equip us to understand the child at this stage of life.

This is a mystery that would seem to go to the very core of child health. Indeed it would seem to have everything to do with the health and harmony of the human being and of the whole universe. Let us therefore try to gain some insight into the mystery of the breath that is being strengthened during this stage of development.

Through our breath we are connected continuously to the outside world and specifically to the atmosphere of the earth from which we draw life-sustaining oxygen and breathe out toxic carbon dioxide. Only during waking hours do we engage with the outside world by absorbing nutrients and sense impressions, by moving our limbs or by communication. Our breath, on the other hand, is continuous – from the moment of our first breath at birth, to our last at death. This continuous and regular breathing activity is critical for maintaining bodily life and health. We can do without water, food, sense impressions and sleep for several days, but not without air for more than about 2 minutes. Thus breathing is the most important mediator between the human being and the outside world.

The brain needs a constant supply of oxygen for it to function normally. When this is interrupted, our health suffers. Every inbreath enlivens the body and every outbreath removes toxic air that would poison the body if not removed.

One can observe that the breathing and the blood circulation are intimately connected with each other: the two lungs embrace the heart like two closely fitted wings that beat once for every four pulsations of the heart. The right side of the heart receives venous blood from two major veins that bring the blood from the left and right halves of the body as well as from above and below; thus blood from *four* quadrants enter the right side of the heart: from 'below', blood rich in metabolic substances and carbon dioxide, and from 'above', blood in addition carrying the imponderable products of cognitive and sensory imprints.

This oxygen-poor blood then flows through one single artery to the lungs, radiating like the finest sparks of fire into the airy, alveolar lung substance through fine capillaries, and meeting the mercurial air sacs of the lungs in intimate embrace. Like dispersing droplets of mercury, the oxygen-rich air, comprising *one* part oxygen to *four* parts nitrogen, diffuses into these blood capillaries at the harmonious rate of *one* air pulse to *four* blood pulses. This blood from both lungs now returns via *four* lung veins into the left side of the heart to be dispersed though *one* major heart artery to upper and lower spheres of the body.

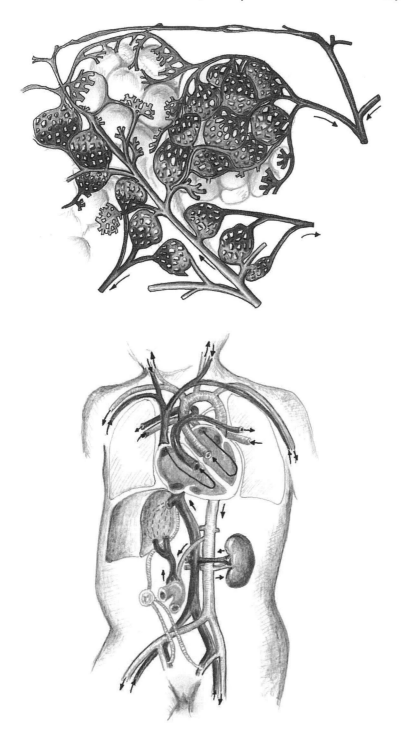

Diagram of heart-lung circulation and the alveolar capillary system

We encounter the ratio of 1:4 frequently in the relationship between the upper and lower sphere. As we saw above, the child strives to attain this ideal relationship between the breathing and the circulatory system and achieves this by the age of about 18. This ratio of 1:4 is as an extremely important indicator of a person's state of health, and deviations from this ideal relationship can point to illness tendencies in a patient. Can it also help us to deepen our understanding of the healing power of breathing?

The breathing and circulatory systems are the central organ systems of the rhythmic system which, as we have seen, mediates between the neuro-sensory system and the metabolic-limb system.

To maintain bodily health, the child absorbs food and drink, digesting and assimilating these nutrients in the form of metabolic products. He must also take oxygen into his lungs. The blood circulation carries oxygen into the metabolic arena where it undergoes combustion as a fuel to drive metabolic processes that maintain all physiological processes in the body. In the process, toxic carbon dioxide and other toxic waste products are produced. These and many other phenomena demonstrate the close connection of the circulatory system with the metabolism. The blood circulation has then to return to the breathing interface to offload its harmful carbon dioxide content and replenish its oxygen supply. With every breath, four pulses of toxic blood are restored to health and renewed with life. It is as if the breathing rhythm continuously tames the circulatory rhythm – as if the breath continuously heals the blood.

Thus the breathing process is intimately connected with the blood circulation and metabolism.

On the other side, the breathing process is also directly connected with the child's neuro-sensory life. Psychologically, the child as he develops his cognitive processes 'breathes in' sense impressions that are also digested and assimilated, and 'breathes out' thoughts and concepts. Furthermore, as we breathe in, more cerebrospinal fluid is pushed into the brain, and as we breathe out it is pressed back into the body. This can be easily observed when a doctor wishes to measure the pressure in the spinal fluid: when a needle is inserted into the spinal canal – a procedure known as a lumbar puncture – and connected to a simple manometer which measures pressure, the pressure will be seen to rise with inhalation and to fall with exhalation. From this it would seem that the breathing rhythm is directly transmitted to the neuro-sensory system.

The neuro-sensory system, as we have seen, is in polar opposition to the metabolic limb system; the former is cool and calm, the latter is warm and active. Likewise the breathing system is cool and calm in relation to the circulatory system, which is warm and active. In the rhythmic system two polar tendencies are brought together and harmonized through the ideal relationship of 4:1.

From this point of view we may regard the breathing system as the rhythmic continuation of the neuro-sensory system and the circulatory system as the rhythmic continuation of the metabolic-limb system. The metabolic-limb system expresses its dynamic activity through the blood circulation, the neuro-sensory system through the breathing rhythm. What happens in the metabolism therefore takes place at least four times as fast as what occurs in the nerve-sense system.

The developmental landscape we are witnessing on our voyage of discovery with the child is at all times an expression of this rhythmic relationship between the life of the neuro-sensory system and that of the metabolic-limb system. An outstanding event is the change of teeth – the culmination of dominant neuro-sensory activity. Here we see the hard, sculpted, spherical head forces of the new teeth dominating over the radiating driving action of the metabolic forces that push the teeth into visible space; having erupted, they stand, if cared for, for the rest of life as rock-hard, immobile bastions of resistance to the constant inflow of living substance. We may recall the nature of the neural system which blocks and inhibits life. Seven years later, when puberty arrives, we can in contrast feel the metabolic forces in ascendance over the neuro-sensory forces, where the life forces appear to have no bounds.

Breathing in Education

In his inaugural lecture to the teachers of the first Waldorf School in 1919, Steiner spoke about the cardinal importance of breathing in the educational process. He describes the two aspects of breathing as relating to primary tasks of the educator.

On the one hand he suggested that the inner breathing or soul functions in the young child are not yet properly regulated and that the breathing process is not yet connected in a harmonious way with the nerve-sense process. We have seen the close connection between breathing and the psyche and have found that the child's soul in the first seven years lives powerfully in his sensory functions; it is as if the *psukhè* – the inner breath – is too powerful in out-breathing or 'sympathy' with his environment. The child opens himself in full trust, in full sympathy with the environment. The one task of education, Steiner says, is '. . . to teach the child to breathe properly . . . to bring the breathing process into a healthy relationship with the neuro-sensory system and . . . thereby draw the soul and spirit of the child into a healthy connection with the physical body.[6]

This drawing in of soul and spirit into the body may be experienced as an in-breathing, inhalation or incarnation. When we wake up, soul and spirit enter the body; we 'breathe' into the body, and during the waking state, soul and spirit reside in it – for during waking life we are conscious of the body and therefore present within it. When we fall asleep, soul and spirit leave the body; we 'breathe' out or excarnate, and during sleep are then somewhere outside the body – we are no longer aware of the body and lose consciousness.

As the imitative faculty declines and cognitive faculties increase, the power of in-breathing and 'antipathy' increases for, as we have said above, wakefulness can be regarded as breathing consciousness into the body and this creates separation and 'antipathy' from the rest of the world. Every time we use our cognitive functions we have to withdraw from the world, and close ourselves off from it in a kind of antipathy. The consistent guiding of the soul harmoniously into the body in this in-breathing activity, will balance the dominant out-breathing tendency of the earlier phase and gradually lead to maturation of the breathing system. The education process must therefore assist in harmonious interplay or 'breathing' between the soul functions of sympathetic sensing and the antipathy of thinking.

Steiner goes on to say that the young child also cannot carry over into his sleeping life all that he experiences during waking life. Exact observation will show that our experiences of the day seem somewhat different when we waken the next day. 'Let's sleep on it', we say. It would appear that something mysterious happens during our sleep to modify our experiences. The child, says Steiner, cannot yet do this. He has a very different waking consciousness compared with an older child: more dreamy, impulsive, non-reflective. He lives strongly in the present and more easily forgets things.

The other task of the educator must be to help the child carry his physical bodily experiences over into the activities of the soul and spirit during sleep.

Every aspect of education will have the effect either of drawing the soul-spirit nature of the child into his body or pushing it out of the body. All activities of the neuro-sensory system, such as observation using thinking and perceiving, abstractions and fine differentiation will tend to incarnate the child; in contrast mobilization of the metabolic-limb system in movement, expansive creativity and pictorial and imaginative work will have an excarnating effect. Rhythmic activities (see below) mediate between these two tendencies and develop harmony.

The breathing process underlies the health-giving nature of all rhythm. And it is in this period of the child's life that he needs to learn the skill of breathing properly; the strength of his future rhythmic life will be determined by the way he learns to breathe now. Pre-disposition for later diseases of the heart, lungs and other rhythmic organs will have their origin in the lack of rhythm during these years. This does not of course mean that children should learn actual breathing exercises. It means that their lives in every possible way should be balanced with healthy rhythms and routines.

Rhythm in the School and Home

It should be a fundamental principle of any healthy education to arrange the curriculum of the junior school in accordance with rhythmic activities. The Waldorf method has evolved out of a deep understanding of these developmental principles. Each lesson, day and term is planned carefully to ensure a healthy inbreath of new experiences and a healthy outbreath of will activity. For instance, the school day may begin by absorbing new perceptions and thoughts.

The child is at rest and concentrating in waking consciousness. This may be followed by some form of rhythmical activity such as music, singing, eurythmy or painting that allows the child artistically to 'breathe in and out', thereby restoring the exhausting nerve- and sense based activity with life-renewing rhythmic forces. The day concludes in 'breathing out' with some practical activity such as woodwork, crafts, gardening, etc. in which the children's limbs are active and mobile. This basic educational principle of working rhythmically with the children can be applied in many creative ways through each lesson and throughout each day.

Do you remember this age of free rhythmical movement in your own childhood?

Do you recall the inner urge to experience life in rhythmic activities? We loved to play catchers, rounders and all kinds of ball games. There were always cyclical crazes and fads happening which had no set patterns, but which seemed to come and go like the seasons; often to do with connecting, collecting and swapping things with other kids: marbles, charms, stamps, transfers, pets, toys, gadgets and other paraphernalia.

Skipping, hopping, swinging, balancing, jumping, tumbling are things we did naturally, any time, on the way to school, in the school break; we rocked back and forth on our school chairs as if we were marking inner time. I loved to sing in the choir with other boys and be directed by the authority of the choir master. I would dance freely and ecstatically to music when no one was watching. I can recall the excitement of reciting 'The highwayman came riding, riding, riding, the highwayman came riding up to the old inn door', and the pride of learning the whole *Ancient Mariner* by heart. I also learnt to play the piano and fly kites during this period.

On the foundation of developing rhythmic life processes, the soul activities of feeling and imagination begin to awaken. The development of both body and soul converge during this time in the rhythmic system, leading to a strengthening and consolidation of rhythmical processes. Thus, both in his body and soul life, the child experiences a stimulation of rhythmical processes and will therefore naturally seek every opportunity to resonate with rhythmical activities. We therefore can readily understand why the child lives so naturally in rhythmical activities during this period.

Rhythmical Movement

To fulfil its life-imbuing function, the etheric body must by its very nature be vibrant, living activity. Working through every cell and particle of the physical body, this dynamic force system transforms lifeless mineral substance into living substance. The most distinctive characteristic of life is movement and a lively child is a child in movement. When movement in living organisms ceases, life comes to an end. It is no wonder then that the etheric body is in constant movement.

To begin with the movements of a young child are fairly haphazard and uncoordinated. With the development of the rhythmic life processes after the change of teeth, they begin to be more ordered. This is why, during this period, the child has a natural desire to move rhythmically.

We have considered the relationship of the etheric body with wider cosmic rhythms: hypothetically we found a connection between the breathing rhythm and the Platonic cosmic rhythm as well as a connection with the sun and the other planets. We may also conceive that the etheric body is formed prenatally out of the etheric forces of the universe, so that after birth the child contains in his life body an image of the cosmos – the world of the stars, the planets and the earth.

If such connections do in fact exist, it is reasonable to conclude that the movements of the etheric body correspond to the movements and rhythms of the cosmic bodies. These cosmic rhythms are precisely ordered, predictable and well researched by astronomical and geophysical sciences. Since Kepler presented his discoveries of harmonic planetary sounds emanating from the velocity of the planets and their planetary orbits, many other researchers have presented similar findings; radiotelescopic research reveals that the universe is full of sound – for instance Jupiter produces a very different sound from the sun.[7]

We saw in the previous chapter that life on earth is completely dependent on these planetary rhythms.

In the course of a day, a child will exercise his will countless times in movements of many kinds. Most will be reflex, and without specific purpose; others will be directed and purposeful; there will also be times when the child has an inner desire to move rhythmically and one may observe then how different these movements appear – graceful, flowing, aesthetic and beautiful. One can sense that the child is striving to imitate and master certain inner rhythms. Could he be trying to emulate the ever-present rhythms of the cosmos?

From time immemorial, humanity has felt and known its connection to nature and the universe. In early epochs, our ancestors lived in intimate contact with these rhythms, observing with great exactitude the movements of the sun, moon and other planets. They could not live without mother earth and father universe, directly and instinctively experiencing these rhythms in dance, song and music. Today humanity has lost this childlike, innocent connection with the world, yet people continue to express themselves through the movements of dance, song and music. Most people are unaware of this primal relationship to the movement of the stars, the planets and the earth, because our evolutionary march towards individuated consciousness requires that we become emancipated from nature and the universe. Nevertheless we can all still feel that such rhythmic activities help to raise us out of our mundane or fragmented existence into a sense of deeper harmony.

Children still feel a natural affinity with dance, singing, listening to and playing music; especially during this period between the change of teeth, they have a deep longing to express themselves rhythmically through these forms of movement.

Although it is not the task of this book to penetrate the nature of dance, music and song in depth, they are so significant during this period of child development that we have to emphasize their essential nature and source. Reference is made to the outstanding contribution that Steiner has made to our understanding of these primeval movements and to the commentaries of Stefan Leber.[8]

Dance, Song and Music, and Eurythmy

We can regard dance as an expression of universal movement through the limbs. When this movement of the limbs flows on into the movements of voice and speech, we arrive at song. When the movement resonates within us we have the origin of music, the world of sound or tone, and we can then make use of a wide range of musical instruments to give this a specific outward expression.

When the movement of speech or tone finds expression through the instrument of the whole human body, in archetypal movements and gestures, we arrive at a new form of human expression which Steiner named *eurythmy*. Here the universal movements of the cosmos inherent in sound and speech find human expression again through archetypal movement and gesture.

Eurythmy was developed as an expressive movement art by Steiner in conjunction with Marie Sivers (later Steiner) in the early 20th century. It is currently used as a performance art, in education – especially in Waldorf schools – and as a movement therapy.[9]

There are many eurythmy ensembles throughout the world that perform locally and tour internationally. Pedagogical eurythmy is included in the Waldorf curriculum and taught in most Waldorf schools, as well as in many non-Waldorf preschool centres, kindergartens and schools. Its purpose is to consciously harmonize and strengthen the etheric body, to awaken the expressive capacities of children through movement, and to bring imagination and ideation into 'vital, moving forms' in physical space.

Therapeutic eurythmy is practised by trained therapeutic eurythmists, often on the advice of a medical practitioner, to support somatic and psychological imbalances and to strengthen the organism's capacity to heal itself.[10] This subject will be dealt with in greater detail in Part 3.

Eurythmy is also used in many social contexts, including workplaces and prisons, to reinvigorate individuals and their social relationships.[11]

Soul Transformation

Let us now accompany the child's journey from the psychological aspect as his soul awakens further.

Whereas in the first seven years the life of will dominated the soul, in the second seven-year cycle the life of feeling is evolving and developing, and characterizes the nature of the child throughout this period.

Feeling

The feeling life of the young schoolchild is awakening from its unconscious working in the bodily realm to become active as more independent and free soul activity. Feelings swing backwards and forwards between happiness and sadness, confidence and doubt, fear and bravado. Thandi loves things – her clothes, food, games, people – and then she hates them; her best friend today is her enemy tomorrow. Our feelings connect us to the most intimate and personal part of our being. What is it that we experience when we open our hearts to a young, trusting child and something like a warm breath of soul seems to flow out from us towards the child? What is it that draws into our inner depths when we disappoint this child and feel ashamed at failing him?

Feelings are a breathing process in the life of the soul.

Recall a happy moment: try to focus on this feeling experience before it provokes a thought or induces an urge to do something. It rests within you in present time, like an inner sensation which is dreamlike, pictorial in nature. It does not take much to go beyond the feeling and do something with it, for feeling is like will held back. Sense how a happy feeling affects the body as an inner sensation: gesture it and observe the expansive nature of your body language. Contrast this with the memory of feeling a sad time, sensing how this changes and moves your body. Gesture this likewise and notice how your body contracts. There are many feelings such as joy, love, warmth, kindness, empathy, courage, confidence, trust, hope, gentleness or sensitivity which expand the soul like an outbreath; other feelings such as sorrow, hate, fear, coldness, cruelty, guilt, shame, anxiety, doubt, mistrust or disappointment contract the soul like an inbreath. There are some feelings such as joy and sorrow that are entirely personal and untouched by other functions of the soul; these remain in the realm of pure feeling. Other feelings are tinged by sense and will activities such as pleasure and disgust; and we may call these sympathies and antipathies. In the former we breathe out a part of ourselves, going outwards in sympathy towards the world like the altruist who is always giving something of himself to others; in the latter we breathe inwards in antipathy against the world, like the egotist who is always taking something of the world for himself. We all do both all the time of course, and 'egotist' or 'altruist' are not intended as value judgments in this context.

When we experience the expansive nature of sympathy feelings, we can find its connection to the expansive nature of the blood circulation and the latter's extension into the metabolic system; it is as if we breathe outwards in sympathy and wish to do something with it, and in doing so move towards the pole of will. When we enter into the contracting nature of antipathy feelings, we can discover their relationship with the contracting nature of the breathing system and the latter's extension into the neuro-sensory system; it is then like breathing in and moving towards the pole of thinking.

Thus breathing is the instrument of the feeling soul.

Maria loved to read fairy tales when she started school. She seemed to live into every character; she cringed and seemed to hold her breath when the wicked queen imprisoned her step-daughter; and visibly breathed a sigh of relief when the prince rescued her from the prison castle. She thrived on all the action, the good and the bad. Puppet shows in the first years of school were a great source of fun and pleasure. Later she listened to the Harry Potter books with bated breathe and the fullest engagement.

Adam in his junior school years was very conscious of his skinny body; he was often anxious and withdrawn, living a secret life to which no one had access.

Thandi was teased for her short, tomboy hairstyle. She felt hurt by these children and reacted with anger and aggression. When punished by her teachers she felt deeply aggrieved.

The child is learning to experience himself in the world of feeling, now in sympathy, now in antipathy. He needs to get to know what it is like to feel shame and sadness, remorse and hurt just as much as he needs to experience pride, satisfaction and happiness. He is exercising and learning to consolidate his rhythmic system and feeling life so that a healthy balance can be created between thinking and will.

The Roadmap

As this middle period of childhood unfolds, a road map outlining the three sub-stages of the journey can help to highlight the essential elements of this epoch.

Seventh to Ninth Year

Can you recall your early school years, the school grounds, the classroom, your first teachers and classmates? Memory pictures of different clarity, suspended in time like a dream in motion, may rise up from a hidden depth when you choose to remember them. What experiences came to your conscious awareness at that time as your soul life was beginning to awaken?

This first phase of middle childhood has its own distinct character and is quite different from the years that follow. These are generally happy, vibrant and energetic years, innocent and uncritical; the child is opening himself to the outside world but is still very dependent on his caregivers for support and protection. He is generally relatively easy to manage, works harmoniously and productively within his group and will often take up community activities or household chores with enthusiasm. It is convenient and easy to assume, now that the child has moved on from being a little child in nursery school and has entered 'big school', eager to learn and willing to help, that he sees the world quite similarly to the way in which an adult views life. Indeed, a modern trend pursued today by the media, politics, commerce and education is to regard the young child as a small adult at an ever earlier age.

Nothing could be further from the truth, nor more harmful to the healthy development of body and soul. Over-intellectual education at this stage will lead to a premature awakening of certain soul functions, a crippling of other faculties, a weakening of life forces and a premature hardening and ageing of the body in later life.

The Swiss psychologist and educationist Piaget concluded that '. . . the thought of younger children is qualitatively different from that of older ones' and that it was essential 'to discover the different methods of thinking used by children of various ages.'[12] The young child experiences the world through an expanded imaginative consciousness. This is a natural and valuable endowment and requires no training to develop. Unfortunately, the ideas and attitudes prevalent in our civilization do not recognize this vital attribute in children and instead feed the child with fixed and ready-made images that damage and inhibit his emerging soul faculties. Martin Large describes how the electronic media, whose fixed images limit the child's fertile imagination, undermine creativity and intellectual development.[13]

In the natural course of development, imaginative pictorial thinking will gradually give way to ordinary intellectual thinking, and the more active and vibrant the imagination has been, the more mobile and creative thinking will become. Therefore the child should be allowed to live undisturbed in his peaceful and dreamlike world of pictorial imagination as long as possible. Abstract and intellectual thinking forces the child to separate himself prematurely from the world and is likely to lead to lazy, weak, static and limited thinking.

With his change of teeth, Adam has actively begun to form his own mental pictures, independent of his sense impressions. On his sixth birthday as he was going to sleep, he casually observed:

> I can see in my mind my new shiny bicycle that I will ride up the mountain, to the sea and everywhere. I feel so excited I can hardly wait to go there!

The will, so dominant in early childhood is carried over into the activity of thinking, but one that is pictorial in nature and imbued with feeling and creative imagination. Such thinking is empowered with living forces for, as we have suggested, these are the same forces that were previously responsible for organic growth and development. Adam no longer needs to see in front of him his shiny red bicycle to evoke his imagination; he can create for himself a memory picture of his bicycle and an imaginative picture of the mountain and sea, a rich, self-contained magical world of moving images and intense feelings. His imagination continues with the following scenario:

> I feel so happy, strong and proud riding up the mountain, but will I be safe all on my own? I know what, I will find an older

friend to go with me. He will look after me. It will be such fun
and we shall take a picnic of juice, sweets and fruit. Maybe I'll
take my dog along . . .

Adam feels secure in this thinking-feeling dream world; in the safe
confines of his own citadel he can fashion and create an imaginative
world that is as real, or even more real, than the other world outside,
and rehearse for the life that awaits him there.

Nothing of this vibrant inner world is visible externally, and if
we are not actively listening for it we can be completely unaware
of its existence and miss a great deal of what is happening inside
the child. We will then tend to relate to the child on the basis of
our own experience as an adult living in the objective world, as
an individual quite separate from everything and everyone. The
modern world also reinforces this perception by giving grown-up,
streetwise children a veneer of adulthood through exposing them to
technology, the media and computerized information long before
they are psychologically ready for it.

I don't believe in that fairytale stuff, I like ninjas, batman . . .
Yet, tell a seven- or eight-year-old child an authentic fairytale, or
let him watch an animated puppet show, and see how quickly the
modern, grown-up façade falls away to reveal a soul hungry for real
imaginative pictures. The child up to the ninth year still feels very
much part of this world. Although he can experience himself as a
separate individual, he cannot yet differentiate himself imaginatively
from the outside world. He experiences impressions in a pictorial
form of imagination and fantasy that connects him directly with the
surrounding world.

At this age he is still devoted to the world of the senses in a
religious kind of way, absorbing impressions and inwardly imitating
them as a natural activity of will. But as feeling life begins to unfold,
this need to imitate the world transforms into a longing for people
from whom he can learn about the world. He will open himself in
devotional reverence to individuals who can tell him about the world
in stories, anecdotes, and images related not in a prosaic, abstract
way but poetically and with imagination.

This is an age where adult authority has its absolutely appropriate
place. Mother and father can become unquestioned authority figures:

My mum is the best mum in the world and my father knows everything.
The child has an insatiable curiosity to learn about the world, is
interested in numbers and letters, wants to read and write but can at
this stage only learn about certain things through a knowledgeable
authority. Thus the teacher assumes a central role of authority in the
child's life, invested with the task of guiding his quest for knowledge
in a rhythmic, health-giving way. The teacher of young children has
an enormous responsibility in nurturing and protecting the child's
imaginative and rhythmic life.

Waldorf Education

An education that is based on an understanding of child development
must take into account the child's soul development at every stage.
One such educational system is the previously mentioned Waldorf
method developed by Steiner and practised in several thousand
Waldorf Schools and kindergartens in sixty different countries. The
Waldorf teacher is trained to understand and respect the unfolding
psycho-spiritual development of every pupil, and endeavours to
meet these needs in every lesson.

Few people who hear about the way these lessons are crafted
and spontaneously evolved are not moved by the truth and beauty
that lives in this method of teaching. The task of this life-based
education is to create healthy balanced children in body, soul and
spirit who will be fully equipped to meet the serious challenges of
a modern society hell-bent on destroying itself through egotism
and ignorance. In a civilization such as children find themselves
today, education will need to be therapeutic in nature, for every
year teachers find that a greater proportion of their students have
physical or psychological problems. Part 2 will highlight these
modern illnesses and dysfunctions in childhood. In Part 3, relevant
therapeutic modalities will be described and an attempt will be
made to highlight the therapeutic nature of the Waldorf educational
system. It would go too far here to describe the curriculum in detail.
There are many excellent books such as *The Recovery of Man in
Childhood* by A.C. Harwood that give a fine overview of Waldorf
teaching.[14]

Between the seventh and the ninth year, then, the child wishes to experience the world in pictures, in the form of rhythm and beat, musically, poetically and artistically, because this is his very nature: he lives and thinks in feeling embodied in pictures, in rhythms, in music and in a world full of living beauty and aesthetics. He therefore has the right to an education that can bring the world to him in this form. An education based on a real insight into the young school child will therefore offer all the raw material of learning in a pictorial, artistic and musical form. These are the years when fairytales, fables, legends, myths and magical realms should form the very core of the child's education.

Stories

Where do stories arise? All stories, whether they be tales, legends, myths, sagas or other narratives – arise out of the human soul and give voice to what is living as pictures and experience in a human being. The great stories that have been carried down first as an oral tradition and later written down, emerged out of the soul life and imagination of people who had deep insight into human nature. The world and the creatures contained in it belong to the human condition. Children from an early age long for the images that express the archetypes that are living in them.

When introduced at the right time, around the age of six, fairytales perfectly match the child's growing consciousness. Folklore tales are a treasure house of truth and morality that can enrich the soul of the growing child for years to come. Their archetypal imagery awakens the living archetypes with which the child is still closely connected, strengthening all aspects of his growing soul functions: his imagination, thinking, feeling and will. They build confidence and inner security by bringing the power and truth of his inner world into everyday life. Later in life, in recalling such stories, individuals can better understand their own personal development, and find in them metaphors for overcoming obstacles and finding inner fulfilment.

In past times, ordinary folk were often unable to think in an abstract fashion: they thought more in pictures, as the preschooler and early school learner does today. The folk legends gave them perennial wisdom and morality in imaginative, archetypal form. Tribal elders still pass on such knowledge, in a similar form, in modern tribal societies today.

Ken Wilbur refers to a 'magical' period in the evolution of mankind when the common folk believed that invisible forces directly intervened in their daily life.[15] We have vestiges of this in common superstitions about lucky charms, Friday the thirteenth and sayings like 'touch wood'. Young children who are recapitulating this consciousness, are mesmerized by magic, naively trusting that what they perceive is real: the egg literally materializes out of the palm of the magician's hand.

The mythical era then followed, when mythical images and symbols were taken as tangible realities: thunder was the displeasure of the gods and Jupiter was the God king who sat on his throne in Olympus. Preschool and early school learners possess a similar naïve mythical awareness which can be positively used to instill good morals, for instance:

Do to others what you would like them to do to you.

In older fairytales, in particular, we find an ancient primeval knowledge of the human body, soul and spirit, of the cosmos and of nature, hidden in the artistry of imaginative pictures. For instance, the beautiful princess represents the human soul, the handsome prince embodies the human spirit, the closed room at the top of the tower is the brain where the princess must spin the golden threads of her hair – that is, spin her thoughts as she develops her conscious thinking.

The folktales collected and recorded by Brothers Grimm and many others from various nations are ideal material for the first year school year (age 6–7).[16] The Waldorf curriculum for the first class uses fairytales as the prime educational resource: archetypal pictures for letters, songs, plays, and for counting and arithmetic.

In the second year of school (age 7–8), the child will be developmentally ready for fables and legends, for as he descends into his earthly body he will want a more human element in stories. In these tales he will meet pictures of animals which personify the virtues and vices of the human soul, and will hear legends of wise men or saints who can tame and master the elements and wild animals.[17]

The fables reflect a stage in the consciousness of humanity when the animal kingdom was regarded as embodying qualities of the human soul: kingly leadership and courage in the lion, crafty intelligence in the fox, contemplative wisdom in the owl, and loyal servitude in the donkey. The saints legends speak of the wisdom and power of the human spirit to overcome adversity. Fables and legends are a natural transition to lead the child from the world of archetypes to an experience of soul-spiritual qualities in the human being and his relationship to nature. They provide easy access to wise moral and social principles that can help children through difficult life situations. In Part 3 we will explore how stories and plays can be used as powerful therapeutic interventions.

Stories depicting the earthward journey of mankind away from paradise are appropriate for the class three child (age 8–9). Epic pictures from the Old Testament are a perfect parallel to the journey through which he himself is now passing. The grandeur of stories about the creation of the world, of Adam and Eve leaving paradise because they ate from the Tree of Life, of Noah who saves the animals by leading them one by one into his ark, of Jacob and his coat of many colours, of David with his psalms, songs and melodious lyre, and of Joshua whose trumpet-call destroys the enemy walls, all help the child discover the awe and beauty of creation, and help engender reverence for the human being's task on earth.

In the following year, the difficult watershed at age 9–10, when the child frequently loses his former natural trust in life and feels cut off from his secure spiritual origins, the ancient myths of different nations can be presented to the child. The Norse legend of Baldur and Loki, for instance, take the child imaginatively through the development of cultures and the battle between good and evil, giving him strength and courage to face the difficulties of this increasingly earthly world.[18]

In the following year the mythologies of ancient cultures such as India, Persia, Babylonia, Egypt, Greece and Africa mirror the expanding, but also ever more earthly consciousness that arises in the soul of the growing child.

As puberty draws close, the child can identify strongly with the stories of the Romans who conquered the world, creating the Roman Empire that brought to humanity an earth-bound thinking, epitomized in Roman Law, engineering and the construction of roads.

The chronicle of stories fills many books, some of which are referenced in the notes to this chapter. For more on storytelling at different ages, I recommend the popular book by Nancy Mellon.[19]

From the Tenth to the Twelfth Year

The tenth year, roughly the central year of childhood, lies at the midpoint of this middle period of seven years. It is frequently a very difficult year in the child's life. Every experienced teacher knows that this year of school is more difficult than previous years. The harmonious, integrated class community can suddenly become disruptive and disunited. Many of the children in the class become more moody, critical and uncooperative. I can recall that my older child was inconsolable on his ninth birthday because he felt he was going to die while my younger child during the same year was terrified that her parents would die. This is the year when a child feels cut off from the protection given him by his secure inner imaginative world, facing the harsh reality of the material world with all the raw vulnerability of his heightened feelings.

Do you remember how this year was for you?

Recall first how you feel when you are frightened or insecure about something. You will probably feel small and vulnerable, as if something big and threatening is pressing in on you. By exercising our 'experience awareness' we can have a vivid experience of the tenth year of life.[20] We may also recall the experiences of the nine-year-old child in Chapter three.

Many children at this age suddenly become fearful of the dark, shy and timid, sensitive to discord, more conscious of tragedy and death, and at the same time more critical and cynical. Unquestioning love and trust for the adult is often replaced by doubt, mistrust and criticism. Children become bored easily, more moody and fussy. It is as if they have fallen out of paradise, cut off from a divine world of living imaginative pictures, and cast into a lonely, harsh world where their feelings are no longer wrapped safely in their former life of imagination.

Feelings have become more objective, and because the child now observes the world more strongly through his feelings, he begins to judge and criticize the world. The defiance and oppositional nature of this year mirrors the terrible twos and threes, only here it is the feelings rather than the will that create separation from the world. For the second time the child becomes conscious of himself as separate from the world; but now he awakens to himself in his feelings, seven years later, as a recapitulation of the will-driven I awakening that took place in the third year.

> I no longer feel safe inside and the world outside is scary; I thought my mother and father were wise and strong but now I know that they too are less than perfect. I am not sure I can trust them fully and I have forgotten the place of trust I came from. I dearly hope that they have something in which they can trust and believe.

This can be a time of great inner pain and sorrow, and it is important that the caring adults can recognize what is happening and support and encourage the child through his experience. It will greatly help the child to know that the adults he no longer wholeheartedly trusts as his higher authority themselves recognize a higher authority, in God, in some kind of divinity, in themselves or in high ethical values.

At the same time as the child becomes aware of himself as separate from the world, he can awaken to the natural world around him with wonder and amazement, beginning to perceive and think about it as a separate reality. Nature is still vibrant and alive for children between the age of nine and twelve. Previously they merged with the world; now they feel themselves, still, at the centre of the universe, but a part of them seems cut off from it.

Nature should therefore be presented to the child in all its beauty and diversity in a direct and living way, with the human being always the central focus and summation of all things. A mechanical, inanimate construct of the world is an untruth for a child of this age. Gardening, farming, bread-making, weaving, home-building, animal studies and mythology provide the right raw material for the ten-year-old child.

By the age of **eleven** the child feels more strongly connected with the earth because his soul and spirit are more connected with the body. His life forces have fully penetrated the rhythmic activities of breath and pulse more fully, and health and harmony is at its height. Children of this age carry themselves with the grace and beauty of young gods and goddesses. They probably experience the world much as an ancient Greek experienced life, who was still connected to the living forces of the world but had made the transition from the picture consciousness of the ancient Egyptian to an intellectual consciousness that gave birth to a new epoch. This may explain why children of this age are fascinated by Greek history and mythology.

Pubescence – Twelve to Puberty

This phase leading up to puberty is characterized by phenomena that once again allow us to witness the working of invisible forces. The sudden growth in the hands, feet and lower jaw that results in the adolescent's often awkward and clumsy movements reveals the life forces that take hold of the limbs at their extremities. The natural rhythm and beauty of the middle phase disappears. The ungainly movements, however active and mobile they are, now seem to be increasingly taken over by the physical laws of mechanics and levers characteristic of the bony system.

The hard, mineralized skeleton is an expression in us of the dead, inanimate and mechanical world of cause and effect. As they engage with this world, the life forces allow the child for the first time to experience this reality and to distinguish consciously a dead from a living world. This is therefore the time when education should introduce the dead mineral world of geology and mineralogy, working always from the whole to the part. For there is a profound difference whether a child first learns about the mountain ranges that are made up of, for instance, granite and limestone, and then comes to quartz and calcium crystal formations, or the other way round. First comes heaven, then the earth, first the embryonic sheaths, then the embryo, first the blood is formed, then the heart. This way of seeing the world leads to an imaginative, creative way of viewing things whereas the opposite, the whole derived from the parts, leads to a reductionist or atomistic conception of the world.

Thus the child's new inner sense and awareness of the mechanical nature of the skeletal system, makes it possible for him now to understand the reality of cause and effect. We can therefore introduce the child at this time to the world of causality, as expressed in nature, science and history.

With the surge in limb growth we can also witness the will swelling in various directions. At the physical level comes the desire for more strenuous physical activity – for joining sports clubs, martial arts classes, bike riding and jogging; and the dance parties begin. This is also when children typically engage most in fighting, innocently or criminally, and when gangs become attractive. If we are to counteract this, we need first to understand why the child at this age gravitates in this direction.

Psychologically, the teenager often becomes more aggressive and assertive, which will naturally depend a great deal on the child's temperament; boys are frequently more outwardly aggressive, competitive and energetic, playing adventure games and seeking daring undertakings such as bungee-jumping, or even engaging in vandalism. Girls are usually more inward, becoming interested in their bodies, in clothes and fashions; they may become socially exclusive, moody, oppositional, and possibly sharp-tongued and verbally cruel to their classmates. We must realize that all these changes in behaviour are a natural and normal process of deeper engagement with their own bodies and the surrounding world and the first attempts to the establishing of an identity.

The will is directed towards conquering the world and this includes conquering the body. For many urban children this is the time for their first body-piercings and tattoos, for cell phones, music players and computerized games. Many children at this age gain a sense of power and control with electronic information and communication. Instead of old-fashioned gangs and outdoor activities, many city teenagers now spend long periods of their free time engaged in organized group-computer games and computer chat sites.

The need to experience one's own power and test this against the world marks this as the beginning of an exploration into new territory; without guiding and protective boundaries this can lead the teenager into dangerous places. These are young warriors who are coming to meet the earthly world in a new way. They are highly energized and hungry for new experiences; their feeling life is intense, and desire has begun to awaken in their bodies. This is all essential, as a teenager who doesn't pass through this difficult phase will find it harder to be or know himself later.

There are many children who feel the new challenges of life intensely but do not have the will to engage either with their own bodies or the surrounding world. These are the children who, instead, withdraw from life. They gravitate to addictive activities and substances through which they can escape from the world.

At this age, teenagers have little life experience and their judgement is not yet developed. Pre-puberty and the threshold of puberty are therefore one of the most vulnerable and high-risk periods of childhood, when children are extremely susceptible to peer pressures and to sensational, commercial or exploitative influences. This brings its own unique crises and challenges as the liberated soul awakens through the force of desire, need for movement, desire to know and a deep longing for love and acceptance. The child may walk a fine line between excessive sexuality, addictive behaviour, striving for power or oversensitivity, withdrawal and depression.

Can you remember this period in your life?

Probably most children try some relatively innocent exploit during this time. I recall borrowing my parent's car and going for a spin around the block with my small sister in the front seat and nearly knocking down a cyclist on the way; I tried out my father's pistol by firing it into the compost heap and I smoked my first cigarette. Many teenagers explore a variety of drugs; some even become addicted – heroin users typically start in their teens. The power-hungry youth seeks drugs such as amphetamines and cocaine, the escapist youth use substances such as cannabis, LSD and heroin. Unhappy youths lacking basic needs such as love, warmth, parental interest and protection can very easily become hooked into many harmful pursuits aside from substance abuse, such as media and cyber addictions, pornography, violence, sexual deviancy, delinquency, gangsterism and others. Children who develop solid foundations in earlier childhood through supportive and caring home environments and a balanced early education, will be far less prone to these excesses.

Unfortunately we are seeing an exponential growth in deviant behaviour in teenagers who either seek to express their vulnerability and insecurity in power-seeking pursuits or by escaping from life in a variety of ways. Part 2 will examine these issues in greater depth.

This untamed exuberance of youth needs to be carefully watched and channelled into healthy activities: there is no better time for a father to take on this challenge by engaging with a teenager in physical activities of his choice. Adventure holidays, organized youth groups, camps and sporting activities of any kind are highly appropriate pursuits during this period.

Horse riding is an especially valuable extramural activity, especially for young girls who taste the first experience of love through bonding with their horse: a teenager can match his strength against the natural power of the horse and learn to cultivate an intimate relationship with another living being.

In the **twelfth year**, the life forces begin to penetrate the muscular system. They first engage in skeletal extremities, then in the muscles and progressively the rest of the skeletal system. Resulting physiological and psychological changes make it possible for the child to relate naturally to the historical experience of the conquering Romans, who engaged robustly with the world in a way similar to that of the child at this age; like the Romans he has his own mind, begins to form his own ideas and wishes to apply them directly to action; he will be drawn to the scientific discoveries and inventions of modern life and the geometrical forms inherent in all living objects. This is an age when learning the art of accurate observation will give children a sense of security in their own, individual and incipient intellectual capacities; but as far as possible this should still be embedded in a holistic sensibility in which art and science can be experienced as one.

During the **thirteenth** year the teenager acquires a new interest in his body and is looking at the world in a new way. This is therefore the right time to teach him the details of human physiology, the mechanics of the human skeleton, hygiene and the topic of sexuality. As the soul awakens to the body in a new way, it will experience itself sexually for the first time; a clear preference emerges for one's own sex. This is usually a normal unisexual orientation devoid of sexual interest. However, according to Kinsey, many prepubertal boys have had some exploratory genital experience with a male partner which does not develop further.

The incidence of homosexuality in men and women is between 1 and 3 percent, and most recall the onset of romantic and erotic attractions for same sex partners only during early adolescence.[21]

Prior to this period, boys and girls mixed fairly freely, whereas now a clear separation develops between the sexes. Boys think girls are inferior creatures, while girls find boys stupid. They both become more self-conscious of their bodies and more secretive about bodily changes. Girls start to mature physically and sexually earlier than boys – between twelve and fourteen – and appear to go through this growth process in a different way from boys. Their physical and emotional tolerance is stretched more than boys: they tire more easily, frequently become anaemic and very moody. This phase seems to coincide with the developing female hormones and sexual organs, and usually passes once menstruation occurs. Boys on the other hand generally mature a year later, have no lack of vitality, generally seek outer action and fall over their own feet in their need to expend energy.

One can literally see boys falling into matter, into the heaviness of their limbs, the growth of their sexual organs and larynx (voice box) and above all in the lowering of the voice. Steiner coined the word 'Erdenreife' which in German means 'earthly maturity', a word that neatly characterizes the stage in a young person's journey when the birth of the soul or astral body takes place.

This phase was described in Chapter four as a culmination of approximately fourteen years of soul activity, during which the soul body works its way systematically down through the threefold organism. During the first seven years it takes hold of the sensory system, developing the soul functions of sense perception and the lower will functions (drives, desires). In the second seven years, the soul body becomes active in the rhythmic processes where feeling life is developed.

While the etheric body partly withdraws from the body (and becomes to some extent free from it at the change of teeth) the soul body is gradually being drawn inwards during this time. Now at the end of this cycle and at the onset of the third seven-year period, it enters the limbs, metabolism and sexual arena, thereby opening up a heightened sentient and sexual awareness; at the same time it enters the nervous system, creating the freedom for the soul function of intellectual thinking to be born. These connections will become clear in the next chapter. Only once the soul body has been completely drawn in, fully penetrating the body, does it come to its full activity when adulthood arrives.

At the age of **thirteen** we may notice a striking change in character, characterized by the teenager fluctuating between outer worldly activities and the seclusion of his inner life.

> Thandi has been busy all week with her new school projects, actively and excitedly researching on the internet, spending hours glued to the telephone speaking to various friends. Then suddenly she has days when she is moody and withdrawn and apparently uninterested in her school work or her social life. She has become more reflective and at times just needs to be on her own. She is more sensitive and easily embarrassed, especially if one draws attention to her bodily development. Her menstruation has recently begun and she has to deal with all its mystery and all the practical issues surrounding it.
>
> Bulani likewise is having to face the overwhelming power of his emerging sexual arousal. It is of great importance to show respect and understanding for this new state of sensitivity.

From now on the development of the soul body occurs in a way that is open to the outside world, just as the physical body at birth continues its development outside the maternal body. Before we conclude this phase of the soul's development and move forward into the next phase, it will be helpful to explore the nature of the soul life and the astral body in more detail.

Soul life – Astral Body*

In earlier chapters we spoke of both the 'soul' and the 'astral body', and they might easily be construed as being one and the same. In anthroposophical and other spiritually-orientated circles there is, in fact, a certain confusion about these two concepts, and an attempt will therefore be made to clarify them.

---

* In anthroposophical literature the astral body is also referred to as the soul body or sentient body

Our experiential research has shown us that our human nature is constituted of three distinct aspects: body, soul and spirit. The soul mediates between the body that is oriented towards the physical, earthly domain, and the spirit that comes from and is directed towards spiritual dimensions.

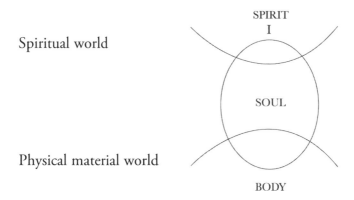

The body provides the foundation for the soul to reside within it; and in turn the latter creates the foundation for the spirit to dwell within it.

The soul or psyche is the generic term to characterize the inner reality that we *create for ourselves* as our own inner world and experience. It is a force that awakens consciousness and awareness out of a state of sleeping unconsciousness. In our journey through childhood we became aware of different aspects of our soul experience: we are most awake in thinking, and reflection and sensing; are partially conscious in a dreamlike condition in our feelings; and are most unconscious in a sleeping state in our will experience.

In our exploration of the journey towards adulthood, we have been following the development of soul life as it interacts with the development of the body. To begin with we allowed ourselves to contemplate the possibility that the astral body is drawn towards the I and spirit germ, anticipating the moment of conception. When the latter occurs, the spirit germ unites with the physical germ, thus initiating embryonic development. The I and astral body complex draws the etheric body into it and these three supersensible sheaths hover around the growing embryo, awaiting the formation of the three embryonic sheaths; then, at approximately day seventeen, they enter the earthly realm for the first time through their respective embryonic sheaths, and remain in this gestational phase until their respective births.

Over the next fourteen to fifteen years, the astral body gradually penetrates the child's physical and etheric body, working on the construction, functionality and maintenance of the internal organs. We saw that the soul life develops in the first seven years through the activities of will and sensing, in the second seven years through the life of feeling, and in the third seven-year cycle through the activities of thinking.

The soul's life now evolves to the extent that the I is active within it, for as the I itself connects with the complex developmental processes of the body, it begins to bring about specific developmental modifications in this soul life.

The **astral body** is the innate power in animals and humans that awakens consciousness of outer impressions while the object is present and disappears again when it is absent. It is a soul force that is not yet influenced by the activity of the I. Thus, the awareness of a fly landing on the skin, or a pleasurable taste in the mouth, arise out of the activity of the astral body; it is responsible for all sense perceptions, sensations, drives, desires, pain and pleasure.

This level of consciousness is the highest level of awareness in animals, and provides for all bodily functions connected with survival and preservation of the species, such as nutrition, protection and reproduction. Soul life here is primarily directed towards serving bodily functions. It does not sustain conscious awareness when the object is no longer present.

But when the activity of the I is brought to bear on the awareness of the object, when it is taken up by the I and made into its own possession, an independent soul life arises whereby consciousness can become permanent.

Maria grew up with a cuddly, soft, warm teddy bear. In her first two years she loved to cuddle it whenever it was in her presence. Her astral body provided the awareness when she perceived the object. It was only in her third year that she would go and look for it when she wanted to cuddle it. This became possible because her soul life enabled her to form a mental picture of the teddy bear whenever she wished. She feels a warm sensation and pleasurable feelings when she thinks about it and she goes to find her 'teddy'.

It is important to realize that these inner experiences may all take place without the presence of the teddy bear. The soul life that sustains all activities at this level of I-awareness has evolved beyond the astral body. Steiner designated this as **sentient soul**. Contained within it are the activities of sensation, the wide range of feeling experience that oscillates between sympathy and antipathy, the will activities such as drives, cravings, desires, passions, as well as the thinking activities connected with forming concepts and mental pictures and naming things.[22]

The soul body and the sentient soul are very closely connected. The soul body creates conscious awareness of the world, the sentient soul gives permanence to this experience. Their intimacy can be pictured in the close affinity that exists between the sword and its sheath, or between the wax and the wax mould.

What is also not generally realized, and which we have alluded to before, is that the 'soul body' is the *finer part of the etheric body* that opens itself through the sense organs towards the outer world'.[23] As such it belongs to the bodily nature of the human being, to the substance of the wax or the vitality of the sword. The sentient soul however is of a different nature: it consists of soul substance which is as different from the bodily substance as dreaming is from deep sleep. As the sheath of the sword holds and contains the potential power of the sword, so soul life contains, dampens down and holds back the vigorous life of the etheric body.

Balance Between Body and Soul

We saw previously that life and vitality diminish as consciousness develops and increases. In the human being it is necessary for the power of life to be contained, at all levels and at all times, by the power of consciousness. We thus see that from the earliest stages of child development, the developmental life-stream of growth is countered by the developmental consciousness stream of soul activities. From one point of view, the healthy development of a child can be seen in a balanced relationship between these two developmental streams.

Numerous examples could be given to illustrate what happens when this relationship is disturbed: A sentient soul that awakens more slowly will result in more primitive and animal-like responses, as seen in intellectual impairment in brain-damaged or Down's syndrome children; on the other hand, a sentient soul that awakens too quickly will lead to precociousness in children and frequently to inhibited physical growth and development.[24]

Lievegoed points out that the child's first soul structure is a provisional one, formed by the environment, through family life, school, society and culture, giving rise to a transitional sentient and intellectual soul.[25] Only later on, in adulthood, will the I have the forces to modify the soul in full accord with the individuality. Between 21 and 28, the I focuses on the sentient soul: between 28 and 35 on the personal/intellectual or mind soul, and between 35 and 42 on the consciousness soul.

Temperament

This stage of the child's journey is not complete until we have met the **temperament** of the child, an extremely useful phenomenological tool for understanding and guiding children especially in the middle period of childhood. Like the constitution that expresses itself primarily in the child's physical appearance in the first seven years (see Chapter seven), the temperament can also tell anyone with a little insight into it a great deal about the child's inner nature. Whereas the constitution tells us much about the physical body, the temperaments inform us more about the way in which the life processes manifest in the body and the soul life.[26] Maria's inner disposition makes itself known the moment she enters the surgery by her light tripping gait, blonde hair, blue eyes and flighty, talkative manner; in comparison, Adam's heavy walk, stooping body and silent demeanour speak of an introverted nature. If we want to get the best out of each child, we will need to understand their different natures and manage them accordingly.

What is it in these two children that determines their very different outward bodily appearance as well as their inner dispositions?

The Four Elements Again

In Chapter three we explored four principal biological systems that constitute the physical and functional body and were able to make some connection to the four primary elements that govern the world of nature and substance. We saw that all the solid material components of the body, such as bones, cartilage and firm tissues, are formed into a biological system that we called earthly because it is connected with the earth element that brings form and structure to matter; the fluid system made up of all fluidic substances like blood and lymph, belongs to the watery element that connects substances and brings them into flow; all the airy substances such as oxygen, carbon dioxide and nitrogen are organized into a gaseous system that obviously has a relationship with the airy element, giving substances mobility and dispersion; and the warmth system consisting of fine variations in degrees of warmth is clearly connected with the fire element that transforms substance and generates energy. We can easily enter the nature of these four elements because they exist within our bodies: we can visualize, sense, feel and gesture the solid element and thereby connect ourselves with its essential nature; we can likewise intuit the other elements.

We also found a relationship between these four elements and the four principal members of the human constitution. The earthly element with its tendency to structure and form clearly underlies the physical body; its main representative system is the skeletal system. The watery element provides the means by which the life body can carry out its life processes; these express themselves physically in the glandular system. The airy element is the medium through which the soul or psyche can engage in the physical world; this aspect of the human finds its physical expression in the nervous system. The warmth element is the only milieu in which the human I can exist in the earthly realm; the blood is the physical bearer and expression of the I. Through experiential awareness, we can find in a similar manner, a connection to the four principle members of the human constitution.

When we now enter empathically into the way in which Adam lives in his body, it is not too difficult to feel the earthly element and the physical body weighing heavily inside him. Likewise, Maria lives in her body in a way similar to that in which the air wafts through her and where her soul life is dominant. In studying children in this way, especially in the years between seven and fourteen, we shall find that they can be grouped into four main types which by tradition have been called the four temperaments.[27]

These were known to Hippocrates, the Greek physician today regarded as the father of modern medicine. In his view the four temperaments were determined by the specific relationship between the four humours – which in our terminology would equate with the four elements – and the four members of the human constitution that work through them. Hippocrates regarded the melancholic person as carrying too much black bile – equivalent in our terms to an excess of the earthly element working through the physical body; the phlegmatic type had a predominance of phlegm which we would equate with an excess of the water element and a pronounced action of the etheric body; the sanguine type had excess blood corresponding to the air element working through an overactive astral body; the choleric type carried an excess of yellow bile that equates to the warmth element working actively through a powerful I.

We can thus regard the child's temperament as an expression of the interaction of these four elemental human forces as they affect the child's body and soul nature. It is not difficult to see how the temperament offers an effective means of moving from symptom to cause, from outer phenomenon to inner causality.

The Bridge Between Heredity and Individuality

The temperament also brings together and makes visible the two streams working through the life of the child, which reveal themselves outwardly in developmental phenomena. In the physical and life bodies of the child, the stream of heredity is acting – specifically through the family line, and through humanity in general in racial and national characteristics. The human genome that maps out the genetic makeup of the individual child has a powerful influence on physical and physiological characteristics. This stream meets the stream of individuality that works through astral body and I in their gradual descent into the earthly world: this is a flow of human life and destiny that develops from the individual's innermost nature, bringing innate capacities and predispositions that are unique for his particular life journey.

These two streams blend together, interacting and colouring each other in the way that blue and yellow merge to create green. The temperament is the mediating link that connects heredity with individuality, allowing the individual child to colour or adapt the characteristics inherited from his parents and their forefathers. It lies in the intermediate region between body and soul, namely, in the sphere of the etheric body.

It takes the best part of seven years for the transformative life forces to work on the model inherited from parents. This is the reason why the temperament only becomes visible after the age of seven years, once the physical constitution described in Chapter seven has matured. By the age of ten the permanent temperament has emerged, but it will still undergo modifications in the third seven-year period.

It is usual for one element to become more dominant than the others, and we can train ourselves to observe these one-sided tendencies in body shape or function, or in the soul expression of the child.

Since we all have a temperament, or more accurately a mixture of temperaments, one of which is usually predominant, the best place to study them is to start with oneself and to observe the way one's body and soul life express themselves in everyday life. We can do this in the way illustrated above, by connecting ourselves experientially to the four elements and the four members of our constitution. The other way is to enter empathically into the child's experience in the manner described in Chapter two. There are a number of excellent books for those readers who wish to explore the topic of the temperaments in greater depth.[28] Below we will briefly outline their different characteristics.

Melancholic Temperament

We can experience the earthly heaviness of Adam's disposition, at the age of 9 or 10, in his thin, tall and drooping body which he seems to drag around with effort, in his downward glance and dull, sad, inwardly focused eyes. This physical heaviness becomes an inner obstacle against which he constantly has to fight, leading to sadness, gloominess and inner soul pain. Because he is always struggling he becomes self-involved, self-conscious and introverted; more than other types he tends to be negative, over-sensitive, over-anxious, critical of himself and others, serious-minded, unsociable, inflexible, demanding, egotistic and to have an imperious sense of entitlement. At the same time he often lacks self-confidence, feels he is not good enough and will often take the blame for things because he feels he deserves to be punished. His cry is often:

Life is so difficult and no one understands me!

Yet, he can also be gentle, kind, helpful and sympathetic, intensely loyal and deeply reflective. He has a tenacious will that penetrates things deeply.

In working positively with the temperaments the cardinal rule is: Work with them, not against them.

Adam needs to feel that we understand how hard life is for him; but life has to go on and there are many people who suffer like him. Empathetic support and firm guidance are the key concepts in helping the melancholic. Thus encouragement, firm boundaries, routines, good planning, openness and honesty help to allay the melancholic's fears and doubts. A range of therapeutic actions can divert his subjective pain to the objective suffering in the world, giving him the feeling that he can do something to alleviate it. These include: caring for the pains and problems of others (pets, siblings, friends), biographies and stories depicting struggle, and cultivating a caring attitude to others.

Sanguine Temperament

In many ways the melancholic is the very opposite of the sanguine. The former is weighed down by the heaviness of earth while the latter is uplifted by the lightness of air. Maria's slender and mobile body shows this lightness flitting nervously around the surgery as her sparkling blue eyes absorb all impressions, and her bubbly light-hearted conversation directly communicates her inner disposition. Because she lives so strongly in her sentient nature and the outer world of sense impressions, she is constantly flitting from one perception, image, desire, idea, person, activity, fashion, etc. to the next. She is therefore changeable, sensitive, flexible, temperamental, superficial, capricious, inconsistent, unpredictable, unreliable, forgetful, impulsive, volatile, scattered and opportunistic. She is always living in the new moment, on the periphery of things and cannot easily hold her centre for any length of time. Maria tells me:

> I always want to do exciting and interesting things otherwise I get bored or irritated.

Her charming manner is very lovable and persuasive and she is well-liked for her optimism, humour, compassion, versatility, positivity and fun-loving nature. Her weak will always lets her down.

We work with what Maria is, not what she is not, very gently steering her towards what she is lacking. Her butterfly nature will best be handled with loving, kind, gentle firmness, never harshly or with irritation. Warmth, encouragement and fun-loving (rather than over-serious) patience work best. If one can awaken love in her, astonishing changes can occur. She will always wish to please someone whom she feels understands her.

She needs to be kept busy by providing a variety of interesting activities for short periods, then removing them so that she does not get bored but will wish to do them again and again. She will gradually learn to complete tasks and to do them well, all of which will strengthen her will. However, helping her to find one special interest that can be sustained can produce miracles in moulding or shaping her temperament. Drama can also be very helpful because she enjoys drama, and the playing of roles that ground her can give her the experience she needs to direct her will accordingly.

Phlegmatic Temperament

Bulani gives one the impression that he is completely at ease within himself. He is a heavily built corpulent child with dull, expressionless features who shuffles in an unhurried manner into my office and parks himself in the most comfortable chair. After a few minutes he calmly takes out a sandwich and proceeds to eat it. He is strongly influenced by his biological functions and the over-prevalent watery element which enhances metabolic processes at the cost of neuro-sensory function. Thus, his glands and digestive functions are usually very active, but he finds it difficult to develop an active thought life.

Let me eat my food and watch the world go by

is his unspoken credo. His biological need for inner comfort and harmony determines every aspect of his disposition and he avoids everything that will disturb his inner wellbeing. He therefore prefers order and routines and dislikes pressure or challenges of any kind. He is undemanding, unassertive, reserved, modest and always cautious, preferring to follow rather than lead.

He chooses the safety of his own self and is asleep to the greater world outside. He lacks imagination and creativity and the will to extend himself beyond his personal comfort zone. He enjoys and excels in eating, sleeping, routine activities and tasks that require little effort. His inertia then disappears and he can be meticulous, dutiful, trustworthy and helpful.

Bulani can best be helped to take an interest in the world if we encourage him to follow by example and praise his achievement. He should be exposed without fuss to the varied interests of other children of like age as often as possible. Giving him things to do that are entirely uninteresting or boring may kindle in him a desire to do more interesting things. His steady, consistent presence may have a stabilizing and calming influence in a group and one can draw on this positive quality to arouse his engagement.

A great deal of patience and creativity are needed for phlegmatic children.

Choleric Temperament

The choleric is the polar opposite to the phlegmatic. The former is impelled by his tempestuous will, while the latter, like a flow of water, always seeks the easiest terrain – of personal ease and comfort.

Thandi informed me from the very first consultation what kind of person she was. She stood in front of her mother, facing me squarely, a small, stocky self-assured nine-year-old, dark hair and jet black eyes flaming angrily telling me that:

I did not want to come here today, she dragged me along!

I could feel the huge amount of power and warmth concentrated in her body and her will, driving her to assert herself in all circumstances. The choleric child is imbued with the power of the warmth element and a strong pulsating blood system that gives him the strength to act. He often has so much power that he feels congested and can at times explode violently.

This power makes him feel self-important, superior, over-confident and convinced he is right. Opposition to his will brings out his defiance, aggression, arrogance, wilfulness and violent temper. He can be highly critical, intolerant, domineering and intractable. When he is given his way he is a natural leader, organizing and directing things skilfully and with innovation. He needs to be the best and to be recognized as such. Then he reveals his tenacity, courage and resilience. He hates being thwarted.

The best personality to balance a choleric nature is someone who at all times is worthy of his respect and whom he regards as an authority. One should never show nervousness in his presence nor allow oneself to be intimidated by him, nor criticize or ask a choleric to apologize. Difficult situations should always be dealt with later when the storm has abated. He always needs to feel appreciated and indispensable. Obstacles continuously placed in the way allow this temperament to work itself out in overcoming the obstacle; he learns to do battle with the objective world, and if the latter proves stronger he gains respect for a higher power.

	Melancholic **Earthly heaviness/** **dominant physical body,** suffering and egotistic, self-centred, depth, introversion, strong will, strong thinking **Empathetic support/firm** **guidance/ helping others**	
Phlegmatic **Watery inner comfort/** **dominant etheric body,** apathy and inertia, intro- version, weak will, weak reactivity **Patient, creative support** **through example**		*Choleric* **Fiery will, powerful** **activity, dominant I** **nature,** strong will, strong reactivity,extroversion **Authoritative calmness/** **appreciation/ create** **obstacles/**
	Sanguine **Airy lightness/dominant** **astral body** flightiness, peripheral, superficial, weak will, strong sensing, extroversion **Kind, gentle, loving** **firmness/awaken love/** **one special interest**	

Four Cardinal Organs

The four principle members of the general human constitution[†] – the physical body, etheric body, astral body and I – engage in the human organism through the medium of their respective elements. The life body, for instance, requires the medium of fluids to manifest its activities. These members also require principle organs as instruments

---

[†] (as distinct from the morphological or physical constitution of the first 7-year period)

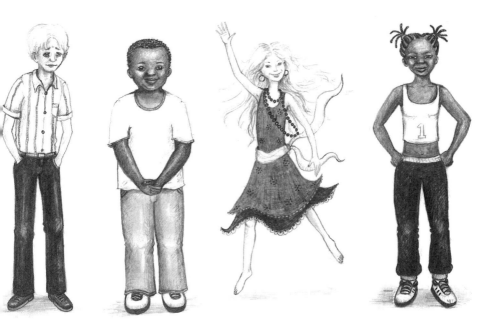

From left to right: Adam (melancholic), Bulani (phlegmatic), Maria (sanguine), Thandi (choleric).

for their specific functions. These organ systems have a structure and function that specifically serve what created them.[29] Thus, the activity of each principle results in an organized functional sphere which has its structural centre in four principle inner organ systems, each with a connection to one of the four elements. These are the **lung**, **liver**, **kidney** and **heart**. Husemann and Wolff describe them as the 'physical regions of receptivity for specific effects of the members of the human being, which work into the organs structuring them, forming substance and directing the elements.'[30] The sphere of functional activity of each organ system extends beyond the finite boundaries of the particular organ. For example, the metabolic functions of synthesis and breakdown of substance in the liver continue in each and every cell.

In studying the temperament of a child, we will invariably find that a dominant organ system corresponds to the over-riding temperament (remembering of course that we usually have an interaction of several temperaments, with one chiefly dominant). Thus the melancholic temperament has a dominant **lung system**;

the phlegmatic temperament has a strong **liver system**; the sanguine temperament has an energetic **kidney system**; and the choleric temperament has a powerful **heart system.**

Insight into these four organ systems can be helpful in forming a clearer picture of the child's overall constitution. The liver for instance is the organ system that governs the watery organism, and understanding its nature will help us to understand why Bulani has such a water-related constitution. This is of particular relevance in understanding and managing pathological disturbances of all kinds, when one organ system becomes over-dominant.[31] For this reason, a comprehensive study of them will be undertaken in Part 2.

Core Picture and Care of Middle Childhood

- Rhythm is the essential feature of this epoch, making it the healthiest and for some the most beautiful period of childhood. It is the time when free rhythmical movement is the natural inclination. It is also the time when we learn to breathe in a healthily regular way.
- Between the age of seven and fourteen the life forces of growth and the soul forces of awakening converge in the rhythmic system. This results in the development and consolidation of, on the one hand, all rhythmic activities, and on the other of all qualities of feeling and imagination.
- The feeling life becomes dominant and passionate, swinging continually between the in-breath of sympathy and the out-breath of antipathy.
- The three phases of this period again mirror the entire journey of childhood and have their own special character:
  - In the first phase the child expresses his feeling life through exuberant and imaginative rhythmical activities, active social interchange and a devotional, uncritical acceptance and need for authority
  - The middle phase is a time of uncertainty and deep feeling where the thirst for knowledge leads to doubt, fear and questioning of adults' authority and knowledge

- In the final phase leading up to puberty, feeling life is experienced in the birth of intellectual thinking, in forming judgements and opinions, strong criticism and defiance. This can only take place when the astral body comes to birth at puberty and enables the child to attain a second level of independence.
- The temperament becomes visible only once the inherited body has been transformed by the child's individual nature after the change of teeth.

By using empathy to enter into the core nature of the child at every stage of his development, we can know intuitively what the child needs for his healthy development.

- Since rhythm is the clarion call of this age one should seek every opportunity to encourage and stimulate rhythmical activities relating to the natural rhythms of the day, week, year and season. Regular times for meals, for work, play, rest and sleep give stability and security. At this age the child has a natural inclination and talent as a dancer, artist and musician. Musical instruments that have a close connection to the breath, such as recorder and flute are especially appropriate for this epoch.
- Ideally every child should have the opportunity to attend a junior school that draws on an understanding of rhythmical activities, which is a fundamental principle of the Waldorf method of education.
- Every effort should be made to encourage the feeling life and imagination of the child, thereby enhancing his health and creativity in the greatest way imaginable. In contrast, all suppression of the imaginative or feeling life of the child should be avoided at all costs at all times. This is possibly the most damaging effect one can have on a child. Part 2 will attempt to show how harmful this is for the child's physical and psychological wellbeing.
- For as long as possible, wonder, awe and reverence should be cultivated artistically, aesthetically, religiously and through respect for people and life in general.

- The inevitable phase of insecurity requires sensitive understanding, encouragement and warm support.
- The critical and rebellious phase around the time of puberty needs to be understood objectively and impersonally as a natural and healthy separation from parents. The fragile independence that develops now needs constant supervision and support from a distance. The teenager wants to feel important and independent but needs to know his parents are there when he needs them.
- Empathetic listening and unconditional respect are the golden key to the heart of the teenager

I open my heart and lungs to the breathing life of feeling and am exhilarated and expanded by my newfound creativity. The sun, and nature, and all the wise people support me, and I trust them implicitly. But then a dark cloud crosses the sun, covers its light and makes me feel cold and afraid. I am in pain because I realize that the world is not always sunny. For the grown-ups the world is also sometimes cold and dark. Can I trust them to care for me? I discover I can think for myself, I can imagine whatever I desire and I can even act out my desires. I know I shall have to find my own truth and my own life and now is the time when I can rehearse in safety.

CHAPTER 9

The Youthful and Truthful Years

The Power of My Thinking and the Strength of My Limbs Impel me on My Search for the Spirit

With the onset of puberty, the enchanted dream life of childhood draws to an end and the stark reality of the material world comes to meet the child. Natural trust and innocent wonder are replaced by uncertainty and questioning. Reliance on authority must be dropped and even rejected in order for reliance on the self to emerge. Old values need to be superseded by new ones.

As the past resonates through his growing soul, we can sense Rajan's feeling of loss and sadness at leaving the warm- and light-filled kingdom that has held and served him faithfully all these years; now, as the future beckons, we can feel his trepidation in stepping out unequipped into an unfamiliar world, but also his exhilaration at the great challenges and adventures that lie ahead.

> If I am to find out who I am and what I am meant to do in life, I must leave the safety and familiarity of my previous life and enter these unknown and uncharted waters.

A new sense of self emerges through interaction with this opening world.

Saskia is discovering her developing body; her newfound sensuality is intimidating but alluring, her flowering sexuality is daunting and exciting. She is making her first acquaintance with older boys. At times she feels frightened and overwhelmed, at other times empowered and liberated.

The ever-expanding encounter with the realities of the world confronts the emerging self with its limitations, bringing with it a range of possible feelings and emotions: loneliness, despair, fear, doubt, shame and intense vulnerability can in a moment change to reactive anger, violence, or just as quickly flow into joy, ecstasy and bliss. These emotional challenges awaken the self's hidden potential, allowing new skills, hopes and passions to emerge.

As the soul awakens, the great polarity of antipathy and sympathy becomes more starkly visible. The soul fluctuates between a new-found cool, abstract thinking and the warmth of passionate feelings, stormy emotions and powerful impulses. Withdrawal and isolation alternate with socializing and the desire to travel; feelings of anxiety and self-doubt compete with boldness and daring. The need to belong will struggle with the need to be individual; and the quest for the ideal will clash with the right to rebel.

As she gradually gains independence, the adolescent progressively frees herself from her former support structures – parents, family, teachers, organizations – and opens up a new world of dependency – the peer group, friends, heroes and new activities. It is the age in which peer pressure plays a powerful role, friendships are born and broken, role models are sought and discarded, and new passions and interests develop.

Rajan experiences an exhilarating new sense of freedom and power as he discovers and explores his newfound independence and creativity.

In this period we see the blossoming and flowering of youth and the dramatic transition into manhood and womanhood. Rites of passage in different cultures – the Bar Mitzvah, confirmation, initiation rites and other ritual events – play an important part in this transformation process.

This is the age when the personality is born and where a troupe of characters explore the roles they will play on the stage of the soul: the narcissist, the proud, or doubtful, or anxious, or arrogant, or rebellious persona, and a host of others. We start to treat the adolescent as an equal, speak to her with new respect and even call on her superior expertise in specific areas of life.

Independent thinking and idealism dawns and develops, and this will lead to decisions and choices that will shape a person's destiny. In fact, as we will see, personal destiny begins at this age. Young people now often develop a very acute sense of justice and injustice, and become very vocal or headstrong in their views.

This youthful phase of development is closest to our adult consciousness and therefore usually most easily remembered. Our growing sense of self during this period allows us to recall the different phases of this time more accurately. Can you remember how your childhood ended, how you journeyed through puberty, your discoveries, adventures, difficulties and achievements? What was the nature of your changing relationship with parents and family members, your community of fellow adolescents and your interaction with school systems and teachers? What were the high points and low points of your secondary school years? End of school examinations and leaving school are memories one usually recalls. Do you remember the flavour of your thought life, your feelings and your actions as you prepared yourself for adulthood as a young man or woman? We can explore the burgeoning experience of the years of one's youth in the same way as suggested in previous chapters.[1]

> I recall a series of pictures from my youth: at 14 I am playing school rugby; I throw the ball to the next player down the line and he catches the ball. At that moment I sense a feeling of warmth pervading my whole body like a shaft of warm sunshine. Now I gesture how it feels and then stand aside and look at this picture. I see unfolding out of this picture a friendship with the player down the line that played an enormous role throughout my adolescent development. This friendship transformed my soul life into a vibrant experience rich in literature, art and new discoveries.

Three Divisions

Late childhood or adolescence spans a period of approximately seven years from puberty to adulthood. Like the previous two periods, it can also be divided into three phases which mirror the childhood journey at a third level of maturity, where the activity of **thinking** is now the dominant element. Once again the first third manifests a very active, will-based phase that mirrors the first seven-year cycle; the second third reflects an intense feeling phase that corresponds to the second seven-year cycle and the third division brings the power of thinking to full expression, highlighting the nature of the third seven-year cycle.

Puberty to early adolescence will phase	– teenager	– 14 to 16 years
Mid to late adolescence feeling phase	– adolescent	– 16 to 18 years
Youth and pre-adult thinking phase	– youth	– 18 to 21 years

Physical Development

The arrival of the physical body marks physical birth, and the change of teeth the birth of the etheric body; now we will view the various manifestations of puberty as marking the invisible birthing and unfolding of the astral body. With each birth we see the emergence of an incisive new era of childhood, which also manifests in physical changes.

As Rajan settles into puberty and adolescence, the proportions of his body become more balanced: his lower arms and legs lengthen so that he becomes more secure in his hands and feet; he grows rapidly out of his arm sleeves and trouser legs. Striking changes take place in his facial features as his personality begins to express itself more strongly: his cheeks fill out, his nose lengthens and his jaw and mouth become firmer and more assertive.

In the middle phase of adolescence growth favours the trunk region – which starts to grow longer and broader – and the physique starts to look more harmonious. The mature form of youth begins to emerge, with prominent shoulders appearing in boys, and broader hips and pelvis in girls.

Finally, in the last phase, the muscles and bones of the lower limbs expand to attain their full maturity.

We also witness active growth in other regions. The enlargement of the larynx and the lengthening of the vocal cords result in a lowering of the voice by an octave in boys and by one tone in girls. At the same time, striking bodily changes take place as sexual characteristics in both sexes develop further. This follows the development of kidneys and reproductive systems that comprise the urogenital system. We shall see that these are the principal organs involved in the adolescent's sentient life and sexuality.

Male and Female Distinctions

Puberty clearly demarcates the two sexes, and if we attend closely to the dynamic of this developmental process we discover striking differences in the whole growth process.

In the male, we find a force of growth pushing powerfully outwards and downwards to create a heavier constitution, a greater lowering of the voice, lower diaphragmatic breathing, the growth of the testes outside of the body cavity, and the sperm cells which are released from the body in seminal emission.

In the female, these growth forces retain their inner metabolic activity in close connection with the rhythmic system; they bring about the regular and rhythmic functions of ovulation and menstruation, internalized reproductive organs, egg cells that are released into the body cavity, rib-chest breathing and a lighter physical constitution.

Boys, as a result, are more physical and earthbound, and therefore connect more to earthly activities; they have to work through matter more deeply and therefore need longer to develop. Girls are more tuned to the cosmos because they live and develop more strongly through their soul life. They are more closely connected to their rhythmic life and therefore more active in their feelings, inner pictures and dream life.

Internally the secretion of male and female hormones in the form of the testosterone, oestrogen and progesterone are an hormonal expression of the 'inner and outer blossoming' and differentiation of the sexes that is so characteristic of puberty.

At puberty, mature ova and sperm cells begin to be produced by the reproductive organs, signaling the achievement of the ultimate physical human capacity to reproduce one's own kind.

Metabolic-Limb System

What are the forces that bring about these changes and that create such a distinct polarity between men and women?

We see from the physical changes that the etheric growth stream has reached the metabolic limb system after working through the neuro-sensory system in the first seven years and the rhythmic system in the second seven-year cycle. It also pushes its way from the metabolism into the limbs, working first into the muscular system and soon after into the skeletal system. The blood is the central component of the metabolic activity underpinning limb development. And the power that drives the blood is the force of the will.

It will therefore be helpful to further explore the consolidation of the metabolic-limb system during this phase of development.

The soul's will activity depends on a functional bodily system to carry this activity into the material, physical world. The systems that generate metabolism and movement best provide the material foundation for all will-based functions, enabling the human being to be active in the outer world.

We have seen that all will impulses such as drives or desires bring about bodily actions through movement of one kind or another, either via the internal processes of metabolism or externally via the motor system. Physical and chemical processes are maintained by the production of energy of various kinds that are generated by metabolic and motor systems. The metabolic-limb system functions like a dynamo generating warmth which provides the basis for energy and other forms of activity sustaining human life.

The word metabolism comes from the Greek *metabolé* meaning change; in German the word *Stoffwechsel*, which literally means change of matter, accurately describes the nature of metabolism. Substances are changed from one form into another and, in the process, a range of life functions come about that enable the will function of the soul to manifest in the material world. One can also characterize metabolism as 'movement of matter' since movement is an innate part of all metabolic-limb activities as well as essential for all change. Indeed, illness sets in when movement in the metabolism becomes too little or too much. Metabolic activity, and the will involved in it, is predominantly unconscious activity. We are completely unaware of what goes on inside our bodies when, for example, we open and close our hand. We are asleep to both the will activity that drives the action and the numerous physiological, biochemical, biomolecular and biophysical activities that occur in the nerves, senses, muscles, joints, blood and other tissue processes.

We can only experience the metabolic-limb system directly when we are fully involved in some activity; the moment we step outside the experience and observe what we were doing we disengage from metabolic experience and enter neuro-sensory experience. Let us for instance observe the process of eating some food: firstly we have the desire to eat something. We move towards, say, a piece of whole grain bread and notice our salivary glands beginning to secrete saliva; we reach out with our hand and place the solid bread in our mouth; we begin to chew the bread with active motion of jaw and tongue. (The moment we observe the activity we must realize we are no longer actually within metabolic activity itself but in nerve-sense activity, which can only describe the dead image of the living activity.) We notice that the bread has changed into a liquid form that becomes sweeter as we continue to chew it. This is because salivary enzymes convert the starch into sugar. We then swallow the liquefied bread, which disappears into our body.

Scientific research tells us exactly what happens next and we have to imagine observing the inner digestive process further: the bread made up mainly of carbohydrates, but also some proteins, fats, vitamins, trace elements and water, is broken down thoroughly and sequentially by the actions and secretions of a number of organs – stomach, gall bladder, pancreas and intestines – into the basic building blocks of food: carbohydrates become glucose, protein is converted into amino acids and fat is broken down into fatty acids, glycerides and phospholipids. These are substances, like the vitamins, minerals and trace elements, that are small enough to pass through the lining of the intestine. By the time the liquefied bread has reached the small intestine, it is completely changed from its original form. It will now become separated into a portion that is absorbed through the wall of the intestine and a portion that is excreted from the body by the large intestine.

The absorbed nutrients now go through further complex metabolic processes: most pass across the intestinal wall into the blood system – the portal system of veins – that transports them to the **liver**. The fatty acids go via the lymphatic system into the general blood circulation and find their way from there into the liver. Here we arrive at the centre of the metabolism where a wide range of biochemical activities process these components further, either into substances that are needed by the body or harmful substances that must be detoxified and eliminated. Glucose for example is converted into a sugar-storage form called glycogen which can be reconverted into glucose and carried to other cells according to the body's need for energy. Carbohydrates, proteins and fats in a form suitable for the human constitution are now built up anew. All these metabolic activities take place in minute liver cells, supported by a great variety of hormones, enzymes, vitamins and trace elements, and are then conveyed via blood, lymph, bile or tissue fluid to their next port of call.

Liver

What makes the *liver* the centre of metabolism? The metabolic-limb system as we have seen is the functional system for sustaining human life. When we examine the liver, we find that it is the central organ of the life body. The genius of language knows of these connections: the concept and the stem word for *life* is embodied in the word for *liver* in many languages: in German: *Leben – Leber*, in Afrikaans: *lewe – lewer*; in Russian, the word for liver is *pyetschen* which comes from *pyetsch* meaning the *stove* or *oven,* the heart and life of Russian culture; while in Italian, *fegato* derives from the word for *vegetable* – and it is true that plants express the nature of the life forces most completely.

All the life functions of the etheric body are strikingly represented by the hepatobiliary functions; its role in fat metabolism and the role of bile in fat digestion connect it to the warmth processes, since fat is the greatest source of warmth. The liver functions optimally at a temperature of 40 degrees Celsius. It has a central role in many nutritive and metabolic processes. Circulatory processes are fully represented by the intricate and unique anatomical arrangement of five circulatory systems: arterial, venous, portal venous, bile and lymph. As a major organ of detoxification and the immune system, it contributes significantly to maintenance processes. Through its assimilatory functions (building up and storage of substances such as sugar) and dissimilatory functions (the breaking down and secretion of substances such as sugar and bile) it is involved in glandular processes. The diurnal rhythm of assimilation (3pm–3am) and dissimilation (3am–3pm) expresses an archetypal day-night breathing process. Finally, the cellular growth and reproductive capacity of the liver is well known: it can regenerate even after seven-eights of the organ has been destroyed.

On the basis of this wealth of life processes, the liver can rightly claim its place as the centre of the metabolic system.

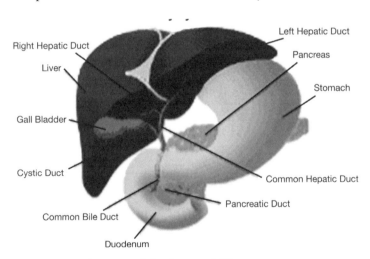

Right Hepatic Duct
Liver
Gall Bladder
Cystic Duct
Common Bile Duct
Duodenum
Left Hepatic Duct
Pancreas
Stomach
Common Hepatic Duct
Pancreatic Duct

Diagram of the hepato-biliary system

An essential aspect of metabolism therefore has to do with the building up of material substance in the human organism. The basic components of protein, fat, carbohydrates, vitamins, minerals and trace elements – products of human metabolic activity – give all tissues their structure. They also make up the cells which determine function, for instance the bone cells that regulate the breakdown and build-up of bone substance, or the blood cells which secrete protein-based antibodies. These products of metabolism thus provide the structural basis for all tissues and organs as well as all the thousands of substances needed to maintain the functions of the body. The tissues are the outcome of sustained metabolic activity, which must also ensure that these tissues are maintained with all their necessary nutrients and constantly built up throughout life.

For instance, the *long bones* are composed on the outside of a hard compact matrix consisting of organic substances, such as proteins and carbohydrates and inorganic elements like calcium, phosphates and other minerals. On the inside there is a cavity filled with soft pulpy *bone marrow* containing numerous blood cells, blood vessels, connective tissue and fat-rich cells. This is the site for the generation of all blood cells: the red blood cells which transport oxygen from the lungs to the tissues and carbon dioxide as toxic waste back to the lungs; the white blood cells which protect the body from alien, invasive and toxic agents; and the platelets which give form to the blood, preventing it from becoming too thin and stopping the blood from bleeding freely when the containing blood vessels are severed.

The **blood** is an 'organ' which belongs predominantly to the metabolic-limb system: it is in constant movement and as we saw is the primal force which moves the heart; its blood cells are being continuously generated at a very rapid rate and it is the carrier of all life processes to all the cells of the body. It carries life-giving nutrients, removes toxic waste, sustains warmth at an optimal body level of 36.5 to 37 degrees Celsius, and regulates the acid-alkaline balance at a very precise and constant level of pH 7.4. It is also, as we have seen, a healing and balancing force which constantly opposes illness.

The **muscles** too belong to the metabolic-limb system. They are the organs that move the body as a whole as well as all the inner organs that are in motion. Skeletal muscles contract and move the limbs under fine voluntary control; cardiac and smooth muscle contraction occurs without conscious thought and maintains the continuous movement of the heart and all other internally moving organs, as in peristalsis of the gastro-intestinal system, the urinary system, the male and female reproductive system, blood vessels, the movement of the diaphragm, the eyes muscles and the fine muscles of the hairs. The muscles store glucose and generate the energy required for movement. It is evident that the muscles carry out the intentions of the will which as we have seen work at unconscious, reflex and conscious levels. They are therefore organs which actively and powerfully serve the will of the growing and developing child.

Metabolism and Will

It will be evident from the above description of metabolism, where verbs – 'doing' words – characterize the process, as well as through directly experiencing its nature as movement, change and action, that the essential element of metabolism is activity. This is also the essential nature of the will.

Warmth is also an intrinsic part of metabolism. It is an element likewise essential for activity. Notice what happens to your body when you cool down. It slows down and becomes less active. If you become hypothermic, body activities reduce further and at the same time life processes become sluggish. When activity ceases, life too ceases. Thus living processes are also a central element of metabolism and therefore belong in the realm of etheric activity.

Since metabolic processes are always characterized by warmth, activity and living forces, we would expect every human cell in the body with a certain level of warmth to encompass a wide range of metabolic activities that are crucial for life. The cells specifically involved in metabolic activities will always manifest greater vitality, replicating and regenerating more rapidly and receiving a greater supply of blood.

There are a wide range of organs specifically designed to carry out metabolic functions.

- Digestive organs – stomach, small intestines, gall bladder, pancreas – involved in the break down and absorption of food nutrients.
- The liver is the central organ of metabolism responsible for the synthesis of the body's essential nutrients – carbohydrates, fats

and proteins – and their breakdown into component elements, glucose, fatty acids and amino acids, the basic building materials for cellular structure and function.

- Excretory organs, colon, kidneys, bladder, lungs, mucous glands, skin – eliminate toxic waste products. These systems eliminate substances that are no longer required, but also absorb products that are needed by the body; for instance, the lungs eliminate carbon dioxide but absorb oxygen; the kidneys eliminate ammonia and other harmful nitrogenous products but also absorb protein, sugar, water and minerals such as sodium and potassium.
- Secretory organs including hormonal glands, adrenal glands, pituitary gland – secrete substances internally that support metabolic activities.
- Reproductive organs – cell division, male and female procreative organs – are directed to the renewal and regeneration of the species.
- Motor organs, skeleton, muscles, joints, ligaments and tendons – enable the body to move around at will.
- The blood moves actively into every part of the human organism, transporting all the respiratory and metabolic products needed by the body, but also the toxic products for elimination by other organ systems.

In contrast to the organs of the neuro-sensory system which transmit information from the outside world inwards, bringing living and active sense impressions to rest so that they can be perceived and made conscious, the metabolic-limb system does the opposite: it brings the human being into the material world by means of warmth and life activities.

Kidney System

Before we explore the soul development of the adolescent, it will be useful to highlight the essential nature of the kidney system. This system is a picture of contrasts and as such tells us a great deal about awakening soul life during this stage of development. The kidneys have the physiological task of excreting unwanted metabolites from the body, but, equally importantly, of retaining and secreting back into the system substances that are needed by the body. Imagine you are observing the stream of fluid passing through the kidneys: you will see it retaining certain substances, and rejecting others. This polar activity of drawing substance towards it and pushing other substances away, is biologically the same activity as the soul function of sympathy and antipathy. We have seen this polarity as the central dynamic of the astral body.

In the morphological structure of the kidney we likewise observe striking contrasts, this time between round shapes and radial shapes:

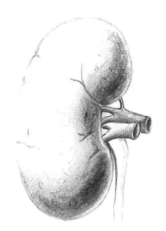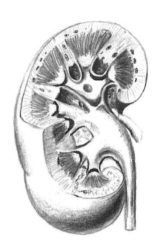

Diagram of Kidney

Attached to the upper pole of the kidneys is the adrenal gland which secretes the hormones cortisol and adrenalin. These are substances intimately connected with human survival.

Cortisol is produced by the peripheral section of the adrenal gland, the adrenal cortex, and has a great deal to do with life-sustaining metabolic functions, such as the production of glucose from protein and fats, protection against injury and the enhancement of healing. These are functions closely allied to the life processes. Like the reproductive hormones which are chemically quite similar to cortisol, we have here a substance that is innately constructive in its nature and that bears the imprint of the etheric body.

Adrenalin on the other hand is produced by the central layers of the adrenal gland, the adrenal medulla, which is closely linked to the action of the sympathetic nervous system. It produces wakefulness, excitement, constrictive action in tissues such as the muscles, blood vessels and glands, and breaks down metabolic substances such as glucose and fatty acids. Here we see a dynamic mediated by the nervous system, which breaks down substance in the service of higher consciousness.

In many respects cortisol and adrenalin are polar opposite substances.

It is important to remember that all soul activities simultaneously require the development of organs that serve as instruments for these functions; thus the metabolic organs that are growing and developing at this time provide the physical, etheric foundation for the soul's will-based activities.

Soul Development

During the first fourteen years, the astral body, contained in its parental sheath, passes through its embryonic and foetal phase of development. Although it is in gestation, it is nevertheless highly active. In the first period it was engaged in sense perception and will activities, in the second period in the development of feeling life. With the birth of the astral body, the soul life awakens on two opposite fronts at the same time. On the one hand it takes hold of the organs of the **urogenital system**, manifesting through emotional, sentient and sexual experience; on the other hand it penetrates the **nervous system**, enhancing alertness and the first experience of independent intellect and critical thinking. Thus, using these organ systems as the physical basis for its activities in the physical realm, the soul unfolds its rich range of capacities that will serve the individual throughout life.

The age of contrasts and polarities has begun. The adolescent swings between the hot, dynamic, passionate blood experience and the cool, quiet, critical nerve-based experience.

At this stage we can observe momentous displays of liberated soul life: powerful emotions awaken through the force of desire as well as through the welling up of feelings such as anger, hate, greed, shame and fear. These emotions are accompanied by the newly awakened phenomenon of movement, as manifest in the need to dance or the desire to travel.

The development of the limbs supports these actions and emotions. Alongside strong feelings, the power of fantasy and imagination grow as a flood of wish-filled mental pictures that anticipate the future. This may lead to the first real love for another person as well as the awakening of sexuality that brings with it all its anguish and ecstasy. On the other hand, the young individual may also feel as though she has been cast out into a hostile world, making her feel alone and exposed.

The feeling that 'no one understands me' expresses the mood of this time. The teenager may become oversensitive and afraid. She may withdraw into herself until she begins to take an interest in the threatening outside world and learns to engage with it; for at this age also, a desire for knowledge and the faculty of logical thinking and judgement begin to emerge. This protects a young person and awakens her interest in learning to master external challenges. However, if her education does not come to meet this need, she may become too self-involved. On the one hand she may fall into excessive sexuality or addictive behaviour, or on the other into a strong need for control and self assertion; this can find expression in a number of psychosocial aberrations such as eating disorders, substance abuse, behaviour disorders and violence in various forms, which will be explored in Part 2.

Thus as the astral body frees itself progressively from its organic activity into more independent life, the adolescent awakens to new experiences and is drawn out into the world. She finds herself on a voyage of discovery, learning and growing through her encounter with the world. New impressions lead to new perceptions and sensations; new desires come to meet the sense perceptions, clothing them with feeling content. On the one hand the soul is awakening in these powerful impulses of will. On the other, it awakens in thinking.

Let us now examine in a little more detail these manifestations of the newly-born soul as it grapples with a world of new experiences.

Desire

Rajan has been friendly with Saskia since junior school. After turning sixteen, he finds himself drawn to her in a different way. When he sees her these days, strong feelings rise up in his soul that move him to want to be with her.

As his awareness of the opposite sex expands, so strong desire and feelings are evoked that drive him to new encounters. Notice what happens when desire enters awareness; we feel impelled to seek out the object of our desire; when we meet it we want it even more intensely and feel happy when we have taken possession of it. Desire ends when these feelings have been satisfied. We may therefore conclude that desire is an impulse of the will at the level of the astral body which, as we have seen above, is active at this time in the maturation of the urogenital system.

Rudolf Treichler succinctly describes the nature of desire and the power it exerts in the adolescent years:

> Desire induces the liberated soul, which is searching for a new connection with the world, to encounter the world through the will. The encounter is experienced in the sensations that arise from this. Perceptions become internalized in the soul; the stilled desire connects itself in sympathy or antipathy with world content. Soul and world arrive at a new union. New desire driving towards new will, awakens in the newly experienced sensations and the striving to a new world encounter. The soul of the young person lives out of such experiences and encounters.[2]

Sensation

Rajan is aware of Saskia even when she is not present. He thinks about her a lot and recalls many mental pictures of past encounters with her. Feelings for her well up in him and his body tingles with delight when he focuses his attention on her.

It is essential to distinguish between sense perception and sensation. Rajan meets Saskia and perceives her directly only as long as she is in his sphere of experience; here sense perception is wholly dependent on the external world – the sense objects and the sensory apparatus. When Saskia departs, Rajan's immediate perception of her ceases, though he retains a memory of the sense perception.

Observe your own sensations and become aware that these are an internal experience no longer dependent on the external world. They arise through external sense impressions that continue to live on as an inner soul activity. Saskia has long gone, yet sensation remains inside Rajan. His interest in her takes hold of his sense impressions of her, arouses feelings of delight and joy, and calls forth mental pictures that live on in his memory. The sensations that he experiences come about through the confluence of desire, external sense impressions and his cognitive awareness of his encounter with Saskia.

Feeling – Sympathy and Antipathy

As Rajan explores his relationship with Saskia, a range of feelings and emotions surge up involuntarily in his soul. He feels full of joy, and at peace in her presence. When he is not with her he is depressed and restless. He longs for her and is impatient for his next encounter. When he sees her with other boys he is jealous and anxious and begins to doubt whether he is good enough for her. His feelings swing between sympathy towards the object of his desire – happiness, joy, love, warmth, patience, longing, hope – and antipathy that draw him away from the object – fear, impatience, jealousy, despair, doubt.

We have seen that feeling is an essential and constant element of soul life. We noted previously that some feelings, such as joy and sorrow, exist completely in present time and are untouched by other soul functions; thus we can call them pure feelings. Other feelings are coloured by desire, sense and will activities, and are connected in some way with past or future; these are the sympathies and antipathies. As we perceive things, we are constantly experiencing feelings of sympathy or antipathy that arise from the impulse of desire. If you follow the inner soul movement of desire that becomes feeling, you can see that feelings are modified desires and as such are closely connected to the life of will. They also make up the inner life of sensation.[3]

Emotions

> Saskia is not yet sure whether she wants to enter into a serious relationship with Rajan. She likes to be with him and feels very happy in his company, but also likes meeting other boys. Rajan cannot bear seeing her with other boys. He either becomes agitated and argumentative or completely despairing. These emotional responses cause Saskia a great deal of sadness.

Feelings need to be differentiated from emotions. Both are connected with the life of will and desire, but as the word infers, emotions carry within them a powerful element of movement. Recall getting angry or very sad – a powerful surge of feeling moves through the body. As the astral body is working its way through the organs of the limbs and the urogenital system, stimulating hormones such as testosterone and adrenalin, vigorous metabolic forces are unleashed in a soul-metamorphosed form. These take the form of desires that come to meet new sense experiences – often giving rise to explosive, passionate or impulsive feelings such as anger, shame, fear, doubt and despair. Movement is a characteristic of the astral body. The latter moves the metabolism physiologically in countless ways, and psychologically moves the soul to encounters with the world. The need for outward movement in the form of sport, dancing and travel is an expression of the emancipated life of soul.

Fantasy and Imagination

> Out of his strong feelings for Saskia, powerful fantasy pictures rise up in Rajan's mind. He imagines himself in a deeply committed relationship with her, enjoying her constant companionship and being sexually intimate with her.

If we have a fantasy, for instance of buying something that we are longing for, we will create pictures in our mind about the object of our desire; we make use of our memory as well our imagination to create the picture of what we wish to acquire. We have seen that our memory is a function of our life forces, while our creative will is connected with our soul life.

After puberty a new and rich life of imagination and fantasy begins. This new capacity comes about as the etheric life forces loosen themselves from the reproductive region in the same way as the forces of thinking freed themselves from the neuro-sensory system after the change of teeth. We may recall from a previous chapter how the natural imagination of the young child is drawn from the abundant creative forces of the etheric body. The astral body, that is also at this time beginning to free itself from the body, takes hold of the life forces liberated from their work in the reproductive region. The biological activity of procreation finds its parallel in the soul as fantasy, either as sexual ideation or artistic, creative imagination. Procreation may be regarded as creative fantasy made physical. This becomes possible at puberty when the astral body is born. We can therefore more readily understand the statement that 'real fantasy is essentially born for the first time with puberty'.[4]

Love

Rajan has fallen in love with Saskia. He passionately declares his love for her and she finally decides that she wants to be with him. He is ecstatically happy. This is his first love affair and it is an entirely new experience for him. His feelings of attraction have become transformed into a heightened experience. He also has some understanding of why he is in love with her.

What is the nature of this first love and where does it come from? Do you remember that feeling of falling in love that welled up in your soul like the rising sun at dawn warming the whole world? It was all-consuming but at the same time self-empowering. Where in our body do we store the living memory of this first love? Can we sense and feel where it resides? And can we find a way of expressing it?

With the birth of the astral body at puberty, soul forces are set free which provide the stage on which the drama of love can unfold: the liberated fantasy, the intensified feelings of sympathy and the awakening of independent thinking, all come together in the new experience of falling in love.

The first expression of love after puberty usually expresses itself in infatuation, admiration or adoration for a hero. We can see this in the adoring fans at rock concerts, the idolization of movie and sport stars but also in the possessive bonds that bind together friends. Parents who understand this phase will have patience with their teenage daughters who sit for hours on the telephone in secret, sharing about their current heart throbs; or with their sons who may be genuinely in love with the heroic qualities of another man but are not destined to become homosexual since the bisexual potential in adolescence is greater than in adult life.

Somewhat later the arrow of eros strikes the heart, filling the soul with needs which only the object of its love can satisfy. Something about this person of the opposite sex resonates with an ideal living deeply hidden in the soul, making it possible, for a short period, for this person to represent such perfection. Before the age of ten, the child has a natural love and trust for authority which is part of the cohesive nature of the will expressing itself in many different ways as the child grows and develops. We can feel that this idealized love of adolescence is a transformation of the former love for authority – which likewise lives as an ideal in the soul of the young child. It is a romantic love born from the highest ideals, as a glimpse of the perfection, which does not yet exist in the human soul. It is therefore destined to fall – as the phrase 'falling in love' suggests – leading to intense pain, bitter disappointment, a feeling of helplessness and a broken heart. If the adolescent can be helped to recognize the real source of this erotic love, she may discover a place in her soul that will never fail her.

The adolescent may also come to experience the love within friendship, which the Greek language calls *philia*; here there is less need for self-gratification and a genuine wish to help and support the other. One takes pleasure in the company of friends and partners, both of the same and the opposite sex, celebrating in their joys and achievements. This is a love free of sexuality, where the expectation of give-and-take creates a more peaceful and stable relationship. Friends can also of course fall in love with each other.

It is usually only with adult maturity that a true and selfless love may shine forth – one which makes the other person at least as important as oneself. This love, known to the ancient Greeks as *agape*, fully embraces the other person and places no restrictions or demands which would limit her freedom.

Sexuality

As their relationship grows both Rajan and Saskia experience a powerful desire to be sexually intimate with each other. Their need to explore this new experience is countered by the fears and guilt that their parents and society have instilled in them. Rajan is desperate to have his first full-on sexual experience, while Saskia wants to wait until she feels certain she is doing the right thing.

As a result of the powerful activity of the soul forces working into the urogenital system from puberty onwards, sexuality as a new impulse awakens in the body and soul life of the adolescent.

What is the nature of this powerful oceanic force that we encounter in our journey through puberty?

Do you remember your first awakening of sexuality? How do you feel about your own sexuality? Do you feel comfortable thinking about this question? It is not something which most people readily speak openly about. It is usually regarded as a very personal and intimate matter that does not need to be shared with other people. Many feel ashamed or embarrassed to speak about it and will also feel uncomfortable speaking about such matters with their children.

The sexual impulse is something very primal, touching the core of our being. It is therefore also an area of great vulnerability for most people, where body and soul meet in exquisite sensitivity. We will only allow the most trusted person to share the intense pleasure or pain that derives from this source.

If we consider that one in three girls and one in five boys suffer sexual abuse in one form or another worldwide, we can understand the shame, guilt and trauma that are often associated with sexuality, making it such a taboo subject. Indeed there is probably no aspect of the personality that is more repressed and less understood than that of sexuality. It is therefore a subject that deserves deeper consideration.

Sexuality can be considered on various levels.

At a *biological level* sexuality is connected with sexual identity and the drive towards procreation.

Sexual identity is the pattern of an individual's biological sexual characteristics: chromosomes, hormones, reproductive organs, external genitalia and secondary sexual characteristics. In the early stages of embryonic life, the embryo is anatomically female. Between the sixth week and third month, differentiation of the male takes place. At this physical and biological level of sexuality, bodily sensation is at its highest and there is probably no greater physical pleasure than the arousal of an erogenous area of the body.

At a *psychological level* sexuality has to do with all matters relating to one's sex or gender, for instance one's gender identity – namely one's sense of masculinity or femininity and one's relationship to the masculinity or femininity of someone else. We examined this in Chapter five. It also includes sexual activity, eroticism, affection and intimacy. Sexuality at this level opens up powerful psychological experiences, providing pleasure as well as pain; many of us will know that deep hurt and grief can be awakened by sexual experiences.

At a *spiritual level* I believe sexuality has something to do with the search for one's own opposite gender – in C.G. Jung's terminology, *animus* or *anima* – as the deeper search for wholeness and for pure love. Sexuality at this level transcends the body, opening the soul to a high peak of human experience where, as neither male nor female, one feels one or united with all things.

Bernard Lievegoed describes sexuality as a given force of nature that we have in common with animals and which we have not yet made human.[5] What does it become when we have fully humanized it? Does it become pure love? At this point in human evolution, love and sexuality are often poles apart. Love is expansive, warming, wants to open up and give to another (sympathy). Sexuality on the other hand embodies desire and need, closes the individual in on himself and wants to take something from the other to satisfy the desire. Once satisfied, the individual closes off from the other (antipathy), unless there is something else to keep the heart open.

In the human constitution sexuality is primarily driven by untamed desire within the astral body. This is the same driving force that exists in the animal kingdom. If sexuality is controlled only by the bodily nature of the will, namely by instinct, drive and desire, sexual activity will be self-centred and socially alienating, contrary to the act of loving.[6] If the self, using the higher aspects of the will (motivation, wish, intention and resolution) can guide sexuality through affection, tenderness and intimacy, it can open the soul to heightened, human experience.

The Development of Sexuality

A child discovers sexuality in infancy when, in the course of exploring the world, she discovers her genitals and may derive pleasure from playing with them. As we saw, gender identity and gender role are usually already present by the second or third year with the display of typical gender behaviour, for instance, identification and choice of toys. By school age the healthy, balanced child will have a stable identity as a boy or girl which remains throughout life. In early childhood there is no preference for same- or opposite-sex playmates, whereas in middle childhood children tend to prefer their own gender groups.

A conscious awareness of sexuality arises in the child's soul some time before puberty in one of the most dramatic events in human development, as the reproductive and sexual organs mature, body hair appears and the voice changes. The teenager becomes curious and interested in the changes that are taking place.

The onset of menstruation is a special and dramatic milestone in a girl's life, initiating the first experience of sexuality and the questions surrounding reproduction. This usually takes place before boys take an interest in sex – although commonly many boys become sexually aware through their first erection and experience of ejaculation or seminal emission (wet dream) during pubescence. During this period sexuality is strongly influenced by the biological processes taking place through the maturation of the reproductive organs as well as by sexually symbolic dreams.

Children frequently begin their sexual exploration through sexual games, where boys and girls undress and look at each other, children play-kiss each other, or, in more sexually conscious settings, give each other oral sex. Innocent interest may however begin much earlier on: I can remember contracting with my six-year-old girlfriend neighbour on the pavement corner to show her 'mine' if she would show me 'hers' – and after she had readily complied I mischievously ran away.

It is important how one deals with these innocent pastimes, since heavy-handed authoritarian responses may create self-repressive and devious reactions. Fortunately for most children most of these games are not discovered and most children grow out of them once their curiosity has been satisfied.

The Secular Trend

Puberty begins about two years earlier in girls than in boys and is occurring at an increasingly early age. Girls, especially, are developing at faster rates and reaching menarche at younger ages.

A major study covering 17,000 American girls indicated that the average age of menarche had fallen from 17 years (between the mid-19th and the mid-20th century) to 13 years; and that one in seven white girls were showing incipient sexual development by the age of 8. In African-American girls this same tendency was occurring as young as 7! By 12 years, 35 per cent of white girls and 62 per cent of black girls had begun to menstruate.[7] Similar studies in other countries indicate the same trend: that young girls around the world are developing earlier than previous generations.

This phenomenon, known as the *secular trend*, has become more prominent over the past fifty years and has been attributed to overweight, hormones and other chemicals in food, poor diets, socio-economic status, excessive physical exercise, better medical services, improved sanitation and health status.[8]

A study by Mattholius in 1977 attempted to investigate the influence of education on the onset of menarche, by choosing cohorts that excluded the above factors; 1175 girls from German Waldorf schools were compared with a similar number of girls from state schools. The average age of onset in the Waldorf girls was 13.25 years, statistically significant compared to 12.63 years in state schools. The latter average age was higher than the average age found in most other studies conducted in state schools.[9]

This trend also appears to be related to the degree to which the child wakes up to the world surrounding her, that is to say becomes *erdenreif* or 'earth-ready' in Steiner's phrase. Dreamier and less grounded children, and those who have been less exposed to sexually explicit movies, videos, rock music and an adult world, tend to have a more delayed onset of puberty.

Most research seems to indicate that the physical changes are accompanied by psychological changes, but there are divergent opinions as to whether the acceleration is positive or negative. Some authors concluded that accelerated development in young people makes them more awake, intelligent and intentional in their actions; most other authors found that earlier developers are generally more anxious, more inclined to conflict, more unstable and neurotic and less emotionally mature. With accelerated growth the development of qualities of heart and feeling, strong will and language abilities seem to be left behind.

One can expect the psychological effects of premature sexual development on the self-esteem and identity formation of teenagers to be significant.

Coping with the Changes

The pubescent child is acutely aware of the other sex. The differentiation of the sexes has taken place. As she searches for her own place in a much larger world, she may often seek out an older person of the same sex for guidance and friendship. During this time she will also tend to mix with same-gender companions. Girls will fluctuate more in their feeling life, either desperately needing to share their feelings with best friends or unable to express themselves other than in the safe world of their diaries. Gradually, biologically orientated sexuality will change into an erotic, intimacy-based sexuality. If this new relationship to sexuality does not occur, loneliness and alienation from the opposite sex may result.

Diaries may take the place of an understanding friend, and are a refuge and solace for the secret world of teenagers. Girls usually start diaries between the age of 12 and 13, boys a year later, and this may continue into late adolescence. This is often the time for romantically idealizing someone of the opposite sex from a distance, which may cause deep suffering and depression.

The extensive physical development that takes place during puberty creates a powerful awareness of sexuality that begins to shape interpersonal relationships. This is also the time when the teenager will discover her sexual orientation, recognizing her dominant sexual behaviour pattern and sexual preference for a person of the same or opposite sex or both. She will want to explore and gratify her sexual needs in a socially acceptable way so that it contributes to the development of her sexual identity.

Many adolescents will have isolated homosexual experiences because of the bisexual potential prevalent at this time. Such young people will often need reassurance that these are normal developmental experiences which do not indicate a dominant homosexual orientation. It is estimated that between 1 and 4 per cent of all adolescent boys and 0.5 to 2 per cent of adolescent girls have determined their homosexual orientation by this time. This is roughly the incidence in which established homosexuality occurs in adults (1 to 3 percent in men, 2 per cent in women). There are no adequate studies to show whether the sexual orientation of young people changes as they grow older. Adolescents who become aware of more permanent sexual predilections will frequently suffer great anguish in silence; there need to be avenues where these young people may receive counselling regarding all aspects of their sexual orientation.

There are a whole range of factors that will determine to what degree and in what way the adolescent relates to sexuality.[10]

- Age: older adolescents are generally more sexually active than younger adolescents.

- Gender: boys generally seem to be more sexually aggressive, become sexually active earlier than girls, masturbate more often, have more sexual partners and have intercourse more frequently. This may be biologically or sociologically determined.
- Family: dysfunctional family life, marital infidelity, absent parents, and parental attitudes to sexuality (either too liberal, or too repressed), lead to earlier and greater sexual activity.
- Socio-demographics: urban adolescents, especially those exposed to media technology, are generally more sexually active than rural teenagers.
- Socio-economic status: sexual activity seems to be more prevalent in lower socio-economic groups (overcrowding, lack of supervision, prostitution).
- Educational status: poor academic performance, early school leavers, limited opportunity generally leads to greater sexual activity.
- Culture: Eurocentric traditions have fostered an attitude of control and suppression of adolescent sexuality which has created a great deal of guilt and repression regarding sexuality; in contrast sexual exploration is encouraged in many traditional African cultures. Western European teenagers become sexually active earlier than American teenagers, who are active earlier than Arabic and Asiatic teenagers; black teenagers in Africa and USA are sexually active earlier than white peers. Since the early 1960s, sexual permissiveness has been encouraged by the student liberation movement in the western world, with effective contraception and medical advances in the treatment of sexually transmitted diseases. Each culture faces the challenge of channelling the sexual needs of adolescents in a healthy manner; physically it must strive to avoid illnesses (sexually transmissible illnesses, HIV/AIDS); psychologically it must seek to avoid excessive preoccupation with sex and interpersonal relationships that would interfere with education and social responsibilities (sexual aberrations, unwanted pregnancies, sex abuse, sexual exploitation).
- Personality factors: self-esteem, inner security and sociability especially in the face of peer group pressure will influence sexual

behaviour. For instance, self confidence will generally create more sexual opportunities than self-doubt and sexual daring may be a way of proving one's character and prowess in the group.

The awakening of sexuality plays itself out between the development of body and soul. There are also other developments which unfold purely in the realm of the soul itself.

Thinking

In Chapter six we traced the development of thinking in the early years of childhood. We saw that conscious thought processes are not yet possible in the first two years, and only arise once the soul activities of memory, speech and imagination are in place. Only then can thinking begin, as a uniquely human function, providing the child with the means to experience herself as a separate individual.

Up to the change of teeth thinking remains closely connected with the body, sense perception and will activity. For instance if you ask a young child to tell you about some object of nature, she will invariably relate it to herself or to what it does. Thus a tree is something *I climb* or that *makes a home for many creatures*. Such thinking is as much a part of the body as any other life function and may be called *body-* or *will-based thinking*.

With the change of teeth, we saw that a part of the etheric growth forces involved in organic function are released and provide the means for a new form of *pictorial thinking*. The child can now create her own inner world of thoughts that are independent of sense impressions; these are pictorial, highly imaginative and clothed in feelings. From the tenth year onwards, as the outer reality of life thrusts itself more into the child's inner imaginative sanctuary, picture thinking begins to be replaced by *intellectual thinking*. The age at which this begins and the extent to which it happens will be determined by the resilience of the child's creative imagination and the intellectualization of the environment in which she is immersed.

With the birth of the astral body at puberty, the soul stream of consciousness reaches into the nervous system – the instrument for thinking – thus setting in motion the development of intellectual thinking. The world horizons of the adolescent are expanding, her desire for knowledge and understanding of the mysteries of life are growing; and coming to meet these challenges is the unfolding of a new power of rational thinking.

The teenager begins to use her own power of judgement, form her own opinions, draw her own conclusions and make her own decisions. Her thoughts arise more and more from her own soul life and less from her bodily impulses, sensations and feelings. She discovers that she can acquire knowledge and express her own opinion, and begins no longer to be willing to accept information on authority alone. The search for truth can now begin in earnest since, through independent thinking, she can attain an inner sense for what is true. The adolescent will now orientate herself increasingly towards the future in her pursuit of the truth.

It was a great moment in Adam's life when he realized his capacity to form his own thoughts and make his own judgements. He steadily discovered his ability to join in a discussion, to voice his opinion strongly. His friends respected his viewpoint even though his detailed analysis of a subject was sometimes exasperating. They thought the way he formed his arguments and made his point was extremely clever. At times, however, he was highly critical and intolerant of other opinions. Adam's ability to think for himself opened up a great interest in learning about the world. He began to read avidly and seek information from many sources on subjects in which he was interested. He wanted to know why things are the way they are and how they work; he wanted to understand the laws that govern life and to explore causes and effects, intentions and goals. He discovered he could enrich his understanding through personal reflection, by asking questions, forming his own judgement and seeking answers that satisfied his sense for truth. He felt a deep sense of satisfaction when he was able to understand something by bringing certain ideas together.

Making the World Whole: Percept and Concept

In Chapter seven an attempt was made to show that an understanding of the world begins with thinking. When we look out into the world our attention is drawn first towards the sense-perceptible world. In a certain sense we are compelled to observe many different sense impressions. Yet until we begin to think, we do not acquire any real knowledge of what we have observed. Our observation invokes our thinking processes and this activity is directed towards the observed object.

Thinking enables us to recognize and name objects so that the world becomes known to us; through thinking we connect sense impressions and create new concepts that unite us with the world. Thinking also helps us to understand the world by breaking it down into parts and building it up again into wholeness. Finally thinking has the power to create new worlds and ideas and to set feelings and actions in motion.

All acts of knowing involve the confluence of perception and thinking. Were we only to perceive things the world would appear to be separate from or outside us; but the perception calls us to find its corresponding concept, and unity is created through our activity of thinking. The I confronts the world first through perceptions, and nature invites the I to take hold of it; but the I wishes to know what nature presents to it, and through its own inner power discovers the other part that bridges the divide, uniting us with nature.

The I has the task of reconciling the realm of perceptions – conditioned by space, time and our subjective organization – and the realm of concepts, thus creating a unified world in our consciousness.[11]

Conceptualizing

What then is a **concept**? We are forming them all the time but know as little about them as we know about our deep sleep. Our world of concepts is formed when, as little children, we confront the world of sense impressions and learn to know what things are. The single concept of tree will encompass every imaginable tree possible.

This concept has come about through the merging of many other concepts such as trunk, branches, leaves, etc.

It is a remarkable fact that despite all our differences, everyone of all ages, cultures, races and nationalities will agree that a tree is a tree. This is because the concept is innately bound up with the objects of the world. It must have an inherent connection with the essence of the object to enable the I to know the object and refer it back to the perception to which it belongs.

Mental Imaging

The universal nature of a concept may become individualized by the personal stamp we give to the object we perceive. If we think about the concept 'tree' we may discover an image of the tree in our mind, that invariably resembles a tree we have seen at some stage in our lives. These **mental pictures** are the after effects of perceptions that remain in our subconscious life. They live somewhere in our organization, popping up when something triggers them. We forget most of the mental images we form and cannot easily recall them.

Observe what happens to something you observed; you formed a mental picture of it, and then the mental picture became for a short while an inner perception, subsequently disappearing into the deep recesses of your subconscious. It is stored as we have seen in our etheric memory bank, where it appears to have an independent life of its own.

Children learn about the world in this way, through the concepts and mental pictures they constantly create.

Concluding and Deliberating

There are other elements connected with the activity of thinking that will help us to understand how children and adolescents experience the world.

An adolescent boy observes someone walking down the road, becomes locked into this perception, recognizes it and instantly **concludes** that it is a girl. He can only do this on the foundation laid by the concept and mental picture that he has already formed for himself.

Conclusions are the most conscious of thinking activities because through them we become conscious of what we perceive. Without the ability to draw conclusions about what we perceive, we could not communicate with each other: in everyday speech we are continually expressing conclusions to communicate our thinking and we are here using the term 'concluding' to refer to our cognitive wakeful recognition and statement of things as a matter of fact.

The boy concludes that it is a girl walking down the road without needing to consider this fact further. But he then has a desire to know more about the girl, so he looks more closely at her and *reflects* on different aspects of her nature. If he is to conclude whether she is pretty or not, he must use other capacities to draw this conclusion. He *deliberates* about the way she looks and out of this he draws the conclusion that the girl is pretty. He has made use of a different capacity of thinking which will expand his mental picture of her. This activity which weighs things up *before* coming to a conclusion is one I here call 'deliberating'.

The capacity of deliberation is awakened by an interest in the world which, as we have seen, can only occur when the soul begins its independent journey beyond the body after puberty. This capacity is an aesthetic, reflective quality of thinking, strongly connected with feelings and wishes.

Steiner stated that the three activities of thinking – forming concepts, deliberating and concluding – are connected with the three realms of the soul and spirit: **concepts** live in the unconscious sleeping life of the will, **deliberations** can only live as habits of judgement in the semi-conscious dreaming life of feelings and **conclusions** should really only exist in the fully conscious waking life of thinking.[12]

Between Description and Definition

If thinking is the starting point of all knowing, it is of vital importance to be aware how children and adolescents form their concepts, and to support the child in the development of her thinking. As they engage with the world, children are constantly forming new concepts, and these will have a powerful formative effect on their bodily and psychological constitutions throughout their lives.

Children who are fed definitions or ready-made 'facts' without thinking about them, and a view of the world that is fixed and rigid – who arrive too quickly at ready-made conclusions and make premature judgements, or are forced to memorize facts in a mechanical manner – develop fixed, immobile concepts which cause their bodies and souls to harden prematurely.

On the other hand, children who learn by hearing descriptions and characterizations of the world that always bear some relationship to the human being himself, who are encouraged to see whole pictures before they make conclusions, and to reflect empathically and carefully before they judge – and who are given information that stimulates their passion and interest – develop living, fluid concepts that keep their body and soul life in a supple and flexible condition throughout life.

In the next chapter we will attempt to shed light on the way in which concepts are imprinted into the human constitution, and to examine how they influence the health or ill health of the human being.

The Roadmap

We have travelled the broad landscape of development from puberty to adulthood. We will now trace each successive annual step of the journey and observe its salient features as a roadmap for our practical orientation and management of this phase of life.

Fourteen – Awakening Sexuality and the Birth of Destiny

The adolescent is beginning to come to terms with her new experiences. She has become accustomed to her rapidly changing physical form and can control her limbs better so that her movements are less awkward. Her altered bodily functions have become more familiar and less mysterious. Saskia no longer feels embarrassed when she mentions her periods and Rajan is far less conscious of his breaking voice. They have discovered their sexual identities and tentatively wish to explore their sexuality further. The world is no longer such a hostile place, because they feel less vulnerable.

They have discovered new capacities of observation, of feeling and of thinking, finding engagement, enjoyment and interaction with people and the world. They sense the beginning of a new-found power and freedom and feel more ready to meet the challenges of life because they feel somewhat more equipped and more resilient than before.

Rajan is no longer regarded as a child, is treated with more respect, is given more responsibilities and enters more consciously into the adult community. However, he seeks his support and refuge within his peer group or close friends, where he shares his intimate thoughts. It is here he discovers his confidence, his sense of new belonging, and his feeling of self-worth. The search for one's own identity and rightful place in the world also often starts here. If the adolescent cannot find her identity during this phase, she may be at risk either of becoming a follower of the herd or a social misfit. Yet even with a strong sense of self, of course, teenagers can still become social outcasts.

The Birth of Destiny

The child with the invisible shelter provided by parents and family has finally disappeared, and an individual who is striving to be free and independent steps forward into the adult world. It is a time of deep and essential truth in the destiny of the adolescent as her true individuality arises like a delicate butterfly emerging from its cocoon. At the same time one can sense her struggle to orientate herself between the various opposing forces that would drive her away from her own true course and the supportive forces that guide her forward towards her true mission in life.

Playing into this are the effects of the past – of parents and their forebears – that structure and shape the physical and life body and play into the temperament of the growing child. There are the powerful influences of the environment – working through the parental home, through language and traditions, through the school community and the larger society – that have imprinted their character into the memory substance of the life body and continue to work on the developing adolescent.

These influences are widely known and recognized. But there are other potential realities, of which mainstream materialistic thinking is unaware, or which are regarded as quaint, speculative and unscientific because they cannot be perceived or proven. Yet for some people these are no less real and have a right to be included in an overview such as this. Readers will of course make up their own minds about what they wish to believe. Such influences include:

- the effects of past lives influencing behaviour and actions
- the direct and continuous workings of benevolent spiritual beings that actively support human evolution
- the effects, likewise, of negative spiritual realities that work at hindering the advance of human striving for their own specific ends.

It is beyond the scope of this book to enter more fully into these forces here. Readers are referred to the appended notes and other references for a more detailed examination of this.[13] The important thing to realize is that at fourteen a young person for the first time becomes the stage and battlefield where this highly complex interweaving of forces begins to work.

The beginning of adolescence and the dawning of the intellect can itself indicate to us the kinds of educational subject matter appropriate for this age.[14]

Fifteen – The Search for Belonging

This is commonly a difficult year for many adolescents, both boys and girls. It is a period of renewed vulnerability brought about by the weight of new-found destiny to which the soul has still to become accustomed. At the same time there is a strong sense of the loss of home, the loosening of family ties coinciding with the unconscious sense of a lost spiritual home. Whereas, two years

before, the adolescent felt cast out of her protected haven, very lost
and confused and without inner bearings, she now feels the burden
of an imperfect world in which she has to find her way, and the
absence of support and protection that she can trust. This calls forth
a desperate longing to reclaim her lost home. The secret longing for
a hero or exemplar rises from this inner yearning of the heart and the
emergence of powerful feelings.

> Rajan befriended a creative writer two years his senior in the
> literary society at school. This was the poetry he wished he could
> write, the man he dreamed of becoming – handsome, confident,
> popular with girls; he looked to him for advice whenever
> possible.

Fifteen is the culminating age for idols in movies, rock music and
sport, cult heroes and older friends who are idolized, as well as
teachers and students in higher grades. I can remember having a
desperate crush on Dalene, a beautiful, lithe, olive-skinned girl
whom I followed around from a distance, never declaring my
adoration – to her or to any one else. It was my secret projection of
ideal love and perfection, in which I transferred divine qualities to a
poor, unsuspecting mortal.

Close friends talk to each other for hours on the telephone and
cling to each other for mutual support, drawing almost spiritual
sustenance from their fused identities. Activities and interests of
various kinds such as computer games, sports or hobbies, as well
as other more dangerous practices such as eating disorders, drug-
taking, sexual activities and different kinds of violence, can likewise
become all-consuming, with a compulsive, even fanatical need to
immerse oneself in it.

The search for what is missing in her life may drive the young
person to seek a false substitute which she finds in the 'perfect'
love or friend, in power or perfection, or in addictions of various
kinds. The spiritual, even religious nature of this age usually goes
unnoticed, but an awareness of it will help us to understand the
difficulties that young people undergo. This feeling of loss makes
them feel vulnerable and oversensitive. Naturally the intensity
of the experience will vary from one child to the next: she may

become moody and self-centred; or anxious and insecure. Deep down there is hope and trust, but at the same time also cynicism, mistrust and the need to reject. Longing and neediness may lead to disappointment and disillusion which in turn may lead to hurt or anger. The fifteen-year-old adolescent can become negative, defiant and rebellious, testing the patience of any parent or teacher. Quite often school performance also falls off.

Powerful contrasts between love and hate, joy and depression, and acceptance and rejection prevail at this age; also between holding onto the past and going forward into the future.

Rajan sometimes expresses himself in a hostile and aggressive manner while feeling terribly unsure of himself. There is little middle ground. The thirst for new meaning that drives him to new experiences and to explore uncharted territory, alternates with lying around bored and indifferent to the world. It is easy to interpret this slackness as laziness or sloppiness, but one should not forget the demands made on the growing body. This is the age when many adolescent girls suffer from iron loss causing fatigue, moodiness and even anaemia.

Thus we see an inner struggle between an insecure youth who still needs support and guidance, but is too proud to ask for it, and a bold, adventurous adolescent who wants to experience her independence now and needs to reject authority. She has to prove she is no longer a child but an individual in her own right who needs to be respected, however crazy her ideas.

The group still plays a powerful role in the life of a fifteen-year-old, who identifies with its current trends, prevailing outlooks, fashions and attitudes.

The young adolescent has a powerful desire to live in the modern world; she will frequently reject all forms of idealism although she secretly longs for it.

For parents it is a time both to trust and also set clear boundaries, to offer patient support and consistency, watching closely to see when they need to intervene. As such, a difficult balancing act is required: of letting go yet keeping a close eye on things at the same time.

Education can play a critical role in the young person's development in this phase; the bold, brash, rebellious and critical spirit can be harnessed by sensitive interaction with subject material that relates to her inward experience and her natural desire for knowledge.[15]

Sixteen – Longing for Truth and Meaning

The shift from fifteen to sixteen can be quite striking. We sense that a definite turning point has arrived for the adolescent. She now usually feels much more comfortable in her body, which has by now attained a size and shape that suggests her future adult stature. She has passed through the tempestuous fluctuations of her unfolding personality, and begins to experience stability and self-control of her emotions as she comes to terms with her sexuality, temperament and unique character. As her personality increasingly asserts itself and people around her affirm her grown-up status, she experiences a greater sense of self-worth and self-respect. Her growing sense of responsibility allows for greater freedom, which hopefully brings appreciation of and greater communication with her caregivers. She commands greater respect from adults and becomes less dependent on parents and peers.

> This was the age when Rajan felt ready to enter into his social life with confidence. He was intensely interested in art and literature and would spend hours discussing with his best friend Akil the books they had read, and the art works they had pored over together. Affirmation of the individual human being, portrayed by Ayn Rand and Dostoevsky, and the spiritual journeys described in the works of Kalil Gabran and Herman Hesse, began to kindle his idealism; he began to search for people with whom he could spend time expounding his visions of life.
>
> He loved nothing better than to listen to the wise words and experiences of adults who were on their own spiritual quest. He had a burning desire to be part of a community of like-minded people. He felt inspired to write poetry and to experiment with different forms of art. During this year he also let go of the artist friend he had hero-worshipped the

previous year. He now became more interested in this friend's younger sister, Saskia.

The Search for Meaning

The same essential themes may be discovered in thousands of variations in the personal biographies of many adolescents. This universal developmental reality we have explored throughout our journey through childhood and adolescence, we meet again here as the *universal adolescent.*

However, as we saw, the experience of the adolescent boy generally tends to be more earthbound and physical, whereas that of the girl has more to do with matters of the heart, soul and spirit. But they will all experience an expanding consciousness and an unfolding of their individuality as their intellect grows, their feelings for others mature and their life skills improve. The world grows larger and richer, and their life becomes more exciting, with deeper troughs and more exultant highs.

The search for truth, new values and meaning takes on many forms and can lead the youngster in positive and negative directions. Wherever they are pulled – towards religion, literature, music, art, science, nature, sport or social initiatives; or also towards the modern media, electronic technology or modern music; or towards the more negative experiences of substance abuse, violence and sexuality – one should remember that behind these pursuits is the longing to find new truth and meaning in life.

This quest is only possible because, somewhere in her being, the young person knows there is such a thing as truth. She lived within it for the first seven years of her life and believed in it through the authority of others for the next seven years; now she has to find it herself – for in our time there are few role models from whom she can really learn about it. And this is also the age where a truth is only acknowledged as such when it becomes an entirely personal experience.

Education continues to play a vital part in meeting the needs of the growing adolescent.[16]

Seventeen – The Search for Self

The older adolescent is moving fast towards becoming a young adult; she feels almost fully grown, has more freedom and responsibilities and may be learning to drive a motor vehicle or have acquired her driving licence. But, though she usually won't admit it, there is still apprehension at being out there on her own. Only the life-tested and street-hardened seventeen-year-old feels completely comfortable free of adult supervision. These youngsters may have left school and be earning their own wages at the bottom of the working ladder, while others drift along unemployed. Those who are still at school or college have the end of their secondary education in sight. All will ask the question: *What shall I do with my life?* This is of course also connected with the other, deeper question: *Who am I?*

Can you recall your preoccupation with these questions? Were they consciously expressed or less consciously experienced as you discovered different aspects of yourself and tried to find out who you were?

Adam had begun to reflect on these questions as early as fifteen and by seventeen was actively engaged in reading and pondering on his place in the world. Bulani in contrast had given little thought to these questions and was not at all clear what he would be doing after school.

Jonathan had a clear picture of himself as a confident and intelligent person and wished to study further to become a leading light in society. Maria on the other hand saw so many sides of her personality that she struggled with her personal identity; at times she was outgoing, self-assured and very sociable; at other times she felt over-sensitive, vulnerable and insecure. She had so many interests that she was unable to say what she wished to do after school.

Thandi, through her choleric nature, often found herself in conflict with others; in subsequent reflection she had the opportunity to face herself and to ask who she was and what she wished to do with her life. Saskia on the other hand would often reflect on why everyone praised and adored her; she could not fully understand what people saw in her because she felt she was lacking in so many areas.

Rajan started to consciously think about who he was when he met Saskia and fell in love with her; he became very aware of his egotistic nature – his fears, doubts, jealousies and possessiveness, but also of his generous, loving and trusting nature. At times he found he could make conscious choices about the direction he wanted his life to take.

In the search for identity and purpose, this question of *Who am I?* rises up into the budding soul of the adolescent in a singularly individual way, giving tentative form and direction to the future that lies ahead.

She will have to look at her strengths and weaknesses and begin to channel her thinking about her future in specific directions. Some students will decide on a career during this year, others later on. It is a fascinating study to explore when and how people determine their vocation and how they discover their true mission in life. I was four or five when I knew I was going to become a medical doctor. Some might say it was because I was surrounded by medical professionals in my family. I suspect that the calling goes deeper than mere environmental influences.

On the one hand life becomes more serious, there are more responsibilities, educational or work commitments and serious life questions to think about; on the other hand, life becomes more playful and adventurous. It is the time for embarking on new exploits and excelling at sporting activities. It is also the time for falling madly in love with an 'ideal partner', when the whole soul is consumed by the passion and infatuation for another human being.

Bulani, who lived in Johannesburg, was so in love with Thandi who lived in Cape Town, that one weekend he hitch-hiked, a distance of 1500 kilometres to be with her for a few days. Sadly for him she was also the love of his best friend Thabo, who won her heart. Despite his deep hurt and disappointment he held on to his love, expressing his feelings in heart-wrenching poetic words. In her presence it was as if the sun rose up in his soul; when he was away from her the sun was dimmed; yet he felt her closeness every moment of the day and in his dreams at night. She became for him an ideal of the feminine, of beauty and mystery for many years to come because he was unable to consummate his love for her. His friend Thabo, however, discovered and spoke to him of the deeply satisfying gift of intimacy, for which he had to wait a little while longer.

Sadly many adolescents get caught up in the competitive race for partners and sexual exploration and lose the exquisite tenderness and beauty of this time of life. This age of romantic idealism can still safeguard adolescents for a little longer from the powerful fall into the physical, sense-perceptible experience that premature sexual activity inevitably brings.

The search for truth and the fervour of idealism remain powerful themes during this year. The adolescent longs to see humanity reflecting his ideals. School life can engage with these themes in many different ways.[17]

Eighteen – Orientation

The self-assurance of adulthood has arrived as the young person in her full flowering stands at the threshold of life and steps out into the world. This arrival is affirmed by modern society which in many countries gives her the vote and/or enlists her into armed forces. Eighteen was always a significant landmark in past civilizations and cultures, when ancient Mystery centres held rites of initiation to prepare young men for manhood.

This is a time of exploration and challenges which spawn a new kind of learning, born of the young person's own life experience. The protected insulation of school life comes to an end and, with the unfolding of requisite strengths and capacities, she finds opportunities to deepen her relationship with the outside world:

I wish to meet many aspects of the world with many aspects of my being.

This inner impulse will express itself in trying out all kinds of new activities and relationships, different jobs and skills, organizing her life in new ways, changing her room and living arrangements, and, for the more adventurous, travelling to different parts of the world in search of new horizons, new impulses and new challenges.

The gap year – a free year before college or university for self-exploration – is a wonderful opportunity for the young adult to explore her own inner life and the outer world. It is sad to see vibrant youth becoming tied down and squeezed into small jobs and career paths or long university and training courses, before they have tasted life in the world. This is still a period of idealism, of hope and of wanting to make dreams come true. It is a precious age that ideally needs to be given time and space, in which the young person's interest in and love for humanity can unfold unhindered. It is more than likely that young people who are given this opportunity will in later life seek out greater social responsibility and commitment.

In opening the door to many challenges, this age has particular resonance with the ancient Greek legend of Persephone.

Persephone, the daughter of Demeter, is an innocent maiden who is seduced in subtle and devious ways by Pluto, the god of Hades. She is taken by him to the underworld and goes through dramatic encounters with despair, death, powerlessness and suicide. Pluto wants her to drink the juice of the pomegranate so that she will forget her previous life and become the Queen of the Dead. To begin with she resists but gradually she succumbs to his fascinating powers and is about to drink the dark red juice when Triptolemos, a young prince, arrives on the scene. He has heard of Persephone's fate from Demeter who, disguised as an old widow, is grieving at the loss of her daughter. He chooses to rescue Persephone rather than claim the crown of his father who has just died. With Hecate's help he breaks into Pluto's realm and calls on Persephone to remember where she came from. In that moment she drops the cup from her lips and is able to leave Hades with her new prince.

Other versions of the legend relate that Pluto seduces her with the pomegranate fruit so that she has to return to the underworld for six months every year.

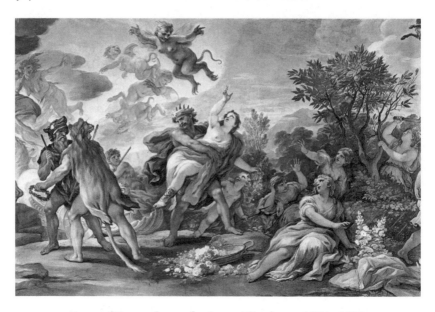

Rape of Persephone, by Luca Giordano, 1684–1686.

These trials of life and death, the power of love and seduction, the search for good and the temptation by evil, come to meet the young adult and will occupy her for many years to come.

Faced with these challenges, the young adult will soon realize that her selfhood is not yet quite ready for the trials that lie ahead and that she still has work to do before she is ready to stake her claim as an awakened I in the world. She may believe she is mature and fully independent, but she still requires the firm and loving patience of adults to support her through this transitional period

First Moon Node

At eighteen years seven months and eleven days an important milestone is reached when the sun and the moon stand in the same relationship to one another as they did at the moment of a person's physical birth. Those who study cosmic rhythms know their significance for human biography. This particular cycle has to do with renewal in the life of the individual; we frequently see major changes, new impulses and resolves, often accompanied by crises connected with relationships or vocation taking place around this time. The editor of this book tells me that it was precisely at this age that he suddenly and 'accidentally' encountered the works of Rudolf Steiner, which were entirely at odds with his conventional upbringing yet gave him the sense of 'coming home' at last.

Nineteen – Consolidation

While eighteen was about orientation and finding one's way in the labyrinth of life, nineteen has to do with consolidation and learning to paddle one's craft oneself. The young person finds out how to use her compass and to hold a steady course. As she gets to know her inner landscape, she starts to feel more sure of herself, her confidence grows and she tastes a sense of empowerment. She discovers she has the strength and the courage to deal with the problems she encounters in life. More and more she learns to trust herself, to know her capabilities and her limitations, and to test herself to determine where she stands in relation to the world.

This is an age when she has to prove herself worthy and capable. At the same time there is still a great longing to explore different pathways and test new capacities. She may embark on outer travels and inner journeys, learn new skills, meet new friends and mentors, and experiment with new ventures – some of which may be highly dangerous. Behind her search is the call for truth, either as a conscious striving or an unconscious impulse that drives her to meet life's challenges, bringing her face to face with the problems that beset humanity.

Some young adults who are only concerned with their own wellbeing will be untouched by these issues. Others will struggle through frustration and disappointment, hurt and sadness, anger and passion, to find hope and the idealistic wish to do something to make a difference. Deep within themselves, these young people feel they are members of humanity and responsible not just for themselves but also for the society of which they are a part.

The young adult will be tested no matter where she finds herself in life, and she will feel that she still has a way to go before she attains full maturity.

Twenty – Preparation for Manhood and Womanhood

This is the third year in which Adam is getting to know the terrain he is travelling, and he is beginning to feel more equipped to face challenges he meets.

At this age a young person is usually well ensconced in her chosen job, study career or profession, feels more secure in relationships and has achieved a certain organizing ability to structure her life the way she wants it. Her parents have come to regard her as an equal, and have realized that the time is fast approaching when she has to look after herself. She is discovering new respect and friendship for adults who have traveled this journey before her and have acquired greater life experience.

As this year unfolds, Adam senses the awakening of a power that is the source of his whole being; he begins to realize that it is here to guide him on his journey through life. This is the power that led him into life at birth and that has been invisibly guiding him every step of the way.

Physical birth is an event we cannot possibly overlook because it brings the arrival of a physical human being. The etheric birth manifests itself far less visibly, with the appearance of new physical teeth. The astral birth takes place much more subtly, becoming visible quite gradually with the manifestations of puberty. The birth of the I however, around the age of 21, takes place without any physical changes whatsoever. It is announced by the adult herself who expresses in her whole being that she has come of age; her physical development is complete and her soul and spiritual development can now proceed consciously because the I – the instrument of self-awareness – has been born. She is ready to receive the golden key that will open the doors to higher consciousness.

Rites of Passage

These rituals or celebratory events marking a stage or a transition in a person's life can be recognized and witnessed by other members of the close community in appropriate ways. Such landmark events have been accorded special significance throughout history to acknowledge the universal reality of important milestones in human biography. Modern cultures and religions vary greatly in their regard and practice of these rites of passage, but almost everyone participates in them to some degree, either consciously or unconsciously.

Childbirth is a universal rite of passage marking the transition from non-earthly to earthly existence. The birthday is a tradition still celebrated by most people to mark the advance into a new year of life. Although not formally celebrated, the significant developmental milestones – crawling, sitting, standing, walking, talking and the change of teeth – are all acknowledged as important milestones along the developmental journey. Coming of age at twenty-one, graduation, engagement to a partner, marriage, weddings and funerals are events that are still universally celebrated.

All religions celebrate rites of passage: for instance, baptism is the ritual act using water and sometimes other substances such as salt and ash, by which the infant child is admitted as a member into the Christian church. Judaism, Islam and other Asian and African cultures circumcise males shortly after birth (*Bris milah* in Judaism), during childhood (*Kitan* in Islam) or around puberty or in adolescence (in African initiation rites). Buddhism practices *shinbyu* whereby parents allow their young sons to embrace the teachings of the Buddha for a certain duration in a Buddhist monastry, in order to gain special grace and virtue from the Buddha. The *Bar Mitzvah* in the boy aged 13 and *Bat Mitzvah* in the girl aged 12, are important rites of passage in Judaism, conferring on the pubescent child personal responsibility for continued adherence to the Jewish faith. Likewise *confirmation* is an initiation rite in many Christian churches to strengthen the bond of the child to the Church; in the Eastern churches it is conferred after baptism, in the West it usually takes place in early adolescence as a more conscious act of commitment towards Christianity.

Three Thresholds

Between puberty and adulthood the adolescent will encounter three important thresholds: With the birth of soul life and the emergence of independent thinking between 14 to 16, the teenager is searching desperately for her identity. *Who am I? Am I male or female? Who do I wish to be? How do I handle my emerging sexuality?* These are questions related to the teenager herself. One can see why close bonding with same-sex friends and the search for heroes is therefore so central during this period. It is a time when the teenager needs to be guided and nurtured through a tempestuous period, when the eruptive power of sexuality can be harnessed and the emotional soil of the soul can be prepared for future loving and intimate relationships. School camps can provide golden opportunities to help address these vitally important issues through appropriately designed rites of passage.

As the adolescent settles into her newfound identity, she will confront a second threshold between 16 and 18 connected with love for and intimacy with the opposite sex. Once again she asks the question: *Who am I?* But now it is *Who am I in relation to You? How do I respond to You? Who are You?* This is the time of fascination with the opposite sex, when boys and girls are attracted to each other and fall head over heels in love with each other. These romantic relationships swing between ecstacy and agony and can be severely challenging for the vulnerable adolescent. This is a time that again requires the steady guiding hand of a caring adult who can offer objective and loving support. During this period the Waldorf School curriculum uses the Parcival legend – which describes the initiation path of the knight Parcival and his search for the Holy Grail – to help the adolescent address many issues of self-discovery, self-awareness and relationship.[18] This story as well as many other great literary works and themes can be used as the basis for consciously designed rites of passage to guide the adolescent safely through these difficult waters.[19]

Having explored her identity and her first intimate relationships, the young person will now encounter her third threshold between 18 and 21, that of her future life task. As she ventures forth into the wider world, she faces the same question again: *Who am I?* But now it is *Who am I in relation to the world? Where have I come from, where am I, and where am I going? What can I do that will have meaning for the world? How can I find a connection to the times in which I live?*

During these years there is usually a strong preoccupation with one's future vocation and purpose in life; now is the time to explore the nature of who one is in relation to where one wants to go. There can be great value in participating where possible in organized rites of passage workshops or courses designed to address the questions of this age.[20] The gap year often serves as a golden opportunity for young people to discover their mission in life.

Most young people today do not have the opportunity to journey through formal rites of passage, guided by a mentor or a seer who has previously undergone the path before them. They are not summoned by their elders or instructed to go through certain trials and rituals. But they still feel the inner urge to test and challenge themselves in different ways. Today life itself offers the challenges of initiation, and a young adult finds herself facing obstacles and working through issues that will shape and mould her developing character. In the coming years this character will be increasingly refined and developed.

Character

In earlier chapters we found that an understanding of the constitution and temperament helps us to understand the child respectively in the first and second seven-year period. Now in the period between 14 and 21, the **character** begins to unfold. Insight into its nature can help us work more effectively with the growing adolescent.

After puberty, soul life becomes progressively more visible and independent as the astral body is born and begins to mature. One manifestation of this process is the unfolding of a particular character or soul type. We can liken this process to the painting of a portrait where the artist uses colour, texture and fine hues to bring out the unique features that reveal a person's essence or inner nature. In this case the artist is the I.

We can therefore regard character as the unique colour and texture of the soul revealed by the I. The light nature of the unfolding astral body after puberty reveals itself in the different 'colours' of the character that come to expression.

The Qualities of Colour

In the rainbow or prism we can experience seven primary colours composing the visible light spectrum. Colour may be said to come about through the interaction of light with darkness. These seven colours are seven primary ways in which light interacts with darkness. Goethe in the 18th century stated that light is 'the simplest, most undivided, most homogenous being that we know; confronting it is the darkness.'[21] Unlike his contemporaries, Goethe did not see darkness as an absence of light, but rather as polar to and interacting with light; he believed that colour resulted from this interaction of light and dark.

In many colour phenomena of nature, such as cloud or smog that overshadows the sunset or sunrise, or the moon against the background of the dark sky, we can see that the darker colours arise where darkness is superimposed on light; the light colours, in contrast, emerge where light is superimposed on dark.

When we allow these seven colours to work on us, using the methodology of experience awareness outlined in previous chapters, and engaging empathically with them, we can start to experience the specific effect of each. Observe the colour red and notice the effect it has on you; compare this with the colour blue and feel the difference. Most of us will agree that red has an activating effect, whereas blue has a calming effect. In everyday life, colours exert a powerful effect on our feelings and actions. We choose the colours of our clothes according to our moods, and paint our homes according to our aesthetic needs.

By allowing such phenomena to resonate within us, we may arrive at an inner experience of the seven basic colours, each of which is distinctly different. These experiences can provide us with a starting point for exploring character types.

The Significance of Seven

It is interesting to discover that many phenomena in the world can be ordered in a **sevenfold** way. Is it a coincidence that there are seven primary colours, seven days in the week and seven notes in the octave? We have seen that our ancient ancestors lived in a consciousness that connected them directly to spiritual realities. They experienced divine beings who ruled the fixed stars – the zodiac – as well as the 'wandering stars' – the planets. These stellar and planetary gods were worshipped by all ancient civilizations: Zeus, Olympus and Thor, for instance, were Greek, Roman and Germanic names for the deity ruling the planet Jupiter. These gods governed various domains of existence: in the cosmos they regulated the world of space and the course of time, resulting in the naming of the days of the week, the colour sphere of the rainbow and the range of musical tones. In the human domain they governed the seven primary organ systems and the seven character types.[22] In the world of nature they govern the seven primary grains and the seven primary metals.[23]

In Chapter seven we examined the seven planetary forces as the source of all life on earth, and their specific influence on the general human constitution. We saw that life on earth is determined by sunlight and sun-warmth, and we looked at the possibility that these life forces were influenced by the other six planetary bodies. Through microcosmic interiorization, these seven planetary forces have become active in the human being manifesting in seven main physiological and psychological domains.

Knowledge of these relationships was still known to the early Christian Gnostics and to the alchemists in the Middle Ages and Renaissance period.

In his work *Harmony of the World,* Kepler, the father of contemporary astronomy, describes seven cosmic intelligences that govern our planetary system according to the harmonic laws of the heavenly spheres, stating that 'The heavenly bodies are moved by spiritual beings, working as instruments in their force fields.' He also makes direct connections between planetary forces and forces of the human soul.[24]

Paracelsus, a doctor and alchemist living in the Middle Ages, intuitively connected the planetary forces to seven primary metals, living processes and human organic and psychological functions.

In our time a conscious understanding of these universal connections has been lost, essentially through a loss of knowledge of soul and spirit. Inevitably this has led to a science that can only regard the human being, earth, nature and the universe from a physical, materialistic, mechanistic and reductionist point of view.

In the first quarter of the 20th century, through his investigations as a scientist of soul-spiritual realms, Steiner was able to bring a renewed knowledge of the connections between the macrocosmic universe, the earthly realm and the microcosmic world of the human being. A study of the phenomena of these different spheres of life reveals that an essential principle runs like a common thread through planet, organ, character type, mythological god, metal and grain. A common law or archetypal principle connects them all as we shall see below when we examine the character types individually.

By entering into the inner nature of phenomena with the same empathy that we use to experience the inner nature of colour, we can discover a singular principle or character living in them; using our accustomed tools of enhanced observation and deepened experience awareness (visualizing, sensing, feeling, gesturing). This is as if we are getting to know a personality living within the phenomena. These seven principles are the same soul forces we witness unfolding in the characters of adolescents as they grow towards adulthood. Using this methodology of both inner experience and outer phenomenology, let us attempt to explore seven character types that evolve from the universal principles governing all existence.

Character Types

According to the dominant forces present in the developing astral body, a specific character type will begin to express itself after puberty. This is a manifestation of the basic life and colour of the soul itself that has come from a distant past, that was organically active for fourteen years and now begins to unfold its nature in free soul expression. The intensity of this unfurling soul life will tend to overshadow the temperament and constitution formed earlier, so that the character becomes the dominant structure during this time. Lievegoed says that the former two become 'more recessive, but continue to make their influence felt in the unconscious layers of the personality. They can also reinforce certain character structure or work against them.'[25]

The Saturn or Individuating Type

> In the colour **blue** I carry my light and my warmth within and behind the darkness. I am inward, I am hidden. I am resilient. I may appear cold, dark and hard on the outside, but I am warm, light and vulnerable on the inside. My warmth radiates through the solar system, through time and space.

The heavenly blue colour expands our gaze and draws the eye ever further out into space.

The planet Saturn, together with its orbit, forms the outer frontier of our solar system and the gateway to the fixed stars.[26] Saturn is the most distant planet, with a distinctly bluish hue that shows very little change. Being the furthest planet from the earth it has the longest orbit (29.5 years).

Lead is a soft, heavy, grey metal. It does not reflect light but has its own inner bluish lustre when cut. Because of its hidden internalized warmth, it is soft, melts easily and conducts warmth poorly. It contains a powerful inner force, great inner resistance and resilience; it resists breakdown by outside elements, including water, and it is therefore used in underwater cables, containers, paints, roof flashing and protective material against radioactive waves.

Chronos was a Greek mythological figure, the father of time. He harvests the ripe fruits with his sickle and also, as skeleton man with his scythe, represents death.

According to Steiner, Ancient Saturn was the first evolutionary epoch of the earth, and essentially therefore the beginning of time.

> Adam is thin, bony and gaunt in appearance and at 16 looks older than his age. He does not take good care of himself, his hair and dress are unkempt and his clothes are unfashionable and dark in colour. He keeps to himself unless provoked and though he has few friends, he is respected for his integrity and individual character; he has very specific and carefully considered views about life and is not shy to present them when the occasion arises. He may come across as critical, dogmatic and intolerant and does not suffer fools easily.

His focus is inward and towards the past, as evidenced by his very strong powers of memory. He is not comfortable in the current world in which he finds himself and seems not to care about the externalities of life. He seems to create barriers between himself and the world. He has a passion for solving mathematical, scientific or philosophical problems and will persevere with his goals until he has achieved them no matter what the sacrifice to his wellbeing. He has a need to understand the laws that operate in the world but is less interested in the little things of life.

His loyalty to his work, to a cause or to a friend who has gradually earned a place in his life, is unquestionable. But he is also egotistic, self-critical, inflexible, moody and intolerant. When he allows himself to look towards the future, he would like to become an actuary, a researcher or an historian, but in his usual, melancholic state of mind he wants to drop out of life and become a hermit.

Because the I works through the medium of the warmth element, its activity will govern all processes of substance formation and dissolution. When the I withdraws from matter, warmth too is withdrawn and substances move towards mineralization and crystallization: from the state of warmth through gas and liquid to the solid state. This is what happens in the mineralized skeleton. When the I enters matter, warmth is enhanced and substances move in the opposite direction towards breakdown and dissolution, as manifest in the warmth of the blood that has the power to dissolve substance, and the spleen, the organ that breaks down blood cells. The red blood cells have no nucleus, live for only 120 days and cannot replicate themselves.

Through its warmth-regulating power, Saturn is the force that governs maturation and aging during life, and also death. Like the orbit of Saturn, it is a principle that lives within long time frames, bearing world memory within it.

Saturn is the force that guides the I into incarnation and life on earth, and that in turn leads the I out of life into death. When the I incarnates from spirit towards the world of matter, individuation, isolation and boundaries in space are formed; when the I excarnates towards spirit, spatial forms dissolve into a world of time where growth and development are expressed through the biography of the individual until separate life is ultimately dissolved at death.

Saturn is the quintessential individual who is faithful to his true origins.

The Moon, or Imitating /Renewing Type

> In **violet** my light and warmth remain partially hidden in the darkness; I allow your light and warmth to express itself through me. I bow down before your greatness. I renew existence in accordance with the universal creative archetype.

Violet provides an excellent backdrop for bringing foreground objects into optimum visibility.

The moon is the nearest planet to the earth, with the shortest orbit. It does not have its own light but powerfully reflects the light of the sun. Its effects on the rhythms of nature and the life of reproduction are well known. Its connection with silver has been familiar to seers, artists and poets since time immemorial.

Artemis was the ancient Greek goddess of the moon and Diana was the Roman equivalent. She carried a silver bow and arrow and her many breasts were a symbol of her great fecundity.

Silver is selfless towards light and warmth, faithfully reflecting light, and conducting warmth exceptionally well. It combines easily with water, forming solutions such as silver chloride. It creates the most perfect mirror and is used in photography to produce a fixed reflection of reality.

> Bulani has a fresh, childlike appearance, round features, full lips and a soft, almost feminine body. He is open, spontaneous and uninhibited in his general demeanour, flamboyant in his speech and dress and takes meticulous care of his health and external appearance. He feels more comfortable following the lead of others and doesn't often have his own opinions. His many friends find him quite gullible and naïve, because he trusts everything he hears and believes what he sees.

He has always had a rich dream life, escaping into a world of fantasy that is full of secret friends, hopes and wishes. He has a pictorial and retentive memory, yet he feels more secure when he records what he hears in class and when he learns things by heart.

He is very family-conscious and upholds the traditions and customs of his culture meticulously. When he returns home from school, he looks after his younger siblings, cooks them lunch, cares for the home pets and waters the garden. He has a natural talent for caring and wants to become a nurse or gardener when he is grown up.

When moon nature is active in the material world, it brings the archetype into manifestation through endless repetition, expressing its nature in cell division, procreation, and the reproductive system, the recapitulation of the species, heredity and the genetic code. The skin is moon's reflective boundary where heredity becomes visible. Moon is the inspiration for the embryonic period and the first seven years of life. In this time of burgeoning life processes, water is the moon element for nascent, generative vitality.

When it works mentally, it acts like a mirror whereby life forces are suppressed and the living creative world is faithfully reflected as an image of the past. Moon is then active in the brain that reflects the external world internally as a picture, and which serves as the instrument for combining thoughts into thought images; and for the intellect that reproduces dead thoughts and provides the basis for materialistic science. Moon is active too in the silver-plated mirror and photographic imagery of silver, in the reflected light of the moon, in the flow of imagination that mirrors creative reality, and in the memory that reproduces the created world.

The moon type is a copier, imitator, actor and faithful servant of original creation. In many respects this is the opposite picture to the Saturn type and can be used therapeutically to address one-sided Saturnine traits in adolescence; for instance we can use moon qualities such as silver in minute doses, foods with abundant life forces and frequent exposure to rhythmic activites, imaginative and reflective thinking and drama work; likewise Saturn qualities can be used in small degrees to address a one-sided moon character:

lead in minute doses, foods with form-giving qualities such as root vegetables and regular exposure to abstract thinking and subjects such as maths and philosophy. As we shall see in Volume 3, each therapeutic modality can be used in a sevenfold (as well as in a threefold, fourfold and also twelvefold manner). Thus we can find in music, movement, massage, nutrition, etc. a moon quality that can balance out a one-sided Saturn character.

By imbibing some of the life-renewing, spontaneous, imaginative and childlike qualities of the moon, Adam can modify his hard, egotistic, over-critical and unsociable nature.

Bulani, on the other hand, requires some of Saturn's self-centred, introverted and serious qualities to offset his gullible nature and excessive concern with external trivialities.

Jupiter – The Thoughtful /Organizing Type

Through **orange** my light and warmth ray out and give shape and order to the world. This is a sovereign power that governs and organizes the world. I become Jupiter when I create order and give form to the world according to higher wisdom.

The planet Jupiter is a prominent, brilliant star that dominates the heavenly skies wherever and whenever it is visible.

Jupiter, Olympus, Zeus, Poseidon and Thor are the mythological deities embodying this planet, and manifest world-creative powers.

Tin is a metal that does not like to surrender its shape, maintaining its form through its hidden crystalline nature; if you try to bend soft tin, it makes known its displeasure with a tearing, screaming sound as the crystals break. It is used as utensils to contain substances, as solders to preserve shapes, as alloys to give other metals the power to maintain shapes, and as tin foil to enfold the shape of objects.

Jonathan is tall, well-built, with strong, handsome features and a striking, broad forehead. He has an unusually commanding presence for his youthful age. From an early age he impressed people with his confident, self-assured manner and his precocious knowledge. He has a highly developed intellect and independent thinking that often gets him into trouble when he challenges his teachers and fellow students in a conceited and arrogant way, believing his opinions are always right.

He has a great talent for seeing the bigger picture, thinking something through in a clear and methodical way and then taking the lead in organizing things through to successful completion. He took on the production of his Class eleven play, organizing and directing the production with aplomb. He loves debating, chess, taking part in general knowledge competitions and organizing projects. His ambition is to become a film producer, a high-powered successful executive, politician or a judge.

Working with the light and air from cosmic heights, Jupiter forms and shapes the head, the brain, the round heads of bones, and the muscles and other organs with convex, rounded forms. Working with the fluid element, it organizes the flow of substances in all realms of metabolism. The centre of its activity is the liver, which radiates chemical actions to every cell of the body. It is a sculptor expressing the ideal in beautiful forms, spiritually as thought forms, in the world of matter as created forms. Through gesture and movement it bring the soul to expression using the flowing, shaping power of the muscles. As character, Jupiter gives shape and order to a person's world in her thinking and actions.

Mercury – The Mobile/Connecting Type

In **yellow** my light shines into the world, illuminating the darkness; it makes visible the diversity of individual forms as well as their unity within the wholeness of the world. I am Mercury when I am imbued with the oneness of life and at the same time can manifest this oneness in the diversity of life. I am the mediator, healer and communicator, bringing people together and creating harmony.

The planet Mercury is the closest planet to the sun. It is therefore seldom visible, and only in the twilight zones of dusk and dawn. As seen from the earth, it performs mobile loops as it dances around the sun.

The shiny metal mercury has all the characteristic of water: it is a fluid at normal temperature, becomes mobile and flowing at the smallest opportunity, is moist to the touch and adapts lovingly to containing surfaces. It can unite with many metals to form amalgams, and dissolves most metals like water dissolves salt.

Like water it assumes a drop form; it easily disperses from one large drop into many tiny drops of different sizes and just as easily coalesces back into one large drop. Its ability to expand and contract readily to changes in temperature and pressure make it ideal for use in thermometers and barometers. In its vapourized form it is highly toxic.

Mythologies depict the force of mercury as Mercury, Hermes, Thoth, Odin-Wotan, Raphael, as the divine messenger connecting heaven and earth and as the representative of healing. He is also depicted as a Robin Hood character who distributes wealth to the poor, keeping the flow of money mobile.

Maria is slightly built, with fine, delicate features, sparkling eyes and wavy hair. She is very perceptive and gives the impression of being constantly aware of everything that goes on around her; she has always been a highly sensitive child, seeing and hearing things that passed others by. She wants to interact with what she perceives, leading to a tendency to be overactive and impulsive. She is very agile, fleet-footed, and dances gracefully. She loves to know what is going on in the world, is very astute, learns easily and is very quick to offer her insights and ideas.

She makes friends easily, is very sociable, fun-loving, and the life and soul of the party. Her friends love her energy and vitality and greatly appreciate her empathy and sensitivity. She has a very flexible nature, likes change and improvization, is full of initiative and is always seeking new knowledge and offering new ideas. When there are personality clashes, she is always the one to mend relationships. When she grows up she wishes to work in conflict resolution or in the communication industry. Her hobbies are magic, dancing and gymnastics.

Mercury knows the ocean and also all the droplets that belong to it. It is connected with the universal intelligence of the macrocosm and in an instant can become the microcosm's individuated diversification, moving mercurially and effortlessly between the two. Like the metal mercury, it connects the unitary ocean with diverse streams, bringing them all together to create a cohesive whole. It stands for 'diversity in unity' as proclaimed by the statue of Mercury on top of the Union Buildings in Pretoria – the seat of government of the Republic of South Africa – whose multiracial democracy is striving for realization of that motto.

Mercury expresses itself in the human body on the one hand through the wing-like lungs that are the most mobile organs in the body, connecting the microcosm to the macrocosm through the medium of the air and made up of millions of air sacs shaped like droplets of mercury bunched together; and on the other through the lymph and glandular system where the diverse life of cells predominates, and where fluid secretions are in constant flow and circulation.

Mercury lives between the two extremes of cosmic expansion and earthly contraction – contraction-expansion/cohesion-dispersion – and constantly strives to reconcile them.

By mediating between extremes and bringing divergent streams together, Mercury is the force of healing as symbolized by the ancient Staff of Mercury, which holds the balance between two opposing snakes – the two polar extremes. Mercury is in continuous sensitive movement between the chaos of diversity and the ordered unity of life.

In many respects, Mercury is the polarity of Jupiter, so that one-sided tendencies in either can be balanced by making use of the other's polar qualities, in the way indicated above. By encouraging the well-formed, organized and grounded nature of Jupiter, one can help Maria to temper her overactive and impulsive nature; this can be assisted by minute doses of tin, well-structured foods like grains, drawing with charcoal which promotes a feeling of inner structure, and therapeutic movements that help to ground her. Jonathan's arrogance and conceit can be harnessed by helping him to become more mercurially flexible and adaptable; homeopathic mercury, painting with water colours on wet paper, encouraging lively and mobile sporting, acting, dancing and therapeutic movements, will benefit him.

Mars – The Active, Masculine Type

> In the colour **red** my light and warmth actively work outwards
> into the darkness and assert themselves powerfully in the outer
> world. I wish to make myself seen and heard on earth. I am
> Mars when I bring the highest creative powers actively down to
> earth.

Red is well known as the most assertive colour, used to attract
attention and to block movement – red traffic lights, red danger
signs, the red colour of fire. Red-coloured cars are apparently the
most accident-prone. One can easily sense a need to defend oneself
against the aggressive action of red.

The planet Mars appears red in colour and is the planet most
similar to earth.

Meteors composed of iron – the metal associated with Mars – are
celestial bodies that fall down to earth.

Mars, the Roman god of war with his iron sword, armour
and shield, is the personification of masculine power and will that
engages actively with the earth.

Iron is a soft, silvery metal that becomes extremely hard when
mixed with carbon, the structural element of the organic world.
Iron is a poor conductor of heat and has a very high melting point.
It does not give away its heat readily and requires a great deal of
outer warmth to change its state. It also has a connection with the
magnetic forces of the earth, as the metal that most easily becomes
magnetized.

Iron is the only metal that exists in material quantities in the
human blood. It is the most abundant metal in the earth, and the
most common of the seven primary metals. Our culture makes use
of iron more than most other elements; it is the scaffold of our
industrialized and mechanized civilization, and also the metal of
war. Our vehicles of iron move us through the world. In our daily
life we make use of iron in a thousand different objects.

Thandi is short, stocky and powerfully built with steely grey
eyes and a strong, firm jaw. She stands firmly on the ground and
walks with a self-assured gait. She gives the impression of being

ready for action at any moment. She is boisterous, enthusiastic, energetic and always the first one in the class to volunteer for work. She is never reluctant or afraid to take up a challenge, excelling in competitive and combative sports such as kick-boxing and karate.

Her classmates are weary of her confrontational nature and impulsive will but respect her strength as well as her passion for truth and justice. Her strong will for action colours her character; she thinks in a precise and practical way and expresses her ideas with powerful conviction. Her feelings are intense, tempestuous and quickly lead to actions. She will take up a cause, pushing people aside in the process and will fight until the job is completed to her satisfaction. In her spare time she teaches youth to defend themselves and plans to develop training studios in self-mastery as her future career.

Mars brings power down to earth. When Mars brings light down into the realm of the human spirit, thinking is imbued with creative forces. Thinking finds its outward expression in the power of speech, through the shield-shaped organ of the voice – the larynx. When Mars carries air power into the realm of the human soul, it lives in the activity of breathing. Through the digestive force of the bile, it brings warmth power down into the realm of living substance: bile digests fats which produce the most warmth in the body. When it carries earth power into the realm of the physical body, it engenders an organ that regulates earthly substance – the lung with its tree-like branching system.

What has the lung to do with the earth? While the airy lung tissue belongs to Mercury, the tree-like branching structure itself belongs to Mars. In the growing embryo, the lungs form simultaneously with the growth of the limbs, with which we make contact with the earth. In the evolution of the animal kingdom, the lungs likewise develop when water creatures, such as frogs, develop limbs to step onto the earth. The regulation of the amount of carbon dioxide expired by the lungs has much to do with the formation of the bony system.

Mars is the bearer of masculine will and guided movement that brings this creative power down to earth and in so doing guides the healing process. When iron is low in the blood, as occurs in anaemic conditions, we feel ungrounded and are susceptible to infections. Iron is an essential element for cellular detoxification. The red blood cell carries oxygen to every cell in the body and makes use of iron to carry out this function. It is the only cell in the body that lacks a nucleus, and the only cell that carries iron in this manner. In all other cells the nucleus acts like a brain to direct cell activities, so we can ask whether iron takes the place of the nucleus in the red blood cell, holding the blood in the earth's orientation like a compass. The iron present in every red blood cell might be seen as the iron sword protecting us against the constant threat of toxicity or infection.

One can imagine the shining sparks of metallic iron in the millions of red blood cells coursing through blood circulation! The picture of Michael taming the dragon with his sword of iron is a powerful picture of the constant healing power of iron in the blood system. The iron closely bound to oxygen also exemplifies the healing power of breathing over the untamed nature of blood circulation.

The glittering falling meteor showers are an outward, cosmic picture of this incarnating and healing principle.

The character of Mars is active will, directed towards the future.

Venus – The Receptive, Feminine Type

In the colour **green**, my inner light rests comfortably in equilibrium with the darkness, creating space to receive and store light from outside. The light from within can commune with the light from without. I become Venus when I open myself with fine sensitivity in the service of a higher principle.

Sunlight captured by the chlorophyll of plant cells creates the green, vegetative world of the plant kingdom. It is a colour very soothing to the eye.

The planet Venus appears in the twilight hours as a bright morning or evening star. It always lives close to the sun. Because of this it also displays different phases, namely full Venus, sickle Venus, etc.

Venus and Aphrodite are the Greek and Roman names for this goddess of beauty and love. In his famous painting of the Venus,

Botticelli depicts her standing sensuously on a kidney-shaped shell, her copper-coloured hair flowing behind as she is blown by gods of the wind and air to the island of Cyprus, the ancient mystery centre where copper was mined.

Copper gives and offers itself selflessly: in its different forms it is an extraordinarily colourful and beautiful metal, easy to work with, malleable and ductile. It conducts heat and electricity very well, combines easily with many substances and sounds melodious when struck. It is used as pipes to convey water, copper wire to conduct electricity, utensils to contain water, nourishment and warmth, and as instruments to convey sound. The family of molluscs and mussels have copper in their blood instead of iron in order to breathe.

> Saskia has a beauty and poise that draws people to her; she has dark and deep liquid eyes, luxuriant hair and a soft, sensuous body that moves quietly and gracefully. Most people love her company because she is unassuming, gentle and so easy to be with; she never pushes herself forward but allows others to have their say first.
>
> She is therefore in the best position to assess a person or situation, and constantly makes judgements about her observations. Some people find her too passive and self-effacing, but they are unaware of the depth of her character. She is very clear about what is right for her. Everyone agrees she is a natural listener. Because of her sensitivity and intuitive feelings she quickly understands what people tell her. Her friends readily confide in her.
>
> She is passionate about many things in her life: she loves to be amidst nature, to tend the garden, play her violin, paint or be with her friends. She is an artist rather than a scientist, thinks imaginatively and acts out of her heart rather than her head. She is always creating beauty in her environment. She has deep feelings for people and is always willing to help when they are in trouble.
>
> She would love to have many careers: nursery-school teacher, gardener, environmentalist, artist; but if she had to make one choice it would be to become a counsellor.

Venus makes space for the spiritual to come down to earth by becoming quiet and by learning to listen with empathy and in selfless devotion. It can care and nurture because it hears exactly what is needed and can also discern what is not needed.

In the human organism it is the receptive power behind all listening and discerning. The auditory apparatus receives and discerns the world of sound, the digestive system absorbs and eliminates the world of substance, the liver takes up substances that it can build up and enliven, and destroys harmful materials; and the kidney excretes what is not needed and absorbs back into the system living substance. Discernment requires clear insight and the ability to judge what is right for any given situation. The body has an innate 'discerning' intelligence to know what it needs to survive, what must be retained and what must be eliminated. Every cell absorbs the exact nourishment that it needs and gets rid of waste material. The venous circulation – the name too suggests its origin – receives lymph and cellular fluid from the tissues and conveys the blood passively back to the receptive side of the heart to be re-energized by the active heart and conveyed to Mars-driven arterial circulation.

In the human soul, Venus is the force behind feeling and sensation, aesthetics and judgement.

She is the silent creative power behind beauty, love, devotion and all the arts. She is the soul that creates a receptive vessel for the spirit. She wishes to dedicate her life to service of the highest things. Venus is the archetypal nurturer, devoted to caring and serving the highest aspects of humanity.

Venus is the opposite picture to Mars, and as such either can be used to balance out one-sided tendencies in the other's character. Saskia's over-caring and over-sensitive nature can lead to frequent exhaustion and overload – which can be avoided by taking on some of the protective qualities of Mars. Small doses of iron, iron-rich foods such as meat, nuts, beetroots, spinach and dried fruit, painting with the colour red and learning to become more assertive, can be therapeutic; Thandi, on the other hand, needs more of the nurturing and warmth of Venus to balance out her over-energetic, aggressive and confrontational nature. She needs more copper substances, vegetables and fruits, the calming colour of green, and needs to be helped to listen to others.

Sun – The Harmonious, Balanced Type

> In the colour **gold**, light and darkness are in singular balance in a way similar to green; the cosmic and the earthly are fully integrated. I am warmth within and warmth without. I am light within and light without. I am sun when I become the highest principle governing the universe and the human being, and the balancing force that harmonizes all polarities.

In the cosmic world the sun is the source of all light, warmth and life on earth. It stands between the three outer planets Saturn, Jupiter, Mars, and the three inner planets Venus, Mercury, Moon. We have seen that the one-sided actions of these planets are regulated and mediated by the sun.

Sun deities are depicted in the myths and mysteries of many cultures: Ahura Mazdao is the Persian sun spirit of light; Osiris, Ra and Horus are Egyptian sun gods; Apollo is the Greek god of light and truth and the creator of harmony in thinking, feeling and will. In the Christian mysteries, the Christ is the bearer of the Sun principle.

In the earthly world gold is a metal that balances polarities. It is able to harmonize heaviness and lightness. On the one hand it is nineteen times heavier than an equivalent amount of water: at a gold-smelting centre, visitors were invited to take home a bar of gold if they could pick it up! At the same time it has a light, radiant colour which gives one the feeling it is warm and buoyant. It has a huge capacity to be stretched and is the most ductile and malleable substance known: one gram of gold can be beaten into an unbroken wire two kilometres long! Gold leaf is so thin and immaterial it allows the light to shine through it, revealing the colour green.

Gold is the symbol and standard of material as well as of spiritual value, and today is still the globally accepted standard for currency; but it is also used in the decoration, adorning and artistic representation of the highest spiritual realities, as seen in places of worship and all great art works.

In the human body the heart, placed at the centre between the arterial system, the capillary system and the venous system, is the balancing organ that maintains the homeostasis of the circulation.

In its systolic contraction it pushes the blood out towards the body, knowing how much force is needed to bring the blood back into active arterial flow after the venous blood, slowed down by the force of gravity, returns to the heart. In its diastolic relaxation it expands its volume and opens itself to the blood flowing back towards it, sensing how much space is needed to absorb the active pressure in the system. It is well known that the blood flows without the presence of a heart, and, as we have seen, the life forces in the capillary system bring the blood into circulation. It is therefore the opposite of a mechanical pump, which can only function in accordance with a preset intention. The heart on the other hand is a highly sensitive vital organ, constantly assessing what lives in the blood circulation and responding accordingly to balance out any disharmony.

This dynamic of systole and diastole determines the arterial blood pressure that conveys oxygen-rich blood and nutrients from the heart to a vast capillary system bathing all the body's cells with buoyant, life-sustaining fluid. It determines the way in which the capillaries breathe out and breathe in their liquid contents, and influences the venous return of blood back to the heart.

We can see the heart and circulatory system active, like an internalized sun, at the centre of our inner solar system, regulating and harmonizing all the forces of the other planets, bringing balance into the life, light and warmth of the whole human constitution.[27]

Rajan is in many aspects a well-proportioned person. He is of medium height, upright posture, walks with measured self-assurance and meets people with an open and friendly demeanour. People describe him as having a sunny disposition. He is warm and positive, cheerful and enthusiastic, honest and generous, loving and compassionate. He radiates a sense of clarity, self-confidence and centredness. One always knows where one stands with him and it is easy to trust and respect him.

He is the most popular person in his class and is frequently chosen to represent his classmates because of his integrity and authenticity. He seems able to hold his inner and outer world in balance, providing what he needs for his own wellbeing and making space for other things in his life.

He enjoys the rhythmic flow and cycles of nature and the outdoor life, art and culture, science and technology, and interaction with people, as much as he enjoys being on his own, learning about himself, searching for truth and studying life. He loves researching the lives of great individuals who have made an impact on the world. After school he wishes to become a medical doctor.

Sun stands at the centre of things, creating balance between the supersensible spirit and sense-bound matter, between cosmos and earth, light and dark, day and night, buoyancy and gravity, form and substance. The sun character is radiant, harmonious, balanced, centred, measured, generous, light-filled, warm and loving.

It may become clear from the above description that a working knowledge of the seven character types may help to shed light on the unfolding soul nature of the adolescent and to understand their one-sided tendencies. All seven principles are latently present and usually one, or at most two, come to prominence. As we have seen in the examples given above, strongly expressed characterological tendencies can create psycho-social difficulties for the adolescent; a sensitive understanding of these seven character types will enable us to work creatively with the young person to draw out other latent soul elements that balance and correct exaggerated character dispositions. There are a range of therapeutic options that can be used to modify extreme one-sided tendencies. These will be described at length in Part 3. The character types can also become a very useful tool for evaluating and assisting pupils pedagogically in secondary school.

In our quest to understand the growing child and adolescent, we have examined three typologies – the constitution, the temperament and the character – as universal principles underlying the phenomena we observe during these life periods.[28] It is important to realize that hereditary tendencies and prenatal influences are powerful pre-determining factors in the sequential development and expression of these three universal elements. As determinants from the past, they are relatively fixed and can be transformed only by the consciously working human I, usually after the I has found its independence, after the age of 21. What is fixed by the past lends itself more to typologies than those aspects of life that are in constant motion and transformation and that have not yet come into being.

The Core Picture and Care of Late Childhood and Adolescence

- During this epoch the etheric growth forces and the astral soul forces converge in the metabolic-limb system, leading to all the phenomena of puberty.
- With the birth of the astral body, the soul awakens on two fronts of experiences: into emotional and sexual will impulses via the urogenital system and into intellectual thinking experiences via the neuro-sensory system.
- This initiates the age of great polarities and contrasts governed essentially by the swing between the hot, mobile, passionate metabolic-blood experience and the cool, quiet, critical nervous-system experience.
- Awakening into independent thinking heralds this age as the epoch of truth, galvanized by a new sense of self and a search for an independent identity. It is the age of idealism, discovery, adventure, striving for knowledge, pushing the frontiers and orientation towards the future in search of truth and self.
- With the unfolding of destiny and the flowering of youth, the character or personality is born.
- Thinking becomes the dominant element of this time, as the adolescent discovers the power of rational and critical thinking, her own judgements, opinions and decisions.
- The childhood journey is again recapitulated in the three phases of this period.
  - In the first phase, the new-found faculty of thinking is tempestuously and explosively influenced by the stormy waves of the emotional life of will activity. Authority is unceremoniously and critically discarded; wonder and trust are rejected for the values of the modern world. Movement in a variety of forms accompanies the wild search for self.

- In the middle phase, the life of feeling evolves in the experience of contrasting feelings and emotions and in the awakening desire for another person; this also colours and strengthens the surge towards independent thinking in desire for knowledge and the awakening of the power of judgement.
- In the third phase, the power of rational, independent thinking comes into its own as the adolescent begins to give structure to her life and future, preparing the way towards adulthood and the birth of her I nature.

The above indications are general principles that can be formulated by a sensitive exploration of late childhood and adolescence; such an understanding will lead to a rational approach to the care of this age period. At the same time, each year of adolescence, as the roadmap reveals, has its own unique character and requires special care.

- A respect for the young person's own sense of truth and voyage of discovery is the essential challenge for caring adults. One trusts that by the time the teenager has begun to withdraw from the protected parental environment, the physical and psychological support provided during the previous thirteen to fourteen years has had a positive effect on the adolescent's wellbeing.
- She must be supported in finding her own truth about her unfolding life, having to learn through trial and error what is and what is not good for her. This applies to every aspect of life: food and drink, physical health, personal life, social life and school life. If the young person feels this respect for truth, she will naturally be more willing to listen to the guidance of a more experienced adult; for while she wishes to discover life for herself, she is also insecure about this new world and wants to learn how things can be done in the most effective way possible.
- In accordance with her development, maturity, temperament and character, one should strive to create for the adolescent a healthy balance between structured boundaries and freedom. The teenager and adolescent generally requires clear boundaries

to her freedom. Most young adolescents secretly value this as the invisible support they need while they are exploring their frontiers. Too much structure or too much freedom can have devastating consequences at this age.

- Negotiation and contractual arrangements are the most effective ways of communicating with teenagers and adolescents. It is essential to engage their thinking, co-operation and active participation in everything that concerns them. We always have to remember, though, that they need to push us away and find their own way forward.

- Space should be given for the young person to exercise her soul life, independent thinking, feelings and need for activity and movement. One should strive to withhold judgement, and to avoid taking her criticism personally.

- Each year will offer different challenges to the caring adult.
    - The delicate unfolding of sexuality and the birth of destiny in the 14-year-old.
    - The intense vulnerability and longing to reclaim her lost spiritual home at 15; idols, cravings and addictions need to be seen in this light
    - The longing to find new truth and meaning in life in the 16-year-old
    - The search for self and a vocation or career at 17
    - The need to orientate, to test and to challenge oneself in the 18-year-old
    - Consolidation and apprenticeship at 19
    - Preparation for manhood and womanhood in the 20-year-old
    - The birth of the I at 21.

Naturally this biographical road map of the adolescent are general indications that will vary greatly in the biographies of individual children.

I feel power in my limbs, in my loins and in my new-found thinking. It makes me feel I am my own self. It gives me a feeling of freedom and a wish to find my independence. Yet as I break through the castle gates, I feel frightened and alone: I have left my home. Where do I belong? I find myself on a painful journey of discovery. I have the power, I lose the power. Who am I? Where am I going? Why am I going there? Gradually I begin to feel safer and more secure; I become someone I begin to trust, I start to recognize my own character. One step at a time, I forge my journey. I test my destiny, my limits and my endurance. I am searching for meaning. I sense the awakening of true power, a power that lies at the centre of my being; a power that has guided me from the beginning of time. I am dimly aware that I have come home.

Chapter 10

The Body-Soul-Spirit Continuum in Childhood and Youth

Three Creative Dimensions of Being Interweave and Interact Throughout Life

We have come to the point in our journey through childhood and adolescence where the individual has been born into the adult world as autonomous ego or I. With this landmark, the journey is in one sense complete.

Looking Back on the Journey

We accompanied the child on his voyage from prenatal into earthly existence, through the creative moment of conception when his physical development began.

We tried to experience the unfolding growth of life forces, first within the neuro-sensory system in the first seven-year period, then in the rhythmical system in the second seven-year period and finally in the metabolic-limb system in the third seven-year period. As mineral substances penetrated these forces like iron filings in a magnetic force field, the physical body assumed its spatial form and dimensions, growing and developing in accordance with the inner unfolding of the etheric body.

This developmental movement proceeds in sequential order from the past towards the future. Simultaneously, we attempted to experience the awakening of conscious soul life, first through the consolidation of the will in the first seven-year period, then through the development of the feeling life in the second seven-year phase and finally through the development of thinking in the third seven-year cycle. We discover when we step into experiencing the awakening psyche of the child, that we are in a different relationship to time compared to experiencing the growing child.

Observe where the will is coming from in the child throwing a tantrum: there is something he wants that he has not yet acquired. Will is a force that comes from and is directed to something that exists in the future: desires, wishes and intentions arise from and flow towards the future; my desire for something pleasurable is for something that exists in the future and that can only be satisfied there. Notice where feelings lie in relation to time: the happy or sad child lives in the present moment only; other feelings, such as hope and fear are influenced by something in the future that has not yet come about, while feelings such as doubt and disappointment are affected by events that have happened in the past; the child's hope for a shiny new red bicycle is directed towards his birthday tomorrow; the child who doubts his abilities and says he can't do sums bases this on his previous experience of not being able to do sums.

Thinking on the other hand is based on mental images and memory determined by the past. Reflective thinking or recollection by its very nature always focuses on events, experiences or sense impressions that have already happened.

We thus notice that when we follow inwardly the developmental movement of the awakening psyche, we move in reversed sequence from the future through the present into the past.[1]

At birth, the physical body was freed from its maternal sheaths to begin its independent life on earth. At the change of teeth in the seventh year, the life body was born out of the etheric parental sheaths, to become freer from its organic functions and to work more independently in the realm of soul and spirit. At puberty, in the fourteenth or fifteenth year, the astral body was released from its parental and community sheath to unfold its independent life in the soul and spirit. With the birth of the I in the twenty-first year, the young adult can step out of the protective I sheath formed by surrounding adults, and forge his own path and destiny.

For the purpose of clarity and understanding, all these processes have been described separately. We now wish to attempt to bring them together and to conceive of the body, soul and spirit as an interweaving continuum of three different realities. We will try to understand how the physical world impacts on soul and spirit, and how the latter affect physical life.

Interplay of Spirit, Soul and Body

When Thandi was fifteen she consulted me with a severe skin inflammation: her arms, legs face and chest were dry, flaming red and extremely itchy. She was not an allergic child and had ingested nothing that might have set off an allergic reaction. On enquiring what was going on at home, she informed me that she had been furious with her parents for the past few days; she was so frustrated because they were not hearing her and she had lost control of her temper – and was grounded as a result for four weeks, unfairly she felt.

One could literally see in this choleric girl the blood surging into the outer perimeter of her fortress, ready to defend or attack as the need arose. I asked her to show me how she felt by expressing herself through her body. We were able to see a visible image of the frustrated hot-tempered person who needed to be heard and treated fairly. Thandi could see this part of herself from the outside and allow this part of her personality to express itself freely. She then offered herself the support that only a best friend could give her.

At the end of this short session her skin looked less inflamed, and symptoms of warmth and itch had receded. In the following days, she continued to process her angry self and give it what it needed and her condition rapidly improved.

It is well known that many symptoms of childhood illness have psychological causes: digestive disturbances, asthma, eczema and allergies may be provoked by emotional factors and may also be alleviated by dealing with these causes. I can remember as a young child bringing on a tummy-ache when I didn't want to go to school; and I would need to empty my bladder frequently when anxious before an exam or running an athletics race.

Can you remember experiences that link emotions and bodily functions? What happens within your body when you are angry, frustrated, worried, frightened, upset, happy, enthusiastic or excited? Feelings and emotions will always bring about some physiological change, much of which can be noticed through attentive observation.[2]

Most open-minded health practitioners will admit this connection, to which the term 'psychosomatic' is applied. However it is frequently used in a somewhat disparaging way to denote a pathological condition where no physical cause can be found. The reality that body and psyche are a continuum is often overlooked. It is clear from its etymological derivation in ancient Greek that this term implies a connection between *psyche*, the soul, and *soma*, the body. The term however needs to be expanded to include the spirit, which as we have seen has an extremely powerful influence on the life of body and soul, and we could therefore coin the term *pneumo-psychosomatic* (*pneumo* means 'spirit' in Greek).

It is evident that the body can affect the soul and spirit just as the latter can influence the body. Physical substances such as grass and pollen, for example, will cause the physical symptoms of hay fever in allergic children, but also the psychological symptoms of irritability and bad behaviour. On the other hand, a sensitive, shy child in an anxious situation may develop an asthma attack, because the emotions trigger off neuro-chemical and immune-modulating substances, which lead to acute bronchospasm.

The relatively new field of **psychoneuro-immunology** attempts to validate these connections scientifically. The interaction between body and psyche has its origins in scientific work done in the early 20th century when it was discovered that emotions could be provoked by stimulating parts of the brain. The word psychoneuro-immunology was coined in 1975 by Robert Ader, who demonstrated that the nervous system can affect the immune system in rats. Candice Pert, the well-known neuroscientist and body-mind researcher, discovered many information substances in the form of neuropeptides and neurotransmitters that communicate between the nervous, endocrine and immune systems. She demonstrated that the emotions and the immune systems are interdependent and that they are modulated by the central nervous system. These discoveries have provided the scientific foundation for holistic and complementary medicine as well as the rational integration of medical disciplines known today as *integrative medicine.*

Psychoneuro-immunology recognizes the difference between psyche and brain, yet still searches for the psyche as located somewhere within the physical body. Even Candice Pert for many years regarded the 'psyche' and 'neuro' as synonymous.[3]

There is now irrefutable evidence that the psyche affects the body: emotions and behaviour have been shown to affect immune function, and immune alterations to induce behavioural and emotional changes. PNI research is seeking the exact mechanisms by which the immune system and brain 'talk to each other'. Much of the research focuses on the hypothalamic-pituitary-adrenal axis (HPA axis) and the autonomic nervous system (ANS). The HPA axis is a complex interactive system between the hypothalamus (a hollow, funnel-shaped part of the brain), the pituitary gland (a pea-shaped structure located below the hypothalamus), and the adrenal (or suprarenal) glands (small, conical organs on top of the kidneys). Together with the involuntary or reflex-acting ANS, these systems have been shown to play a major part in the neuro-endocrine system that controls reactions to stress and regulates many body processes, including digestion, the immune system, mood and emotions, sexuality, and energy storage and expenditure.

The functions of the soul we have been considering throughout this book – cognitive, affective and volitional responses – are for the most part still regarded by science today as an outcome, be it in some bio-molecular or bio-energetic form, of the neuro-endocrine system. There is very little research indicating that these neuro-hormonal responses are physical reactions to interdependent soul activities.[4]

The idea that the soul is an independent entity and not part of the body is difficult for Western medical science to conceive because it cannot be scientifically proven. Science prides itself on its objectivity, which requires that the personal subjective element, namely the psyche, be removed from the field of enquiry. This mode of observation is appropriate when one is investigating the physical world, but is totally inappropriate when one wishes to know something about the psychological dimension. The psyche is inevitably subjective and personal. To investigate this domain, therefore, one must turn an objective eye upon subjectivity. We have attempted throughout this book to place the phenomena of soul life on the research table and examine them like any other object of observation.

Pneumo-Psychosomatic Factors in Child Health

In our journey through child development we have discovered the close correspondence between biological and psychological function. The healthy development of each system and the healthy functional relationship between biological and psychological systems has major implications for the child's future health.

The Neuro-Sensory System

We have seen that the neuro-sensory system as the child's information-receiving system provides the biological basis for the psychological functions of thinking, sensing and therefore all cognitive learning. Sensing needs the apparatus of the sense organs, which are extensions of the nervous system, while thinking requires the instrument of the healthy functioning brain (see Chapter six, p. 158ff).

A child will be able to sense and think effectively only when he has a strong and well-developed neuro-sensory system; healthy sensing and thinking will in turn develop this system.

Accordingly, strengthening the child's nervous system will create a firm foundation for healthy cognitive functions. One therefore wants to give the child an environment that can stimulate the senses in a healthy way, and avoid over-stimulation of the neuro-sensory system by abstract intellectual learning and excessive TV or computer viewing.

The Rhythmic System

This is made up of the integrated totality of all rhythmic activities in the human organism. The primary rhythmic organs comprise the cardiovascular-respiratory system, which, through the rhythm of contraction and expansion, bring harmony to the breathing and circulatory processes. The integrated rhythmic system is the basis for all biological rhythmic functions and is finely tuned to the life of feeling. We have explored the effect of the breathing and heart rhythm on the life of feelings and emotions. Research into this system will naturally require a study of rhythmic processes. An experience of the rhythmic system will naturally only be possible in the experience of rhythm itself, which, as we discovered in Chapter eight, exists in the momentary interval between rest and movement. What is the experience of this interval, this ever-present moment? Perhaps it is the realm of pure feeling. Perhaps we can only experience rhythm through tuning to it in our feeling life.

If healthy rhythm and feelings are intimately connected, one may presume that the healthy development of feeling will support a healthy rhythmic system, ensuring strong heart and lungs. It also means that a healthy rhythmic system is the best foundation for healthy feelings.

Allowing a child to express his feelings actively, and providing established routines and rhythms in his life, will therefore strengthen all rhythmic organs and functions.

The Metabolic-Limb System

This system makes use of the metabolic-motor organs to generate metabolism and movement, which bring the child into physical contact with the outside world. These organs are the power stations generating the energy needed to activate all physical and psychological functions. We have seen that the will forces needed to perform any function, mental or physical, arise out of the generating activity of these organ systems. We can only research metabolic processes by directly experiencing the activity of some living process – for only then are we engaged in will activity itself. The moment we withdraw from this will-based experience and observe the phenomenon from without, we have left the realm of metabolism. Therefore a science that prides itself on its scientific objectivity and proclaims this as the benchmark for real science, inevitably excludes all phenomena that concern the will, metabolism and rhythmic processes.

This relationship between metabolic organs and the will infers that a healthy life of will leads to strong metabolism and muscular-skeletal system, which in turn provides a good foundation for creativity and for the life of will. Encouraging healthy movement and active exploration and creativity will therefore strengthen the individual's metabolic and locomotor systems.

Body-Soul-Spirit Continuum

Let us now explore the pneumo-psychosomatic connection and continuum further. We return to our first premise: that the child's emerging soul exists and develops between the body and spirit. The body is a product and extension of the world of matter, while the spirit is a representative element of the world of spirit.

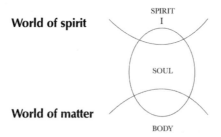

During waking life, our soul life becomes active: the outer world generates sense experiences which make up a great content of our soul experiences. Sense impressions are received at the frontier between body and soul, through the twelve sense organs that mediate the sense-perceptible world in different ways.[5] These sense impressions set in motion an instant communication between body, soul and spirit, where activities such as desires, sensations, feelings, mental pictures and thought processes ultimately lead to actions that are carried out at a physical, psychological or spiritual level. Or else soul life is activated from within through desires, sensations, feelings, mental pictures or thought processes, and this can lead to actions at the level of body, soul or spirit.

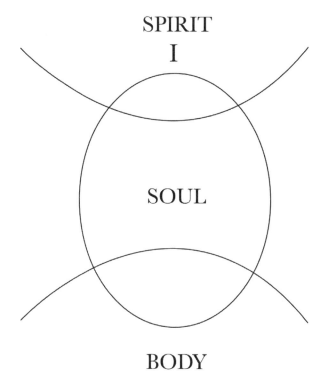

SPIRIT

I

SOUL

BODY

Body–Soul–Spirit Continuum

Experiencing the Pneumo-Psychosomatic Continuum

We can verify for ourselves the nature of this continuum between body, soul and spirit by exploring one of thousands of soul experiences that take place daily in our lives.

We can become aware of something that gives pleasure or displeasure: for example, fragrant, strong coffee in the morning, the anticipation of relaxing after strenuous activity or having to face some difficulty at home or at work. The I, which belongs to the realm of spirit, becomes active in the sensing of the coffee aroma. The olfactory sense organs, which belong to the body, convey impressions from outside into inner soul experience. The sense impression pushes through the boundary between body and soul without us having any control over the process.

With careful observation one will notice that two things appear to happen simultaneous with the sense perception.

Firstly, something from within immediately comes to meet the fragrant scent of the coffee. In the moment that the sense impression enters the soul, we are drawn towards it by a force that impels us to take an interest in it. When we trace this experience we find that **desire** or **interest** for the coffee rise up from some unconscious realm of the *body*. Desire meets the sense impressions at the boundary of the soul as they enter through our sense organs; this desire takes hold of the sense experience and changes it into a **sensation**. The body tingles with anticipation of the coffee.

Instantly we feel pleasure and delight in the experience. We connect the sensation with a pleasurable and sympathetic feeling experience. Someone else however might dislike this experience and feel antipathy towards it. We see that as soon as desire emerges, feelings arise. If the **feelings** alone satisfy us, the desire subsides and disappears; if not, the desire continues. The more the desire swirls around the soul, encountering sense impressions, the more sensations arise.

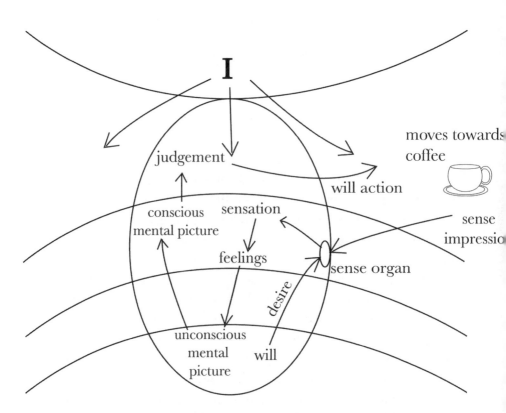

Body–Soul–Spirit Continuum experiencing coffee

The I then becomes engaged in the will; we make a move towards the coffee.

Thus, the sense impressions awaken desire, which creates sensations and feelings, which lead to a **will action**.[6]

Secondly, and simultaneously, we experience the need to know what we perceive. From the more conscious realm of the *spirit*, where thinking has awakened, thoughts grasp hold of the perception or sensation of the fragrant coffee to form a concept or mental picture. The I now becomes active in deliberation or judging; this leads to a specific mental image and to cognitive understanding of what has been perceived.

I love that scent of the coffee and I must pour myself a cup.

The memory of previously enjoyed coffee may now unfold through the release of previous mental images that were locked up in the etheric memory resonance bank.

We thus see that certain soul elements appear to arise within the soul itself, whereas other elements have their source in the body or spirit; the two elements belonging specifically to the soul life are feelings – including sympathy/antipathy – and deliberation or judging.[7] All other elements either come from without via the body or from within via the spirit.

Effects of the Body-Soul-Spirit Continuum in the Life of The Child

In early childhood the soul is deeply submerged in the body, and therefore what evokes the soul life will have a direct effect on the body. Thus sense impressions which enter the body from without through the sense organs, lead to sensations such as warmth or pain. At the same time, bodily experiences such as hunger or thirst will lead to feelings of discomfort and displeasure. These sensations and feelings activate the life of will, which as we have seen is deeply rooted in the body in the young child, leading to the desire for food and the appropriate call to satisfy this need. The desire and interest for something may also enter the soul through contact with the outer world. The child sees his milk bottle and wants to drink it. We thus see once again that desire, which belongs to the life of will, is closely connected with sensory experiences.

Whether desires or needs are satisfied or not will make a great difference to the child's wellbeing.

Let us imagine a child who needs attention. When the desire for affection is directly met, the child is happy; the desire ends because it is satisfied and in its place a feeling of pleasure arises. On the other hand, when the need for affection is not met, the desire continues and the child is unhappy. Unfulfilled needs or desires and associated negative feelings of pain, guilt, loneliness, fear, doubt, hatred, etc. will have a damaging effect on the child's physical and also psychospiritual health.

As the soul life develops, other elements begin to awaken and gradually, around the time of puberty, begin to emerge from their physical containment. Mental pictures begin to play a significant part in the child's soul experience. Judging and other feeling-related experiences will influence the life of mental images which will feed the imagination and fantasy.

We notice that these mental images, like desires, appear to have a life of their own. Just as we cannot easily control our desires and do not know where they arise from, so we cannot always bring back a previously created mental image, and are unaware of where they disappear to. Steiner informs us that a great proportion of our store of mental images continue to live unconsciously in the life body and are brought back into consciousness at given moments only with the I's participation in the act of remembering. The I must form an active connection with the life body. Memory is thus the process whereby the I enters the etheric body and casts the mental image from the past upon its inner mirror.[8]

When these images cannot be brought back into consciousness, they continue to live an independent existence in the unconscious etheric depths of the soul, where they may exert a negative effect on the physical body.

Let us imagine a child has experienced his violent father abusing his mother. The sense impressions and judgements made by the child create mental images of these frightening experiences; they sink down into unconscious soul life where they are stored as a cluster of vibrating experiences in the etheric body. According to their nature they will resonate with a corresponding frequency. These images left unattended are the causes of the deepest suffering and ill-health, both to the child's body and soul, and continue to exert their effects well into adult life. To transform these images in an appropriate way will be of great help to the child.

Desire, for example for affection or attention, which remains unsatisfied, and mental images of negative experiences that are locked away in the life body's unconscious memory, are the source of a great deal of physical and psychological illness. Part 2 will focus on physical and psychological disturbances in childhood, where these effects and their therapeutic correction will be examined in detail.

From the realm of the spirit, the I is active wherever it is needed: in the body-based sensory world where perceptions and sensations are experienced; in the life-based etheric world where mental pictures are remembered; in the soul-based feeling world where sympathy or antipathy and judgements are experienced; and in the spirit-based reflective/cognitive world where conclusions are formed.

It is an extraordinary human phenomenon that all this occurs in a flash outside space and time, in the blink of an eye, and happens thousands of times every day! With every perception or mental picture, desires, interest, feelings, judgements and mental images are evoked without us normally being aware of them!

Soul Pictures During Childhood and Adolescence

Let us now consider the soul experience of children at different stages of development.

- Two-year-old Thandi before she attains self-awareness in the third year of life
    The soul forces of a child at Thandi's age are primarily active in her body. Her life forces are working on the development of the brain, nervous tissue and sense organs, growing and developing these organs so that her soul can make the best use of them. In

her soul life she has become wholly sense experience, absorbing every sense impression through her twelve sense organs.

These sense impressions coming from the outer and inner world actively engage her will; with passionate desire and interest for the smallest detail, she drinks in the sensory world, thus forming sensations that her body likes or does nor like. Her I is actively involved in her sense experience and her will activities. Her feeling life is strongly linked to these inner bodily sensations. The untamed, animal-like sentient body devours the sense impressions, pushing them down for further processing into the bowels of the etheric body. Here, on the impressionable, wax-like matrix of resonant life forces, these sensations are imprinted for future reference as unconscious memory.

Thandi thus becomes a master imitator, since everything she has experienced is now drawn out of her life body and reflected back to the world. She has learned to walk and to talk by

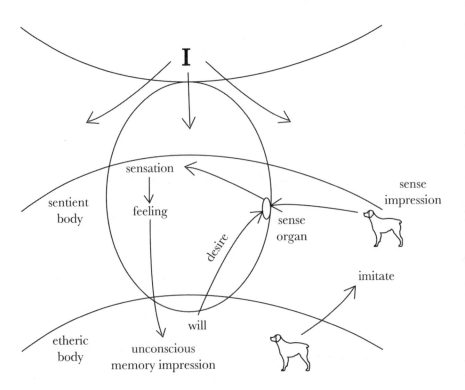

Body–Soul–Spirit Continuum before third year of life

observing walking and talking in her environment, and acting out what is living in her life body. There is no discerning or protective power available to her, no capacity of reasoning or memory that can counteract or adjust the compelling nature that the body and the outer world exert on her.

- Thandi after she has become aware of herself as a self-contained individual

  Thand's I can now engage in the unconscious activity and begin to exert its individual preferences. For instance, when she sees a fluffy dog, her current sensations create a new etheric image which stimulates the old images she has experienced of

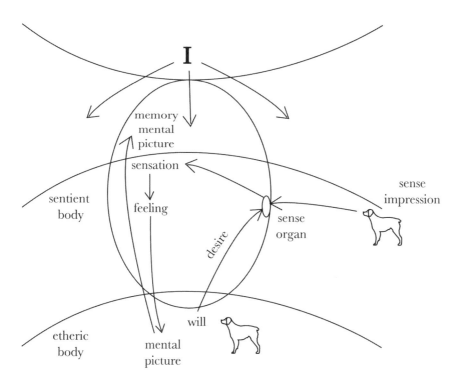

Body–Soul–Spirit Continuum after third year of life

fluffy dogs. Now the I can dive down into the etheric body and reflect back the image as a mental picture. She remembers the dog and can consider whether she wants to play with it. She has begun to use her reasoning faculties because her I is available for this participation. The dawning of choice and freedom has begun.

- Adam when he was a nine- or ten-year-old child

 With the change of teeth, some of Adam's life forces became available for body-free thinking. The life forces still bound to the body are actively working in the rhythmic functions of the body and the soul, as we saw in the development of all aspects concerned with the life of rhythm. This rhythmic activity allows the soul to awaken the faculty of feeling.

 When Adam finds a shiny new bicycle waiting for him on his tenth birthday, his desire for it calls up powerful rhythmic sensations in his body which are translated into strong feelings

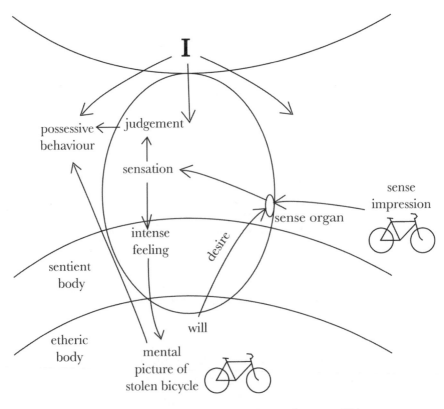

Body–Soul–Spirit Continuum in tenth year of life

of delight and happiness. His I engages in his feelings and his reasoning, judgement and behaviour are strongly influenced by these feelings. For instance, he becomes very possessive and more caring of his bicycle and decides to look after it more carefully than the last one that was stolen. This attitude is also strongly motivated by the memory he has of the stolen bicycle and the sadness that it caused him when he lost it.

- Rajan between the age of 15 and 16

  We should remember that Rajan has gone through puberty, and that his soul life is beginning to open out towards the world. His life forces are freer to work into his feeling life, and the life forces still working organically are now engaging in his metabolism, limbs and reproductive organs.

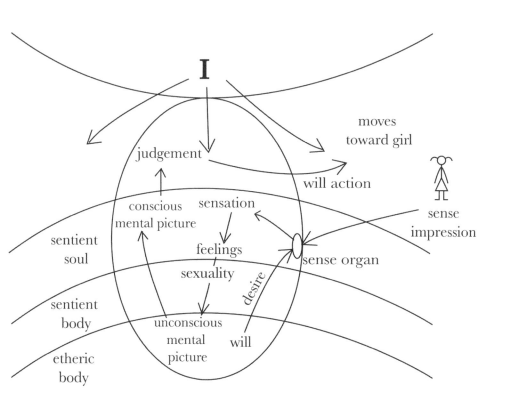

Body–Soul–Spirit Continuum in sixteenth year of life

Rajan notices Saskia, a beautiful girl in his class; he is especially attracted to her green eyes, black hair and slim body, and feels the urge to get to know her. The I active in sensing goes out to meet the sense impressions arising from her attractive face and sensuous body, and his bodily sense organs convey impressions from without which penetrate his inner soul experience. Rajan is drawn towards Saskia by his desire which arises from the body. At the boundary of the soul, desire fuses with his sense impressions, changing it into sensations of a sensuous and sexual nature. His heart beats faster; his blood pulsates through his body. He feels pleasure and delight in what he has experienced. He connects the sensation he experiences with a pleasurable and sympathetic feeling experience. These sensations may at first be unfamiliar and difficult to master especially as the new experience of sexuality awakens. He may experience any of the wide range of adolescent feelings such as shame, doubt, fear, hope, boldness, disappointment and nervousness. His I has now become active in feeling. His judgement and feeling responses expand his imagination and fantasy. Next his I becomes engaged in his will and he may move physically towards the girl because he wishes to interact directly with her. At the same time, a need arises to know what he perceives; he inwardly judges and then becomes conscious that *this is a pretty girl whom I would like to get to know*. He moves towards meeting her as the memory of previous acquaintences unfold through the release of mental images.

- Maria at the age of 19

The life forces are nearing the completion of their bodily work, having grown the limbs, consolidated the metabolism and matured the reproductive organs. These life forces are becoming more available for the full activities of Maria's soul life as they express themselves in independent thinking, feeling for others and actions that will determine her future life.

She is in a meaningful relationship with her boyfriend and is faced with the dilemma of going away for the weekend with him or studying for her university examinations. Her desire to go with him surges through her when he tries to convince her to come. She is aware of how she is sexually aroused by her feelings and inner sensations. Her I surges down into bodily and

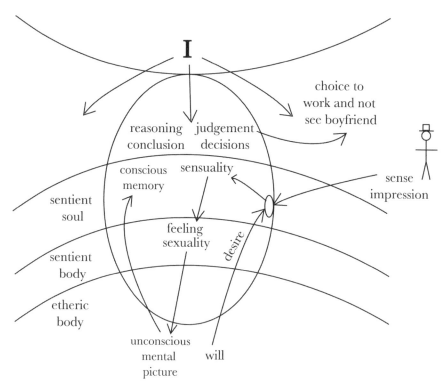

Body–Soul–Spirit Continuum in the adult

emotional places. However, she is able to turn away from this awareness and consider her responsibilities. She remembers her commitment to her studies. Her I flashes into reasoning and judgement, calls up a mental picture that reminds her of her responsibilities, arrives at a conclusion and makes a decision not to go. The I is moving towards its independent life when it can make choices not merely for transient pleasure, but ones that are true and good for the bigger picture of life ahead.

Summary of the Continuum

From our experience thus far, and with the examples given, we can state the following:

The body conveys sense impressions via our sense organization, and, via our will organization, pushes desire into the realm of soul where it is experienced as sensations, feelings and mental pictures. The spirit dives down into the will and sensory life of the body, into the feeling and judgement life of the soul, and into the memory bank of the life body to retrieve unconscious etheric images. The sensations, feelings, judgements and mental pictures of soul experience can work down into the body through actions of the will or up into the spirit through actions of the I.

In every moment of the child's life, this continuum of body, soul and spirit is happening all the time in continuous interaction. Outer events leading to bodily changes influence the life of soul and spirit; soul experiences interact with body and spirit; spirit activities penetrate soul and body. Every aspect of child development may be considered from this point of view. One thereby gains a new perspective and depth of understanding that equips one to care for the child in a responsible way. This can also provide one with new possibilities for addressing, supporting and where necessary correcting problems and difficulties that the child encounters.

But how do the different members of these three realms – body, soul and spirit – convey their information content to each other? How for instance does the sentient body pass its bodily awareness to the sentient soul so that it becomes a soul experience? To put this more tangibly, how does the desire for a cup of coffee and its rich aroma and taste turn into a deeply satisfying and pleasurable feeling? Or how does the experience of sentient soul transform into awareness in the body? How does a feeling such as anger instantly move the blood and cause heat and redness in the face, a rise in blood pressure and a racing heart?

And how does the I as a spiritual entity bring about instant changes in the body or soul when it senses, feels or acts in a particular way? How does the I, when it feels deeply hurt and humiliated by something, move the body so quickly and powerfully to carry out a violent act? Or how does it stop the overwhelming impulse of anger and prevent harm to human life?

A new medicine based on the body-soul-spirit continuum has its foundations on insight into these questions.

The questions above locate the interfaces between the three realms of body, soul and spirit. Now let us examine these interfaces more precisely.

Soul and Body Interface

On the one hand, the astral body mediates between body and soul. In our study of the developed astral body we found that it is composed of sentient *soul* and sentient *body*. We learned that the sentient body is the finer aspect of the etheric body, and provides us with the means to perceive and sense the outer world. The sentient soul on the other hand is that part of the soul where inner experience begins and where sensations, sympathies and antipathies, feelings and mental picturing are experienced.

It is within the astral body – the body of consciousness – that the sense impressions are experienced and immediately imprinted onto the wax-like matrix of the life body.

This is how sentient life gains access to the physiological processes of the body.

For instance, a child experiences violence; the sense impressions, mental pictures and anxious feelings are mediated by the sentient soul to cause the sentient body to resonate in a particular way; this may result in asthmatic breathing constriction. Soul experience thus becomes body experience.

The process can also flow in the reverse direction; a high pollen count may trigger an asthmatic attack which results in feelings of anxiety; the resonating sentient-etheric body can thus invoke a soul experience in the sentient soul.

Through this intimate interface between the sentient body and sentient soul, we discover that all the physiological processes mentioned in Chapter seven have their corresponding psychological processes.

The life process of breathing regulates breathing at all physiological levels – sensory, respiratory and circulatory; at the soul level it regulates 'breathing' in feeling life; thus excessive in-breathing of the soul manifests in fear and anxiety, whereas excessive out-breathing comes to expression in anger. Fear and anxiety at the psychological level will translate to restricted asthmatic type breathing at the physiological level, a correspondence that is frequently found in asthmatic children.

Likewise the dynamic life process of secreting works physiologically in the glandular and eliminating functions of the body, and psychologically on the individual's ability to express himself freely.[9] Thus children whose free soul expression is blocked frequently display symptoms of glandular congestion or digestive obstruction, such as sinusitis, adenoid congestion and constipation.

And the same is true of all the other life processes.

The table below schematically represents these connections.

Life process	Physiological function	Psychological function
Breathing	Respiration, circulation, sensing	Emotional in-breathing – fear or out-breathing – anger
Warming	Warmth processes	Warm or cold personality
Nourishing	Nutrition, metabolism	Soul digestion – well digested or undigested experiences
Secreting	Glandular, elimination	Soul expression – blocked, rigid or open
Maintaining	Immune functions	Soul maintenance – care or neglect
Growing	Growth and development	Personal growth – stagnation or progression
Reproducing	Reproduction, cell division	Creativity – artistic, spiritual

Soul and Spirit Interface

The personal or intellectual mind-soul mediates between the soul and spirit. This is the aspect of the soul that brings the rational, cognitive life of the spirit into the soul realm. Deliberations, judgements, ideas, conclusions, decisions and resolves that are taken up by the spirit can have their expression in the workings of soul, and thence also in the body. In the example above, Maria is tempted to spend the weekend away with her boyfriend; the feelings and sensations arising from her soul and body experience pull her in this direction.

However, from a realm free of the body and the psyche, the I brings down truths that go beyond the transient pleasures of satisfying body and soul needs. Her motivation, wishes and higher intentions to develop her career and to fulfill her life destiny, determine her resolution and actions. To be sure she has to struggle with the forces rampant in her soul but in the end her spirit wins the day and she is able to subdue her feelings with logic and good reason.

Interface of the Elements

Early on in this book we drew on experience awareness to explore the realm of the four elements and discovered that our human bodies are composed of four elemental systems: a solid organism composed of the body's solid matter, a fluid organism composed of various fluids, an aeriform organism containing all the body's gaseous contents, and a warmth organism consisting of the body's varied and differentiated warmth components.

We also found that it is possible to observe and think in four different, element-related ways if we allowed the essential nature of each element to permeate our mode of observation and thinking. Likewise we discovered that each of the four members or sheaths which make up our human constitution is connected with a specific element.

Earth	Solid system	Solid substance	Earth observation	Physical/ mineral body	Lifeless corpse
Water	Fluid system	Fluid substance	Fluid observation	Etheric/life body	Sleeping living body
Air	Aeriform system	Air substance	Aeriform observation	Psyche/soul	Dreaming awareness
Warmth	Warmth system	Warmth substance	Warmth observation	Human I	Conscious awareness

In our voyage through childhood, we found that the body's twelve sense organs – nine of which can be located at the physical level and the higher three at a supersensible level (see note on the 12 senses), are the instruments which enable us to sense the world.

The life body, working through the fluid organism, is the vehicle for the conceptual thinking process, and is made up of the four ethers – life ether, sound or chemical ether, light ether and warmth ether. Sound ether is primarily active in the fluid organism. We discovered in Chapter seven the essential nature of the four ethers in our thinking, see page 185ff.

The astral body works through the air element, thereby creating the instrument for feeling. Light ether is especially active in the air organism. We have seen repeatedly that feeling is an essential element of soul life.

The I organizes our 'warmth body' into a highly differentiated configuration and activates it. Working through the warmth ether, the I activates our will, setting in motion all the diverse will impulses: both those rooted in the body – instinct, drives and desires; and those formed in the spirit – motivation, wish, intention and resolve. And as we have seen it is the will that moves the body, the soul and the spirit.

How does the I activate the will? And how does it drive these will impulses so that it can work right into the human organism? If we can understand how the will interacts with the human constitution we will be closer to understanding the body-soul-spirit continuum.

The I can unite these impulses of will and direct them into the organism through the pivotal fact that the will works primarily in and through the warmth organism.[10] Warmth is the bridging element that participates in body, soul and spirit: it can warm the body through physical warmth, warm the soul through warm feelings, and warm the spirit through high ideals and noble actions.

Only warmth penetrates all levels of existence. It lives as a state of warmth independent of the other states of matter – solid, liquid and gas. It lives in the warm air we exhale, the warm blood, and in the warmth of our skin. It also lives, via the light ether, in the warmth of our feelings, via the sound ether in the warmth of our thinking, and via the life ether in the warmth of our sensing. And it lives as pure warmth as will activity.

In these ways, via the warmth organism, the I sends the will down into the air organism where it can affect any aspect of this organism – for instance the breathflow, or at a soul level, the feeling life. It can descend deeper into the fluid organism where it affects any function of the fluid body such as blood circulation, the flow of secretions or the faculty of thinking. Finally it can enter the realm of the physical organism where it has an impact on all solid, material structures of the body.

At the same time one can say that through the impulse of will, the I enters the warmth organism, and can thereby penetrate the air, fluid and solid organisms of the human being.

Physical Body	Sensing	Earth organism	Life ether
Etheric Body	Thinking	Fluid organism	Sound ether
Astral Body	Feeling	Air organism	Light ether
Human I	Willing	Warmth organism	Warmth ether

The Vital Role of Warmth

Returning to the question of how body, soul and spirit communicate with each other – how does body intelligence become soul experience, how does soul experience become body awareness? We can now see this from the perspective of the elements.

Someone once told me how he kept himself warm during a snowy night in subfreezing temperatures. He had with him a small gas cooker, a sleeping bag and a hot water bottle. He boiled up some snow in a pot, turning it into liquid water, then boiling water and then placed it in the hot water bottle where it kept him warm throughout the night.

Through the activity of warmth, solid ice changes into liquid water. With further warmth, liquid is transformed into air, and the air can be converted into heat. It can go the other way too – when warmth is withdrawn, it reverts back to air, liquid and solid substance.

Just as warmth changes ice into liquid water and steam, so if we take the *warmth* of desire for a cup of coffee (desire is will working through warmth) and combine it with *sense impressions* of fine taste and aroma (sensing takes into the body a fixed 'icy' image of the outer world) we get a pleasurable warm feeling both before and during drinking (feelings are mediated by the air). Warmth changing ice into water and steam therefore has a soul parallel in desire (warmth) changing sense impressions (ice) into sensations (liquid) and feeling (air, steam).

When a high degree of warmth is added to fluid that is at body temperature, the fluid is immediately mobilized and becomes warmer; and if the utensil holding it conducts heat well, it too will become hotter. The same happens when the will-warmth of anger dives down into the blood: the blood heats up, and moves around the body in a flash, causing the heart to beat faster and the body to become warmer. The increased heat may in turn fire up the will to act violently unless the I, working out of the cool regions of the rational mind, brings calmness to bear on the fiery will.

When warmth is removed from a fluid, the latter cools down. Likewise when a child's soul life cools down – when, for instance, he is anxious – tissues contract, blood flow is restricted and the body temperature cools down. The child becomes sick and we say the child has 'caught a cold'.

Pathology of Warmth and Cold

From these examples we can see how insight into the relationships between the four elements and the four human sheaths working within the body-soul-spirit continuum, can help us to understand the connections between the latter three realms, manifesting in both health and illness.

In Part 2, we will draw on these insights, and our experientially developed awareness, to explore pathology at a psychological, functional and structural level. We will see that the excessive warmth of unsatisfied desires, or the crystallized icy images incarcerated in the etheric body as a result of sustained fear, cause aberrant behaviour in a young child. If nothing is done to help, the psycho-emotional disturbance will result in functional changes such as appetite loss, or disrupted sleep or growth . If the life body continues to resonate in a disturbed way, physiological changes due to disturbance in one of the seven life processes become noticeable. For instance glandular secretions seen in a runny nose or cough become more prominent, liver and digestive congestion expressed in tummy aches, nausea, vomiting and diarrhoea occur, blood flow is increased in certain areas causing recurrent inflammations such as sore throat and earache, and the immune system is weakened, resulting in frequent infections.

If the problem continues unaddressed, the functional syndrome moves further into structural manifestation with the production of more permanent or chronic physical symptoms such as adenoid swelling, pneumonia, obesity, arthritis, or even cancer.

We can regard health as the balanced and harmonious interaction of the four human sheaths as mediated by their four elemental agencies. All pathology can be viewed as a disturbance in the relationship and interaction of these sheaths and elements. Healing must therefore be seen as the restoration and correction of a healthy balance between these sheaths and elements.[11]

Above and beyond the workings of all the different aspects of body, soul and spirit, it is the I alone, the core of our essential spiritual identity, that has the power to traverse all barriers and enter whichever realm the developing human individuality requires at any moment in time.

In the next chapter we will examine the nature of the human I in greater detail.

Awakening to the I

I am the Quintessential Source and Activity that Integrates and Guides the Human Being Towards his Chosen Destiny

The Nature of the I

On many occasions in preceding chapters, mention has been made of child's I. What do we understand by this single letter, which we make use of many times each day to refer to ourselves, and without which no one could communicate intelligibly?

From the moment we are aware of ourselves in the third year of life, we use this most modest of words to represent ourselves to the outside world. It is the only word in all languages which I use to refer only to myself, and that you use to refer only to yourself. Although it has a relationship with the physical, psychological and spiritual aspects of the human being, it exists as an I in its own realm, and with its own imitable activity.

I am an I to myself alone.[1]

What we have called the I can therefore only refer to an aspect of self that stands at the very centre of one's being. Although this term may be unfamiliar as an objective concept in itself, it accords with the designation every conscious human being uses for this human reality. Some readers may find it difficult to name it in this way; this may touch an ancient chord in the soul, for at one stage in humanity's evolution the name of the omnipotent God could not be uttered or written down. To this day Judaism forbids writing down the holy name of God, using only vowels to refer to it. The I is certainly connected with and related to the divine in us. Though we name it and refer to it many times a day in this small vowel, what do we consciously know about it?

Where in human experience is the I to be found and how can we experience it? If the I is the core of my being it must be closely connected to my experience. I cannot find it below the threshold of my consciousness; I must search for it in my waking, conscious experience.

There is a reality within me which, hundreds if not thousands of times every day, meets every perception that floods through my senses. This reality can grasp hold of the perception and internalize it through sensations; it can also mobilize the forming of concepts or mental pictures that allows me to be conscious, to think, and to give meaning to what I am perceiving or sensing. It can likewise activate the vast, musical range of feelings; and is also the reality underlying the exercising of will in countless different ways.

The I must be active in every such experience, as the common reality integrating them all. Imagine how busy and active it must be! In a flash it moves from perceiving to feeling to thinking to acting. In the words of a doctor I once knew, the I is 'pure activity'.

If the I is the core of my being it must also live in the body and soul and be innately involved in their nature and activities. It must be able to enter the realities of the physical, etheric or astral dimensions and operate in accordance with the laws of these realms.

Modern science would have us believe that what we name as I is, like everything else in our systems, a kind of material product of the body, like a neuro-chemical secretion or a creation of the human genome that somehow leads to experiences of the kinds mentioned above. Such a viewpoint subjugates and demeans the highest reality of every human being to a factor determined by the material world. In this scenario there would be no possibility of human freedom. The greatest human discoveries, creativity and expressions of moral individuality such as love, loyalty, faith and goodness would all have to be regarded as material products of the body. The human being would have no free choice and therefore would have no choice of freedom. Yet our experience tells us that we do have choices. Indeed we can decide to oppose the needs and desires of the body and soul, and act in a way that we believe is good and true. And in so doing we discover we have the potential for freedom.

This is a viewpoint that regards the I as an inner authority that can make choices which change the future. As such it can give direction to body and soul and thereby determine physical and psychological outcomes. We can come to see the I as a source and not the end result of our life here on earth. In our journey through childhood, adolescence and youth, we can therefore regard the I as the wellspring rather than the result of this developmental journey.

The Embodiment of the I

This book rests on the viewpoint, confirmed by experience, that a child is a physical-spiritual being. On this basis the question as to the origin of the soul-spiritual reality of the child and its connection with the physical dimension was examined in Chapter three. As suggested in the foreword, until our own conscious awareness can give answers to these questions, a description such as that put forward by a modern spiritual scientist of the calibre of Steiner may be taken as a starting point for awakening our inner understanding of these matters.

In accordance with this view it is the eternal I being of the child that, at a certain point in time, elects to return to the earth as part of a human evolutionary process that can take place only on our planet earth. The nature of the I partakes of a reality that is very different from the earthly dimension, and, if it is to become the main actor on the earthly stage, it must acquire the appropriate support for its brief sojourn on earth. It will have to acquire a human physical body, brought to life by a life body and given consciousness by a soul organization. It thereby clothes itself in a manner appropriate for human existence on the earthly plane.

Before conception, as we saw, the I has much to do with the shaping of the future earthly body, in the construction of the spirit germ and the drawing together of astral and etheric bodies. For the first two to three weeks after conception, the I, together with astral body and life body, is active outside the embryo, preparing the embryonic sheaths that will serve as the portal of entry and the creative working centre of the respective human members.

We saw that the I has a great deal to do with the development and the functions of the placenta; through the latter it is able to guide and direct the unfolding human drama of the ultimate creation – the physical body – using the astral and etheric body to help produce and develop the archetype or idea that underlies this creative process.

I am convinced that any person privileged to witness even a small phase of the exquisite precision and perfect synchronization of the nine-month embryonic process will experience a reality as close to perfection as they will ever discover. One is easily tempted to speak of a divine hand that guides this creative process. In the journey of the child towards human life on earth, we may regard this guiding hand as the child's own I, that wills the newborn baby into physical existence and inaugurates her life as a citizen of the world.

Before the I can take its rightful place as the conscious forger of its own destiny on earth, it must create the organs that make this possible. In the first two years, before the child is aware of herself as a separate individual, it has to achieve the three tasks that were described in Chapter five. These are the three fundamental functions that allow the I to reveal itself here on earth: the human faculties of walking, speaking and thinking.

From the moment the child is born, the I is actively at work in developing the organs of movement that will ultimately result in her learning to stand and walk. It will guide her through an intense learning experience from uncontrolled and uncoordinated movements, to controlled, purposeful movements: she learns to move the parts of her body, and her body as a whole, according to her needs. Gradually the I moves the child to find her equilibrium in space, through positions of horizontality to a position of verticality, which is an essential human prerequisite for her free movement in space and the further unfolding of her will.

Having found the means to move freely in the world and to meet her fellow human being with free and open arms, the

I moves the child to learn to speak so as to communicate with her fellows. Through this rhythmic interaction with people, she develops her organs of speech and at the same time her rhythmic system, which provides the physiological foundation for her organs of feeling.

With the first impressions that flood in through one or more of the twelve sense organs the I, through the etheric body, begins actively to shape the brain so that it can become the organ for cognitive human awareness and thinking that will allow consciousness to develop.

Only when these three human faculties are in place can the first awareness of oneself as an I take place in the third year, when the child first begins to use the word I. It is this event more than any other that so distinctly separates the first three years of the child's life from the rest of childhood – and indeed from the rest of her life. The child who is unaware of herself as an I is a very different human being from one who is conscious of herself as a distinct human individual.

It does not require special human faculties to recognize the unique nature of the child before she names herself I. Observe a healthy one- or two-year-old at any moment of her waking life and you will be struck by the extraordinary vitality and energy, powerful wilfulness and connectedness to all things that flow through the child. This is a consciousness that is at one with all things and which ends when the child becomes aware of herself as a separate entity. It is a state of being that those questing for higher consciousness strive to attain throughout their lives. Some say this is the goal of earth evolution: to bring those forces working in early childhood into full consciousness.[2]

During the first three years of the child's life on earth, while the I is actively preparing the instruments through which it will work into the world, the child is imbued with the universal power of the I which is still closely connected with those realms it came from. However, once the I has created the appropriate organs, it will progressively connect itself with the earthly realm and begin to work through the instruments it has created.

In the further developmental process we start to see many manifestations of the I's embodiment in the earthly world. Here are a few examples from each of the three stages of child development, which the reader may be able to add to from his or her own experience.

Expressions of the I

- The individual naming of objects and the making up of words expresses the unique way each child perceives her world.

- The first period of obstinacy and defiance in the third year is a picture of the early resistance of an unsure I to a potentially hostile world. By allowing the I to assert itself wherever possible, the child gains in confidence and soon moves on to other learning situations.

- In the world of play the I explores the world and gains a more continuous sense of itself. It enters the living world of fantasy and imagination, thereby generating the foundations for a creative life of soul, and rehearsing for the child's future life ahead.

- Making conscious choices, setting specific goals, expressing one's own view and elective respect for authority, are further evidence of the I's gradual embodiment as the child prepares for school. By the time she enters school, a sufficient continuity of self-awareness has been achieved to facilitate formal learning and the first stage of independent thinking.

- The change of teeth heralds the birth of independent thinking and memory, when the I can begin to engage with the world beyond its bodily limitations. For the next two or so years, this thinking is imbued with a dream-like feeling content that creates for the I a kind of safe haven protecting it from the harsh reality of the outside world.

- In the tenth year, this feeling of safe protection ceases and is replaced by heightened feelings of vulnerability, loneliness, isolation and fear. The I awakens to a renewed sense of being separate from the world, as it did in the third year. Now it feels far more alone and unprotected. It passes through a second phase of defiance and opposition as it struggles to come to terms with its growing engagement with its own body and the surrounding world. With the proper support and care, the I adjusts to its stronger earthly connection and begins to prepare itself for its mature connection to the earth, which takes place at puberty. Lievegoed describes this phase of the journey that begins with the nine-year-old crisis and continues until puberty, as a feeling experience of the I. It must experience itself in the grace and beauty of pubescence, but also in the awkwardness and secretiveness of puberty.[3]

- With the emergence of sexuality, the I has to confront a plethora of new emotions and feelings before it discovers who 'I am' at the level of sexuality. It discovers that it has the use of powerful instruments, a robust and sexually mature body and a burgeoning creative mind, and can actively engage in life. Thus it sets off on its first of many conscious journeys of exploration into a highly seductive world. The search for identity and a rightful place in the world has begun at the very time when the birth of destiny takes place. This confrontation with an unsympathetic world and the unfamiliar burden of destiny brings about the third experience of separation from the world (at around the age of 15).

- Between the fifteenth and sixteenth year, the I again dives into an experience of vulnerability, loneliness and yearning for home and a hero. But it will also need to experience the contrast of boldness, sociability and independence as it strives towards truth. Gradually, the I begins to experience a greater stability and control of self. It becomes conscious of an emerging personality which brings with it a new sense of self-worth, confidence, responsibility, independence and freedom. The search for truth and meaning becomes more intense and will continue in the years to come. In its quest to know who I am, the I continues to throw itself into new adventures and new explorations; but life is also becoming more serious as the question of vocation and serious relationships become relevant issues.

- At eighteen the I is ready to meet the challenges of life on its own, no longer needing the support or protection of parents, school or friends. This year marks a threshold for the I. It is a time of self-orientation as the I prepares for its adult life ahead; it is ready and able to make choices and decisions that will have a bearing on its future life. The I faces the world in a new way, searching for meaning and connection that can lead to the fullest self-expression. Lievegoed describes this as the beginning of self-realization, a new awakening that will express itself in the resolutions, values and idealism that manifest during this time. As the I consolidates its forces, it longs to prove that it is a powerful and worthy member of the human race. This may lead to new trials that test commitment and responsibility, sometimes even to the point of ending this earthly life. Many are the youthful soldiers that have given their lives for the ideal of protecting their nation.

The final leg of the twenty-year journey of childhood and youth has arrived, and we can witness the birth of the I as the unique core centre of the child's being.

In reviewing the panorama of this first stage of life, we can say that the I's long period of gestation has to do with preparing the human constitution as a suitable instrument for carrying the awakened I into the world. This preparation is the goal and purpose of childhood, adolescence and youth, to provide the physical and psychological foundation for the I to fulfill its destiny on earth.

What is this destiny? Clearly, it is different for every individual. Yet, common to all seems to be the evolutionary task of discovering *who I am*, ultimately coming to a conscious understanding and experience of the I. It is the I itself that prepares the human constitution for this task. The physical body is fully grown, the etheric body has completed its work on the three principal human systems – neuro-sensory system, rhythmic system, metabolic-limb system – the astral body has unfolded its activities of will, feeling and thinking. Now the I – the crowning glory of the human being – can be born.

The Mission of the I

With the birth of the I, the true mission of the human being can begin to unfold. This is a theme that could fill many books and much indeed has been written about this subject. I would venture to say in the words of John the Evangelist 'that if they should be written every one, I suppose that even the world itself could not contain the books that should be written.' (John 21: 25) Here we will touch on certain aspects of relevance to this book.

Throughout humanity's long ages, the seeker embarking on his journey of initiation has always heeded the admonition 'Know thyself'. The journey of preparation through childhood, adolescence and youth brings the individual to the point where she can consciously hear within herself this same challenge: *Who am I?*

Earlier we asked how we can experience the I. There are many different spiritual paths to attain or acquire this. It is my conviction that one of them is the journey involved in understanding and caring for the child, adolescent and youth.

Recollecting

In the course of our journey from conception to adulthood, we have accompanied all the developmental stages of the I's embodiment with our own personal experience. We can retrace each of these stages through an I experience and become conscious of our original experience as a child. To do so we have to practise actively recalling and reviewing our past journey, thus awakening to our own inner child and adolescent. Recollection of our evolving I may then bring an awareness of our own I as a part of a world or universal I; we may experience our own I as a drop in the ocean of the universal I. We can thereby gain knowledge of the universal child and adolescent. We can for example rediscover that sense of being at one with everything as the experience of a state of being that characterizes the young child. This in turn can remind us of the words: 'Except ye become as little children, ye shall not enter the kingdom of heaven' (Matthew 18: 3).

Empathic Listening

Insight into the nature of the child and the developing I will allow us to hearken to the child or adolescent in a different way, to sense and feel what is taking place in her soul and to be mindful of 'where she is'. Thus we can come to know the child in our care in a very deep way, discovering elements of her true nature. All this has to do with the practice of empathy.

When we make use of rhythm and breathing in the practice of empathy – by 'breathing' with one's feelings into another's soul and then 'breathing' this experience back into one's own soul – we create harmony between two souls and can experience the I being mirrored back to us through the I of the child – which is why we feel so enlivened and uplifted when we interact openly with children. We experience our own I as part of the world I, through participation in the I of every other human being. Somewhere, at some level, we can identify with the experience of every person. This gives reality to the words 'Inasmuch as ye have done it unto one the least of these my brethren, ye have done it unto me' (Matthew 25: 40).

Creative Caring

By remembering or retracing the I's embodiment through the developmental journey, and by being mindful of where the child is through empathy, we are best able to help her. This will also give us an intuitive sense of what the child needs to be best cared for and supported. Do I need to offer her the loving care of a mother, the protective support of a father, the loyal and trusting hand of a friend or the guiding help of a teacher? I can be any of these and more for the child, because they all exist within the creative layers of the human psyche. This is where creative resourcing comes into play. Thinking about a situation creatively may lead to new possibilities that result in miraculous outcomes, even in the most difficult situations. The soul is the stage where life unfolds in a myriad of possibilities. I discover what the child truly needs so that she can find greater freedom in her life: 'And ye shall know the truth, and the truth shall make you free' (John 8: 32).

Meditative Verses

Words which Steiner offered at Christmas 1923 in Dornach, Switzerland, capture in a deeply contemplative form the experience of the I as it lives through the human being's three soul spheres (thinking, feeling, will). The pertinent verses are presented here.[4]

> Soul of the individual human being!
> You live in the limbs,
> That bear you through the world of space
> Into the ocean-being of the spirit:
> *Practise spirit recollection*
> In depths of soul,

Where in the working of world-creating life
Your own I comes to being in the I of the divine;
Then in the universal human being
You will truly live.

In these words we may hear the heavenly and 'golden' moral being of
the child (see Chapters 6 and 7) in the first seven years, who lives in the
will that is most active in the limbs; and we can hear a call to our own
intuition to remember our own original experience of childhood.

Soul of the individual human being!
You live in the beat of heart and lungs,
That lead you through the rhythmic tides of time
Into the feeling of your own soul being.
Practise spirit mindfulness
In balance of the soul,
Where the surging deeds of world evolution
Unite your own I with the I of the world.
Then in the working of the human soul
You will truly feel.

Here we can sense the inspiration that lives in the beautiful and
healthy being of the child in the second seven years of life (see
Chapter eight), dwelling in feeling as she breathes through the
rhythms of heart and lung; and likewise we can sense here the power
of true listening that lives in empathy.

Soul of the individual human being!
You live in the resting head,
That unlocks for you universal thoughts
From the wellsprings of the eternal.
Practise spirit vision,
In quietness of thought,
Where the eternal aims of the divine
Grant light of world being
To your own I
For free and active will;
Then in the foundation of the human spirit
You will truly think.

Here, through the truth that comes through thinking, we can sense the guiding force that lives in the developing I in the third seven-year period (see Chapter nine); and can visualize the immense imaginative power that works through our creative resources.

No Knowledge Without Self-knowledge

In the awakening of the I we find out who we truly are; we also awaken to an understanding of child health and to a rational approach to caring for children. Experts give all kinds of advice about the best way to care for children. A certain amount of practical advice has been given in this book about various aspects of child health. This is all based on personal experience; in some cases it may concur with other opinions, in other cases it may completely disagree. In the final analysis we all have to form our own experience and be guided by our own truth.

The three principles that have been continuous motifs throughout this book – trusting our own long journey of original experience, learning the art of empathy and discovering the enormous power of creative resourcing – can become powerful tools for each of us to forge our own experience and arrive at our own truth. By experiencing the I, we can come to know, love and care for the child within and without.

Our hope for the future must be that children are increasingly understood, nurtured and protected. It is up to us to ensure that this happens.

CHAPTER 12

For Mother, Father and the Universal Child

The Power of Mother and Father Within Me are the Forces I Need to Nurture and Protect Myself

With the awakening and emergence of the I into adulthood, the journey of childhood and youth has been accomplished. However, a book about child health would not be complete without consideration of the role played by the mother and father in the life of the growing child. The child's journey on earth is intimately bound up with his relationship with his mother and father. In some ways it is the most intimate relationship of all. In this final chapter we will explore the eternal covenant that exists between mother, father and child.

In Chapter three we ventured imaginatively into the prenatal voyage towards conception and birth, and entertained the possibility that the child's higher self seeks out a mother and a father to provide a physical body in which earthly development can occur. The universal child has a connection with the universal nature of the mother and father. Accordingly, every child will receive the inherited imprint of both a father and a mother, and embark on a new life on earth with this strong imprint on his destiny. The relationship naturally follows a path unique to every child: some will experience the presence of both mother and a father throughout or for part of their childhood; others will know only a mother or a father; some will have to experience losing one or the other during childhood; and some will have no experience of either. Whatever the circumstances, this fundamental relationship will have a powerful and significant influence on the life and soul of every child.

In every individual mother and father, there likewise lives the universal mother or father underlying all individual parental variations and potential. This ideal reality of the mother and father, and likewise their ideal relationship to the child, is imprinted in our collective memory as a legacy of our evolutionary process and can be accessed imaginatively in the manner described throughout this book. Each one of us can find our own personal relationship to the child, the mother and the father within.

The following description is my personal experience of this relationship.

I enter the new world as a stranger, needy and vulnerable; my body and soul need nourishment and warmth; my spirit needs space to unfold its potential. I seek out those individuals who will nurture and care for me. I need to be reminded of my true intentions. I need to be protected. My inner activity propels me forward to take hold of this world and to forge my destiny. I have a clear mission.

First I need to create a secure home in a strong body and to make it my own; it must work well for me so that it can serve me all my life. My senses inform me about this new world and thus help to form my body. They need to be nurtured by a healthy environment. I need to be touched and rocked, to taste sweet mother's milk, to hear reassuring sounds and to sense that I am safe. My will needs freedom to unfold, to move and to find my orientation in space and time; yet it needs to be contained in a health-giving way.

Then I need to build a vibrant soul life, to experience the world in a healthy and creative way, to encounter the symphony of my feelings and to express them freely and in total safety.

Finally I need to discover my Self so that I can re-unite with my lost home. My life of thinking needs to be reflected back to me so I can learn to discover this gateway to my spirit. I know I cannot do this alone, I need people to care for me and protect me. As I walk the journey I will feel small, lost and frightened a hundred, a thousand times and more; I contract and become little when I am cold and hungry; I feel crushed when I am alone and uncared for; I feel diminished when I doubt that I can do something; I feel unworthy and undeserving when I dislike who I am; I want to run away and hide or pretend I am strong.

When I feel small there is always something around me that is huge and dangerous, hostile and threatening, always ready to pounce and squeeze me into small spaces. The world can become menacing, demanding and unfriendly.

I have the right to call for help! It is my mother who will nurture me! It is my father who will protect me!

I am your Mother, the uncompromising love who nurtures and cares for you. Since earth's beginnings I have always been present; I am the power of mother nature that is all-providing; I am the reverberating force of all mothers who bear the growing seed of children. You grow within my womb so close to my inner core, and your awesome corporeal creation I carry within me until you are ready to enter the world; I follow your path through life with joy and sorrow. It is my nature to give to you, and your right to take from me; I am there to warm and feed you; I embrace you with my bodily warmth; I give to you the nectar food of my body and later provide you with the earthly gifts of nature. I will always accept you for who you are; when you are sad and dejected, I am there to comfort and love you; when you feel lost, I hold you close to my heart. I am always there for you, mostly when you need me, but also when you go your own way. I hear who you are!

I am your Father, your unconditional protector who guards you and gives you shelter; since cosmic beginnings and time immemorial I have always been present. I am the resonating power that guides and drives the universe; I am the propelling force that activates the seed of children and sets in motion all growing processes. Throughout your life I am the steadfast rock that supports you and that enables you to unfold your life in freedom; I guide you and give you direction, and contain your exuberance and excessive will. I will always support you as you are and for your unlimited potential. When you feel weak, I can hold you in my strong arms; when you feel frightened, my courage will give you strength; I can keep away the threatening monsters, I can shield you from the pressures of life; I can carry you across the stormy oceans; and when the waters are too deep I will hold you on my shoulders. I hear who you are!

Yes, I feel the loving care of my mother who warms and nurtures my body and soul; I grow peacefully and happily in her heart-felt embrace. When I am sad and lonely she listens to my cry, and comforts and consoles me in fullest trust. She accepts and believes in who I am; my body absorbs it, my soul thrives on it; I see the way of love and trust and feel how it works its magic in me.

Yes, I feel the protective support of my father who strengthens and guides my unfolding spirit; my body feels strong, my soul feels safe as I absorb the power of his steadfast support. When I am frightened and under attack he shields me; when I am crushed and depressed, he lifts the heavy load. He never lets me down, he trusts in who I am; he is always there when I need to be protected. I see the power of strength and authority that gives me confidence and security.

As I travel this voyage of discovery, through all the stages of childhood and adolescence, absorbing and learning the lessons of life, my mother and father are always present. When I play with my imaginary friends, my playmates or my pets, I invoke the power of mother and father. I imbibe and imitate their nature, so that their nurturing care and protective power grow into me and become part of who I am. And so, when I arrive at a sense of myself as a free and independent being, I discover that these forces of the mother and father are there within me, like the gift of speaking or the aptitude for thinking. I discover then that I can become my own mother, my own father; and I can call on these powers to care for and protect me whenever I need them. I realize that the universal mother and father are within me and I am never alone.

As we accompany the child through all phases of his journey, from birth to adulthood, we can therefore honour the great service of motherhood and fatherhood in providing indispensable resources for the child that will allow him ultimately to nurture and protect himself. These are the gifts that also eventually make it possible for each child to develop the resources to nurture and protect their own children.

This book is an endeavour to awaken to the reality that every child at all stages of his growth and development has a unique story to tell and an important message to give the world. It is vital that the world hears it. We as mothers, fathers, teachers and carers need to find the will and strength to hear this story. Only then do we gain insight into and respect for those who entrust themselves to our care. Only then can we become worthy custodians and advocates for children. Only then can we nurture and protect them in the way that we ourselves would wish – or would have wished – to be nurtured and protected by others.

Childhood

Childhood is a time for learning about the essentials –
About the heavenly world and the earthly,
About goodness, beauty and truth.

Childhood is a time to be loved and to love –
To express fear and to learn trust –
To be allowed to be serious and calm
And to celebrate with laughter and joy.

Children have a right to dream,
And they need to grow at their own pace.
They have the right to make mistakes
And the right to be forgiven.

Children need help to develop self-mastery,
To transform themselves and bring forth their highest
    capacities.
Children have a right to be spared violence and hunger
To have a home and protection.

They need help to grow up healthily
With good habits and sound nutrition.
Children need people to respect,
Adults whose example and loving authority they follow.
They need a range of experience – tenderness and kindness,
Boldness and courage, and even mischief and
    misbehaviour.

Children need time for receiving and giving,
For belonging and participating.
They need to be part of a community, and they need to be
    individuals.
They need privacy and sociability.
They need time to rest and time to play,
Time to do nothing and time to work.

They need moments for devotion and room for curiosity.
They need protective boundaries and freedom for
    creativity.
They need to be introduced to a life of principles
And given the freedom to discover their own.
They need a relationship to the earth –
To animals and to nature,
And they need to unfold as human beings within the
    community.

The spirit of childhood is to be protected and nurtured.
It is an essential part of every human being and needs to be
    kept alive.

International Alliance for Childhood
Joint Working Group – New York 1999

Notes

Chapter *I*
The Universal Child

1. To avoid the awkward use of both genders, I will alternate from chapter to chapter.
2. N. Postman, *The Disappearance of Childhood,* Vintage Books, New York 1982.
3. P. Aries, *Centuries of Childhood*, Vintage Books, Random House, New York 1962; J. H. Plumb, 'The Great Change in Children', *Horizon*, vol. 13, No 1, Winter 1971.
4. S. Freud, *The Interpretation of Dreams*, Wordsworth Editions, Ware, Herts 1997.
5. J. Dewey, *The School and Society*, University of Chicago Press 1899.
6. As far as I know Steiner does not specifically refer to the 'universal child' but speaks generally of the 'universal human being'. We can assume that this concept includes that of the 'universal child' as well.
7. See www.allianceforchildhood.net/
9. N. Postman, *Amusing Ourselves to Death*, Heinemann, London 1986.
10. S. Palmer, *Toxic Childhood. How the Modern World is Damaging our Children and What We Can Do About It.* Orion Books, London 2006.
11. J. Garbarino, *Raising Children in a Socially Toxic Environment*, Jossey-Bass 1995.
12. O. James, *Affluenza,* Random House, London 2008.
13. M. Large, *Set Free Childhood*, Hawthorn Press, Stroud 2003.
14. The Book of Tobit: The apocryphal texts which appear in some Bibles between the Old and New Testaments.

Chapter 2
Meeting the Child

1. **Regression Therapy** is a method used by various psychotherapies such as hypnosis, gestalt psychology, psychodrama and body therapy to access past experiences hidden below the level of conscious awareness and affecting the client's wellbeing. Early pioneers and authors in regression therapy include J. L. Moreno, M. Netherton, H. Ten Dam, R. Woolger and A. Tomlinson. It has also been integrated as part of traditional medical treatment by various medical practitioners such as Drs M. Simoes, T. Okuyama, P. Gyngazov, N. Kondavati and J. Peres. Regression therapy has proven helpful in dealing with issues of self-esteem and personal empowerment, and residual scars from adult or childhood sexual abuse. It has provided swift and effective release of deep emotional blockages, states of anxiety, depression, phobias, inexplicable chronic pain and persistent symptoms of post-traumatic stress disorder. W. Blake Lukas in her book *Regression Therapy* Vol 1&2, Deep Forest Press, USA 1993, draws together the fruits of research of many authors and practitioners.

2. **Psychophonetics** as a methodology of experience awareness was characterized in the notes and references to the foreword. It was originally called *philophonetics* and was evolved by Yehuda Tagar during the 1980s as a modality of personal development and performing arts based on anthroposophy, psychosophy, humanistic psychology and the expressive arts. It was originally developed as a method of deep observation of the interactive dynamics of body, psyche, consciousness and spiritual awareness for the purpose of the performing arts, for a deepening of adult education and for the experiential study of anthropsophy and psychosophy. It later evolved in the 1990s into applications for counselling and psychotherapy. In 2003, the latest forms of philophonetics counselling were re-named psychophonetics.

3. The profession of psychophonetics is determined and defined by the Persephone Institute of Psychophonetics, which offers a number of professional courses.
    *   Foundation Year in Personal Development and Counselling Skills. One-year course for self-management, healing, transformation, communication, counselling and deep leadership skills
    *   Graduate Diploma in Psychophonetics. Two-year course building on the Foundation Year leading to qualification as a professional practitioner
    *   Postgraduate Diploma in Advanced Psychophonetics. One-year training following the graduate diploma, in psychophonetics-based relationship counselling, group work, workplace consultancy and special topics

Graduation qualifies practitioners for membership of the International Association of Psychophonetics Practitioners. Short courses, workshops and lectures are offered on a wide range of topics that include: personal development, parenting skills, relationship and sexuality, vocation, recovery from addiction and abuse, inner child, the healing power of sounds, counselling skills, care for the caring professionals, stress management, humanizing the work place, the seven conditions of sustainable human development, introduction to psychophonetics and introduction to psychosophy, deep leadership skills. Courses are currently run in Cape Town, South Africa, Stroud, United Kingdom and Melbourne, Australia. Contact addresses and telephone numbers can be obtained from **www.psychophonetics.com.**

4. Exercises will be given in some chapters for those who wish to revisit their biographies in this experiential way.

5. We here approach the threshold that Steiner describes in a number of texts as *Imagination, Inspiration* and *Intuition.* See the following books.

   • *Theosophy: An Introduction to the Supersensible Knowledge of the World and the Destination of the Human Being* (1904) Anthroposophic Press Inc., New York 1961.
   • *An Outline of Occult Science,* (1910) Anthroposophic Press Inc., Spring Valley, New York 1972
   • *Fundamentals of Therapy, An Extension of the Art of Healing through Spiritual Knowledge* (1925) Rudolf Steiner Press, London 1983

6. Advanced Diploma in Psychophonetic Counselling / Internal Training Material of Persephone Institute of Psychophonetics

---

7. *Try visualizing a lemon, then sensing and feeling it (noting the difference between these two); then find a gesture, movement or sound to express the experience of the lemon; and finally let go of the gesture, movement or sound and observe the experience as an after image in imagination.*

---

8. R. Steiner, (1924) *Eurythmy as Visible Speech,* Anthroposophical Publishing Co., London 1956.

9. The term *inner child* may have been coined for the first time in 1963 by W. Missildine in his book *Your Inner Child of the Past.* Generally it is used to denote the subjective childhood experiences which remain imprinted in the psyche. Popular psychology sees it as the childlike aspect of the human psyche. The inner child concept has been popularized by the American pop-psychology educator and self-help movement leader John Bradshaw in his books: *The Family* (1986), *Healing the Shame that Binds You* (1988), *Homecoming: Reclaiming and Championing Your Inner Child* (1990), *Creating Love* (1992), and

Family Secrets (1995). Healing the inner child is an essential stage in the twelve-step programme for recovery from addiction, abuse, trauma, or post-traumatic stress disorder. Transactional Analysis calls it the 'Child'. C. Whitfield names it the 'Child Within'. A number of other authors who have developed the concept include P. Mellody, L. Hay, L. Capacchione and Dr M. Paul.

Chapter 3
Where Do I Come From?

1. J. Bockemühl, C. Lindenau, G. Maier et al, *Towards a Phenomenology of the Etheric World,* Anthroposophic Press, Inc., USA 1985.
2. Ibid. One can observe this world of matter in accordance with its elemental nature in the manner described by J. Bockemühl.

> **3.** *We can arrive at a deeper experience of these four elements and four systems by moving our awareness from outer observation through inner visualizing to sensing, feeling, and then gesturing or moving one's body accordingly, and finally observing our body as suggested in Chapter Two. For instance, after observing the flow of fluids externally, we can visualize the flow of fluids through the body, then attempt to sense and feel their flow inwardly; we can form gestures and move the body in the nature of streaming fluids, and then observe the after-image of the body position created. By this means we can experience entering into the nature of the fluid element and the system of bodily fluids. In a similar manner we can arrive at an experience of the other elements and bodily systems.*

4. R. Steiner, *Theosophy: An Introduction to the Supersensible Knowledge of the World and the Destination of Man.* (1904) Anthroposophic Press, New York 1971.
5. In seeking new insights it is necessary to adopt a completely open attitude whereby we actively put aside our preconceptions and prejudices and allow new information to resonate in our soul, then observe our own inner response.
6. R. Steiner (1912–13), *Life between Death and a New Birth* Anthroposophic Press, New York 1968.
7. Steiner used the word *Ich* in German to designate this core component of the human being. Its only real equivalent translation is *I* but traditionally the word ego has been used instead. I have chosen not to use ego because English readers may confuse it with the term *ego* that has been used historically to translate Freud's description of *das Ich.* For Freud *das Ich* or *I* was that part of the mind which contains consciousness and specifically those psychic functions such as judgement, tolerance, reality-testing, control, planning, defence, synthesis of information, intellectual

functioning and memory. (R. Snowden, *Teach Yourself Freud,* The McGraw-Hill Companies Inc.)

8. R. Steiner (1922), *Geistige Zusammenhänge in der Gestaltung des menschlichen Organismus Berlin* 7.12.22 GA 218 Rudolf Steiner Verlag, Dornach, Switzerland 1972.

9. R. Steiner (1923), *Man's Being, His Destiny and World Evolution*, Oslo 17.05.1923 GA 226, Anthroposophic Press, New York 1966.

---

10. One may come to such an experience of the male and female principles when one visualizes, feels, senses and gestures the nature of the masculine, then the feminine; and then stands outside the experience to observe the after-images created.

---

11. See note 6 above.

12. K. König, *Embryologie und Weltenstehung:* Verlag die Kommenden, Freiburg I. Br. 1966; T. Weihs, *Embryogenesis in Myth and Science*, Floris Books, Edinburgh 1986; F. Wilmar, *Vorgeburtliche Menschwerdung*, J. Ch. Mellinger Verlag, Stuttgart 1979; K. Appenzeller, *Die Genesis im Lichte der menschlichen Embryonal Entwickelung*, Zbinden Press, Basel 1976.

13. R. Steiner, *An Outline of Occult Science*, Anthroposophic Press Inc., New York 1972.

14. Op. cit., note 12 above.

15. See note 4 above.

16. Op. cit., note 12 above.

17. R. Steiner, *Rosicrucian Esoterism*, GA 109, 111, (7.6.1909) Anthroposophic Press, Spring Valley 1978/*The Theosophy of the Rosicrucians* GA 99, (29.5.1907) Rudolf Steiner Press, London 1981/ *Man's Being in his Destiny and World Evolution* GA 226, 17.5.1923, Anthroposophic Press, New York 1966.

18. S. Drake, *The Path to Birth*, Floris Books, Edinburgh 1979.

---

19. One may start with an imaginative picture of the growing embryo and foetus; this picture can give way to a feeling awareness and sensation within the body, and this, in turn, can be precisely translated into a gesture, movement and sound; the after-image observed may bring to conscious awareness an inner experience of intra-uterine life.

---

20 C. Stark, M. Orleans, Haverkamp, J. Murphy, 'Short- and Long-term Risks after Exposure to Diagnostic Ultrasound in Utero', *Obstetrics and Gynecology* 1984, 63:194–200; J.P. Newnham, S.F. Evans, C.A. Michael, F.J. Stanley, L.I. Landau, 'Effects of Frequent Ultrasound during Pregnancy: A Randomised Control Trial', *Lancet* 1993, 342:887–891.

Chapter 4
The Journey

> **1.** *We can reflect on any growth activity using fluid thinking, whether we observe something external such as the growth of a plant, or the growth process of a painting or sculpture, or an internal process such as studying a course and ultimately achieving the qualification certificate. Using the methodology of experience awareness described in Chapter two, we can use visualization, body sensing, feeling and gesturing/movement and sounding to access deeper levels of awareness of the growing and maturing, experience of gestation until it culminates in the birth experience. The latter is invariably accompanied by a sense of liberation.*

2. The buds for the permanent teeth are formed already during the third month of foetal development, lying alongside and inside the deciduous teeth, but they remain dormant until approximately the sixth year of postnatal life. The deciduous teeth are fully formed before birth.
3. R. Steiner and I. Wegman (1925) *Fundamentals of Therapy. An extension of the Art of Healing through Spiritual Knowledge*, Rudolf Steiner Press, London 1983.
4. Schools based on the educational ideas of Rudolf Steiner.
5. *Morphology* refers to the branch of science that investigates living forms.
6. *Metabolism,* from the Greek word *metabolè* = change, refers to the processes of chemical change and exchange in an organism. When we do see symmetry in the organs of metabolism, we find that the dynamic of the neuro-sensory system has entered the metabolic realm, for instance in the dual kidneys, which have the round shape of the head and the finely structured nature of the nervous system. The kidneys are furthermore very sensitive organs with a rich nerve supply. Embryologically they have their origin in the head region, and have an oxygen need similar to the brain.

> **7.** *One can visualize, sense, feel, gesture, move and sound the inner dynamic of the compact, cold and constricted neuro-sensory system, then contrast it with the expansion, dispersion and warmth of the metabolic-limb system and finally experience the balancing, mediating experience of the rhythmic system.*

8. L.F.C. Mees, *The Human Skeleton, Form in Metamorphosis*, Anthroposophic Press, Spring Valley, New York 1984.
9. R. Steiner (1917), *Von Seelenrätseln,* Rudolf Steiner Nachlassverwaltung, Dornach 1976, translated as 'Riddles of the Soul'.

Chapter 5
Citizen of The Earth

> 1. **One can use imaginative awareness exercises to deepen experience of the birthing process. By concentrating on the inner imaginative picture one may enter, as it were, the birthing child's feeling and sensory experience. Our body can find gestures and movements to express the nature of the birthing process, and also sounds which express the inner experience of the birthing child.**

2. Water birth: Indigenous tribal communities are known to use water for birthing. In the 1960s, the Russian researcher Igor Charkovsky studied the possible benefits of water birth. Leboyer in the late 1960s developed the practice and Michael Odent took this work further. By the late 1990s this practice had spread to many western countries. There is considerable research that promotes the safety of water births. A large-scale study in the UK (1994–1996) showed a decrease in perinatal mortality (1.2 per 1,000 for waterbirth vs. 4 per 1,000 for conventional birth during the same period), a decreased risk of tearing and a zero episiotomy rate (surgical cutting of the birth opening) (Harper 2000; Gilbert 1999; London: Office for National Statistics 2005). There are also no documented reports of water aspiration or inhalation or increased risk of infection.
3. Frederick Leboyer was the first obstetrician to first popularize gentle birthing techniques including water birthing in his book *Birth without Violence*, Knopf, New York 1975.
4. R. Goldberg, *Caesarean Section. Is the Rising Incidence a Cause for Concern?* Dreamcatcher Publications 2002.
5. D.P. Behague, C.G. Victoria, F. C. Barros, 'Consumer demand for Caesarean section in Brazil', *British Medical Journal*, 2002: 324: 942.
6. L. Snyman, *Is the high caesarean section rate a cause for concern?* Review Article, Department of Obstetrics and Gynaecology, University of Pretoria 1999.
7. K. Efekhar, P. Steer, 'Caesarean Section Controversy. Women choose Caesarisection', *British Medical Journal*, 2000: 320, 1073.
8. R. Al Mufti, A. McCarthy, N.M. Fisk, 'Obstetricians' Personal Choice and Mode of Delivery', *Lancet*, 1997: 347: 544
9. Snyman, op. Cit.
10. J.S. Bell, D.M. Campbell et al., 'Do obstetric complications explain high Caesarean section rates among women over 30?' *British Medical Journal*, 2001: 322: 894–895.
11. C.M. Glazener, 'Sexual function after childbirth: women's experiences, persistent morbidity and lack of professional recognition', *British Journal of Obstetrics and Gynaecology*, 1997: 104: 330–335.
12. E. Hemminki, 'Impact of Caesarean section on future pregnancy – a review of cohort studies', *Paediatric Perinatal Epidemiology* 1996: 10: 366–379.

13. E. Hemminki, J. Merilainen, 'Long term effects of caesarean sections', *American Journal of Obstetrics and* Gynaecology, 1996; 174: 1569–1574.

14. G. Paxelius, K. Hagnevik et al., 'Catecholamine surge and lung function after delivery', *Archives of Diseases in Childhood*, 1983; 58: 262–266.

15. A. Hollmen, M. Jagerhorn, P. Pystenen, 'Influence of labour and route of delivery on the frequency of respiratory morbidity in term neonates', *International Journal of Gynaecology and Obstetrics*, 1993; 43: 35–40.

16. M. Enkin, G.J. Hofmeyer, *A Guide to effective care in Pregnancy and Childbirth*, Oxford University Press 2000.

17. Ibid.

18. R. Lilford, H. Van Coeverdern de Groot, Moore et al., 'The relative risk of Caesarean section', *British Journal of Obstetrics and Gynaecology*, 1990: 97: 883–890.

19. R. Oliver, 'The ideal caesarian delivery', *Journal of Prenatal & Perinatal Psychology & Health*, 2000:14(3–4), 331–334. Oliver suggests only using regional anaesthesia, creating the right mood in theatre and allowing labour to begin prior to surgery; then performing a transverse incision which may reduce the chance of future deliveries being automatically delivered by Caesarian section; the amniotic sac is only ruptured once the baby's presenting part has been gently elevated and the nose and throat is gently aspirated, without pulling on the head. Having delivered the body, the baby can be gently compressed by the warm, wet hands of the obstetrician to simulate vaginal squeezing and the cord is only clamped after the cord stops pulsating. The baby is then handed to mother and father while the paediatrician decides whether stimulation of the breathing is needed. The obstetrician awaits the delivery of the placenta, instead of pro-actively pulling it out, after which the uterus and abdomen are closed.

20. A.L. Shapira, a Masters student in psychology presents an interesting review of *The Emotional Ramifications of being born in a Caesarian Delivery*, Santa Barbara Graduate Institute, 2008. She provides the following references: J.B. English, *Different Doorway: Adventures of a Caesarian Born*, Earth Heart Publishers, Point Reyes Station 1985; J.B. English, 'Being born caesarian: physical, psychosocial and metaphysical aspects', *Journal of Prenatal & Perinatal Psychology & Health*, 1994: 7(3) 215–229; L. Feher, *The Psychology of Birth: roots of human personality*, Continuum, New York 1981; S. Ray and B. Mandel, *Birth and Relationships: How your birth affects your relationships*, Celestial Arts, Berkeley CA 1987; T.R. Verny and P. Weintraub, *Tomorrow's Baby: the art and science of parenting from conception through infancy*, Simon & Schuster, New York 2002.

21. K. König, *Brothers and Sisters*, Floris Books, Edinburgh 1984.

22. Bert Hellinger, a German psychotherapist, is the principal developer of a therapeutic method best known as *Family Constellations* and *Systemic Constellations*. There are several thousand professional practitioners worldwide who use his insights in a broad range of personal, organizational and political applications. Some reference works include:
  • B. Hellinger, G. Weber and H. Beaumont, *Love's Hidden Symmetry: What makes love work in relationships*, Phoenix, AZ: Zeig, Tucker & Theisen 1998.
  • D.B. Cohen, 'Family Constellations: An innovative systemic phenomenological group process from Germany', *The Family Journal: Counseling and Therapy for Couples and Families*, 2006: 14(3), 226–233.
23. Ibid.
24. R. Steiner (1904), *Theosophy: An Introduction to the Supersensible Knowledge of the World and the Destination of the Human Being*, Anthroposophic Press, New York 1971.
25. Secretariat, World Health Organization *Infant and Young Child Nutrition: Global strategy for infant and young child feeding*, World Health Organization. WHO Executive Board 109th Session provisional agenda item 3.8 (EB109/12), 2001-11-24.
26. M. Glöckler, and W. Goebel, *A Guide to Child Health,* Floris books, Edinburgh 2000.

> **27.** *Using the methods of experience awareness one can place oneself imaginatively in the position of a completely trusting and vulnerable newborn child, visualizing, sensing, feeling and gesturing her nature. One can then step out of this position and observe the picture of the newborn child that is visualized in the after-image. See how this image affects you. What kind of birth reception would you wish for this child and what kind of living environment would be right for her? Imagine such a reception and such an environment. When you can visualize the environment in a symbolic representation, then sense, feel, gesture and become it for the child. One may then inwardly welcome the child into the world in a manner that one would wish to be welcomed.*

Chapter 6
The Heavenly Years

1. R. Steiner (1919), *Study of Man*, Lecture 4, Rudolf Steiner Press, London 1975.
2. Steiner describes *motivation* as an aspect of the will unique to the human being. Animals have instinct, drives and desires but cannot have motives because they do not have a self-reflecting capacity which the I confers: the I can transform instinct, drive and desire into

motivation. For example, I am motivated to lead a healthy life which will harness and direct my instincts, drives and desires in this direction. *Wish* underlies all motivation. It is a force that perceives what lives in the future that has not yet come into being in the present. Our wishes can be determined by our desires or can transform our desires; the wish to do things differently or better next time is an expression of the I transforming the soul life of desire. *Intention* is a wish which takes on a clearer and more specific, tangible form. For example, one has a clear picture of how one would do things better next time. The I here, according to Steiner, has changed the drives of the will into something spiritual. *Resolve* is, in a sense, the highest form of will. Here Steiner says that the I has freed the soul completely from the physical body.

3. Anna Jean Ayres (1920–1989) was a developmental psychologist who formulated the theory of sensory integration dysfunction, a term she coined in the 1960s. Although controversial, her theories and conclusions regarding SIT are currently popular in occupational therapy and developmental psychology. She is the author of several books including *Sensory Integration and the Child*, Western Psychological Services 1990.

4. These are: the *interoceptive sense,* referring to the sensory system of internal organs; the *tactile sense* processing information about touch and warmth, primarily via the skin, the *vestibular sense,* which gives information about movement, gravity and balance, and the *proprioceptive sense,* which gives awareness of body position and body parts.

5. R. Steiner (1910), *A Psychology of Body Soul and Spirit*, Anthroposophic Press, New York 1999; R. Steiner (1916), *Menschenwerden, Weltenseele und Weltengeist,* GA 206, Rudolf Steiner Nachlassverwaltung 1967; R. Steiner (1920), *Geisteswissenschaft als Erkenntnis der Grundimpulse sozialer Gestaltung,* GA 199, Rudolf Steiner Nachlassverwaltung 1967.

6. *Direct your attention to each of the twelve senses. In sensing the four lower senses, touch, life, movement and balance, our own immediate physical bodily environment becomes the object of perception. We discover something new about the condition of the body. Through our perceptions of warmth, taste, smell and sight, we project ourselves beyond our physical body into our close surroundings and actively enter the polar nature of our soul life, (warmth-cold, light-dark). When we focus on the four higher senses, we become aware of higher supersensible reality that has to do with the nature of spirit. Become aware how each sense impression impacts on your sensing organism. With your inner sense of life perceive this resonance and then express it through gesture or movement. When you observe the after-image, you will notice that it is your personalized imitation of the object perceived outwardly or inwardly. For example, a sharp object touched may lead to a gesture of recoil, but sensing the I of another person may lead to the same gesture.*

7. Quoted by A. Soesman in *The Twelve Senses,* Hawthorn Press, Stroud.

8. Ibid.

9. R. Steiner (1919), *Study of Man,* Rudolf Steiner Press, London 1981.

10. See note 5 above.

11. J. Salter, *The Incarnating Child,* Hawthorn Press, Stroud 1987.

12. Labial sounds *b, m, p, f, v,* – dental sounds *d, t, s* – velar or palatal sounds *k, g, ng* – lingual sounds, *a, e, i, o, u, l, r,* – nasal sounds *n, m.*

13. K. König, *The First Three Years of the Child,* Heil- und Erziehungsinstitut Bingenheim/Friedberg, 1957; T.F. Gross, *Cognitive Development,* Brooks/Cole Publishing Company, Monterey California 1985.

14. D.A. Louw, D.M. Van Ede, A.E. Louw, *Human Development,* Kagiso Publishers, Cape Town 1998.

15. R. Steiner (1923), *World History in the Light of Anthroposophy,* Rudolf Steiner Press, London 1997.

16. Plato and Steiner after him indicated that the child derives his concepts from his store of spiritual experiences, brought with him from a time before he can form his mental images.

17. R. Steiner (1922), *Knowledge of the Human Being According to Body, Soul and Spirit.* Lectures to the Workers of the Goetheanum. GA number/publisher/date?

18. N. Doidge, *The Brain that Changes Itself,* Viking Press, USA 2007.

19. S. Goddard Blythe, *The Well Balanced Child,* Hawthorn Press, Stroud 2004.

20. M. Large, *Set Free Childhood,* Hawthorn Press, Stroud 2003; K. Buzzell, *The Children of Cyclops,* The Association of Waldorf schools of North America, Fair Oaks 1998.

---

21. *Focus your empathic attention on the mental picture of a young child who surrenders his soul to the outer world. Sense, feel and gesture this experience, then detach and observe the after-image. Now focus on different sense impressions that impact on the child. One can be quite specific and enter in the same way as above into specific impressions – for instance untainted mother's milk, poor nutrition, loving parents, toxic fumes, warm clothing, vaccinations, sounds of nature, loud TV stimuli, secure home life, harsh emotions, etc. Following this, let the impressions impact on the after-image of the child and imaginatively observe the effect.*

---

22. R. Goldberg, *Infectious Childhood Illness – A Developmental Challenge for Life,* Dreamcatcher Publications 2004; R. Goldberg, *Immunisation. Should I vaccinate my child?* Dreamcatcher Publications 2004.

23. R. Goldberg, *Fever A Gift of Health,* Dreamcatcher Publications 2003; R. Steiner (1907), *Education of the Child in the light of Spiritual Science,* Anthroposophic Press, USA 1996.

24. M. Glöckler, W. Goebel, *A Guide to Child Health,* Floris Books, Edinburgh 1990; R. Goldberg, *Creative Nutrition for Healthy Children,* Nos. 9 &10 in the series *Awaken to Child Health,* Dreamcatcher

Publications 2005. The wide range of childhood disturbances common in our time will be the subject of Part 2.

25. J. Salter, *The Incarnating Child*, Hawthorn Press, Stroud 1987; M. Glöckler, W. Goebel, *A Guide to Child Health*, Floris Books, Edinburgh 1990; S. Maher, Y. Bleech, *Putting the Heart back into Teaching*, Novalis Press, Cape Town 1998.

Chapter 7
The Golden Years

> 1. *Our memories of childhood in these first seven years provide us with rich material for accessing the child's nature at each phase of development. Using the methods of experience awareness we have described, we can visualize a memory, and allow this picture to call up a feeling which touches the body in some place as a sensation that can be expressed as a gesture, movement, sound or speech. By detaching oneself either through physical or conscious repositioning, one is able to observe the child (oneself) physically as well as emotionally. New insights regarding childhood experience will thereby emerge that equip us to better understand the child, and if necessary to support and care for her in a new way.*

2. Formal schooling starts at different ages in different countries. Although children start school at 'rising 5' in the UK, the Waldorf system which this book advocates, and many other countries, do not begin formal schooling until this age.

3. R. Steiner (1921), *Cosmosophy* Vol 2 GA 208–29. 10. 1921, Completion Press, Gympie, Australia 1997.

4. It is a phylogenetic phenomenon that as consciousness increases in the animal kingdom, life potential decreases: as the nervous system develops through the nematodes, fish, reptiles, mammals and humans, so their reproductive and regenerative capacities diminish. The neuro-sensory functions provide the foundation for consciousness – perception and cognition – precisely because vitality is reduced in these organ systems.

5. In the organs of metabolism and locomotion, vitality is dominant and consciousness is diminished.

6. As developed for instance by a path of spiritual training. See R. Steiner, *How to Know Higher Worlds. A Modern path of Initiation*, Anthroposophic Press, USA 2006.

7. Michaela Gloeckler, 'Knowledge gained through practical engagement with anthroposophic research findings, illustrated by the dual aspect of the human's being etheric organization', Dornach, Switzerland 2008.

8. R. Steiner (1920), *The Bridge between Universal Spirituality and the Physical Constitution of Man*, Anthroposophic Press, USA, 1979.

9. E. Marti, *The Four Ethers*, Schaumberg Publications, USA, 1984.

10. R. Steiner (1907), *The Education of the Child in the Light of Spiritual Science GA 34*. Anthroposophic Press, Spring Valley USA 1996.
11. Ibid.

> *12. Through visualizing, feeling, sensing and gesturing the nature of a small child we enter deeply into her experience. Then, stepping outside of this role, we can observe how the world streams into her and how she then imitates what she has perceived. We can go further and re-enter the child at a deeper level, imagining that we become the dynamic, mobile etheric body itself as it receives the imprint of sensory impressions. Thus imprinted the body will imitate accordingly, through gesture or movement.*

13. B. Lievegoed, (1987) *Phases of Childhood*, Floris Books and Anthroposophic Press, Great Britain 1987.
14 U. Grahl, The Wisdom in Fairy Tales, New Knowledge Books, East Grinstead 1972
15. Brothers Grimm, (1975) *The Complete Grimm's Fairy Tales*, Routledge, London 1975.
16. R. Steiner, *Kingdom of Childhood*, Anthroposophic Press, New York, R. Steiner, *Practical Advice for Teachers*, Anthroposophic Press New York 1937, R. Wilkinson, *Interpretation of Fairy Tales*, Henry Goulden Publications 1984.
17. Sally Goddard Blythe, *What Babies and Children Really Need*, Hawthorn Press, Stroud 2008.
18. C. Violato and C. Russell, 'A Meta-analysis of the published research on the effects of non-maternal care on child development' in C. Violato, M. Genuis and E. Paolucci (ed.) *The changing family and child development*, Ashgate, London [in press.]
19. P. S. Cook, 'Rethinking the early childcare agenda. Who should be caring for very young children?' *Medical Journal of Australia*, 170, 1999: 29–31.

Chapter 8
The Beautiful, Healthy Years

> *1. One can stay with the feelings and notice how the body responds; one may sense some change in a part of the body, for instance a change in the breathing or the pulse or the tightening of muscles; one can listen intently to these subtle changes and then allow the body to express them through a gesture or movement, staying there long enough to experience something of the memory picture that now takes form. One then moves physically out of this position and observes where one has arrived. Do you see the child in this after-image before you? Do you see where the child is, how he or she is: do you see the context?*

2. Besides breathing, the others are: nourishing, warming, secreting, maintaining, growing and reproducing. Cf. R. Steiner, *Riddles of Humanity*, GA 170.

3. W. Hoerner, *Zeit und Rhythmus*, Urachhaus, Stuttgart 1978.

4. In actual fact the sun returns to a point that is slightly different from the previous year as a result of its movement within the solar system, a phenomenon called the procession of the equinoxes.

5. These exercises can be studied in Steiner's works: *Knowledge of the Higher Worlds and its Attainment* GA 10 and *An Outline of Occult Science* GA 13, Anthroposophic Press, Spring Valley, N.Y. 1972.

6. R. Steiner (1919), *Study of Man*, Rudolf Steiner Press, London 1966.

7. J.E. Berendt, *Nada Brahma The World is Sound*, Frankfurt a.M. 1983.

8. Ibid.; and R. Steiner, *Eurythmy as Visible Speech / Eurythmy as Visible Sound*, Anthroposophical Publishing Company, London 1955.

9. A. Stott, *Eurythmy: its Birth and Development*, ISBN 0954104846.

10. M. Kirchner-Bockholt and Wood, *Fundamental Principles of Curative Eurythmy*, ISBN 0-904693-40-6.

11. T. Poplawski, *Eurythmy: Rhythm, Dance and Soul,* ISBN 0-86315-269-4, pp. 80–4.

12. J. Piaget, *The Child's Conception of the World*, Routledge & Kegan Paul, London 1928.

13. M. Large, *Set Free Children*, Hawthorn Press, Stroud, UK 2003.

14. A.C. Harwood, *The Recovery of Man in Childhood*, Anthroposophic Press 1958.

15. K. Wilber, *Integral Psychology*, Shambala Publications, Boston and London 2000.

16. *Grimms Fairy Tales*, Routledge, London 1983.

17. J. Streit, *Animal Stories*, Walter Keller Press, Dornach Switzerland 1974; C. Kingsley, *The Heroes* William Clowes & Sons, London 1985.

18. Ancient myths: J. Streit, *And there was Light* (Bible Story companion for Class 3) Private publication 1978; Walter de la Mare, *Stories from the Bible*, Faber and Faber 1977; R. Querido, *Creativity in Education*, San Francisco, Dakin 1982.

19. N. Mellon, *Storytelling with Children*, Hawthorn Press, Stroud 2000.

20. *Vividly recall an experience which caused anxiety; sense what happens in your body, especially when the visualization is intense. Feelings also arise and the sensations will be experienced in a particular part of the body. Allow the body to respond to these sensations – usually it will tense up, withdraw or feel as though it is growing smaller. If you now exit from this stance/gesture you will be able to observe the after-image, which may appear like a small and vulnerable child. If you now try to observe what is causing the child to cringe and withdraw, you are likely to sense 'something big and threatening pressing in on you'.*

21. Kaplan and Sadock, *Synopsis of Psychiatry,* Lippincott Williams & Wilkins, London and New York 2003.

22. The confusion that has arisen, at least in anthroposophical circles, relates to what constitutes the **astral body**: Steiner sometimes refers to the astral body as the soul body or sentient body, (R. Steiner, *Education of the Child in the Light of Spiritual Science,* Anthroposophic Press, New York 1996; and at other times he refers to it as the combined soul body and sentient soul (R. Steiner, *Theosophy An Introduction to the Supersensible Knowledge of the World and the Destination of Man,* Chapter 1. GA 9, Anthroposophic Press, New York 1971).

    I choose to see the astral body as a development in consciousness in time. In the animal kingdom and in early childhood, the astral body can be regarded as the same as the soul body. As the I awakens to the world, the awakened astral body unfolds its inner soul life and the sentient soul comes into being as the first transformation of the soul by the I. Now the astral body takes on the nature of the united soul body and sentient soul.

    Later in adult life, the I may have the opportunity to work further on the subjective life of feelings and of desires, purifying and transforming the astral body into a second soul transformation; spiritual science refers to this as the 'spirit self', and in eastern traditions it is known as 'manas'. The ancient Greeks called it the golden fleece. Artists traditionally represented this purified soul in the halo surrounding the head of saints.

23. S. Leber, *Kommentar zu Rudolf Steiner's Vorträgen über Allgemeine Menschenkunde als Grundlage der Pädagogik Band III: Der leibliche Gesichtspunkt,* Verlag Freies Geistesleben, Stuttgart 2002.

24. With the birth of the etheric body at the change of teeth, certain life forces were freed from organic processes to become forces available for memory and conceptual thinking. Now, with the birth of the astral body at puberty, other life forces are liberated to become part of the soul life that the I has created. The I can now begin to work on these liberated etheric forces.

    These forces freed from the nervous system form the soul's foundation for the intellect. Steiner called this the 'intellectual soul'; it may also be translated as the personal soul. The forces freed from the rhythmic system create the soul foundation for social life. This soul aspect can be called the mind or heart soul (*Gemuetseele*). Later in life the I can begin its work of transforming the etheric forces into what spiritual science calls the 'life spirit' and what eastern spiritual traditions calls 'buddhi'.

    To complete the picture, the I can also work at transforming the physical body, making these forces available to the soul. This results in the birth of the consciousness or spiritual soul, which in adolescent development can take place only in its most germinal form and which in a distant future may be further transformed into spirit man or atman. (R. Steiner, *Theosophy An Introduction to the Supersensible Knowledge of the World and the Destination of Man,* Chapter 1. GA 9, Anthroposophic Press, New York 1971).

25. B. Lievegoed, *Phases of Childhood*, Floris Books, Edinburgh 1987.
26. B. Lievegoed, *Man on the Threshold: The Challenge of Inner Development*, Hawthorn Press, Stroud 1985.

> **27. The four temperaments can be experienced best when one enters the nature of the four elements: earth, water, air and fire through our now accustomed method of visualizing, sensing, feeling and gesturing/moving. For instance when one experiences the fixed, cold compact nature of earth and expresses it in a gesture, one will observe in the after-image the picture of a melancholic individual. Likewise for the other three temperaments. Thereafter it may be easier to enter into the nature of the four members of the human constitution and to experience the predominance of one, which leads to the manifestation of a particular temperament. Thus by experiencing the nature of the earthly element as described above, one can experience the dominance of the physical body and thereby discover the inner nature of the melancholic temperament.**

28. B. Staley, *Between Form and Freedom*, Hawthorn Press, Stroud 1988; R. Steiner (1908), *The Four Temperaments*, Anthroposophic Press, N Y 1976; K. Koenig, *The Human Soul*, Floris Books, Edinburgh 1973.

> **29. From everything that has thus far been said about the four members of the human constitution, one may form an inner picture of each in turn and allow this mental imagery to create inner feelings, body sensations and outer expressions for its dynamic activity. This may be expressed through movement, painting, modeling or other artistic modalities. If one now attempts to concretize these activities one can arrive at an experience of the four cardinal organs as the functional centres or instruments of these members.**

30. F. Husemann, O. Wolff, *The Anthroposophical Approach to Medicine. An Outline of a Spiritual Scientifically Oriented Medicine*. Vol 2 P 197 Anthroposophic Press, New York 1987, 12534 USA.
31. Ibid., and V. Bott, *Anthroposophical Medicine; an extension of the art of healing*, Rudolf Steiner Press, London 1978.

Chapter 9
The Truthful Years

> **1. If one wishes to explore one's youth, many mental images will appear with varying intensity. One may focus intently on a particular memory picture, and observe that a feeling connected with this time will often arise; the feeling may lead to a body sensation for which one can find a gesture or movement whose after-image can be observed.**

2. R.Treichler, *Soulways, The developing Soul Life Phases. Thresholds and Biography,* Hawthorn Press, Stroud 1989.
3. R. Steiner, *A Psychology of Body, Soul and Spirit,* 1–4 Nov 1910, Anthroposophic Press, New York, 1999.
4. R. Steiner, *Soul Economy and Waldorf Education* 13th Lecture 4th January, 1922, GA 303 Anthroposophic Press, New York 1986.
5. B. Lievegoed, *Phases: Crisis and Development in the Individual,* Rudolf Steiner Press, London 1979.
6. W. Gädecke, *Sexuality, Partnership and Marriage from a spiritual perspective,* Temple Lodge, London 1998.
7. M.E. Herman-Giddens, et al., 'Secondary sexual characteristics and menses in young girls seen in office practice: A study from the pediatric research in office settings network', *Pediatrics* 1997, 99(4).
8. Weight-gain: There seems to be a link between overweight and obese children and premature sexual development; early breast development may be stimulated by a protein produced by fat cells called leptins which are essential for the progression of puberty. Higher levels of insulin present in overweight girls, stimulate sex hormone production.
    Hormones and other chemicals in food: Growth hormones and steroids given to cattle and pigs may stimulate early sexual development. Pesticides such as DDE – a breakdown product of DDT and other chemical pollutants in the food chain such as Bisphenol A – a chemical cousin of oestrogen – mimics sexual hormone activity.
    Poor diets, extreme exercise and athletic exertion will accelerate sexual maturity.
    Higher socio-economic status, moderate physical exercise, better medical services, improved sanitation and health status, will delay sexual maturity.
9. H. Mattholius, 'Der Einfluss der Erziehung auf die Akzeleration des Menschen' (The influence of education on the acceleration of youth) *Beiträge zur einer Erweiterung der Heilkunst,* Issue 4, 1997.
10. D.A. Louw, D.M. Van Ede, A.E. Louw, *Human Development* Kagiso Publishers, Pretoria 1998.
11. R. Steiner, *Philosophy of Spiritual Activity,* Anthroposophic Press, New York 1986.
12. R. Steiner, *Study of Man,* GA 293 Lecture 9 Stuttgart 21 Aug–5 Sept 1919 Rudolf Steiner Press, London 1981.
13. Notes from '*The Birth of Destiny and the Transformation of the Human Heart*' References:
    *   R. Steiner, 26 May 1922, 'The Human Heart in relation to the life before birth and after death' in the volume GA 212, The Human Soul in relation to World Evolution
    *   R. Steiner 1908, *The Influence of Spiritual Beings,* GA 102., Anthroposophic Press USA
    *   R. Steiner 1919, *Lucifer and Ahriman,* Rudolf Steiner Publishing Co, Canada 1954

- B. Lievegoed, *Man on the Threshold*, Ch 8, Hawthorn Press, Stroud.

14. The birth of independence and the expansion of horizons opens up the needs for more specialized subjects. Modern and political history, and the great revolutions in thinking, science, history and discovery are especially relevant, for instance the Industrial Revolution, the French Revolution, and the wars of liberation in all countries, journeys of discovery and exploration, and the invention of the telephone and steam engine. A more conscious aesthetic appreciation of poetry and drama becomes appropriate and vital too, for instance Byron's passionate craving for excitement and fullness for life, and Shakespeare's comedies, with their lyrical language, intricacies of plot and wellspring of emotions. With the awakening of independent thinking, mathematics – algebra and geometry – and mechanics provide the confidence required for self-reliant thinking. Moving on from more localized geography, world geography now allows the adolescent to encompass the whole globe in his thinking.

15. As thinking develops, the history of art offers vivid illustration of the evolution of mankind in its descent from heaven to earth; and the study of ancient history, with the birth of thinking in humanity, will mirror the adolescent's own journey. Greek and Shakespearian tragedy can help the adolescent comes to terms with her own inner concerns, doubts and anxieties. On the other hand Romanticism in literature can support the heart in opening to the world, nature, and other human beings.

16. As the search for truth and meaning becomes more urgent, the educational process can provide an indispensable platform for the restless soul of the adolescent to grapple with real issues. The drama of the human soul can find rich reflection in the struggles of nations and individuals as depicted in history, philosophy, science, literature and drama – for instance in the conflict between the church and paganism, the crusaders, Arthur and his Knights of the Round Table, the search for the Holy Grail, the Parcival legend and many other similar themes. Drama during this time may be of great help as the adolescent experiments with different roles, emotions, identities and life situations. A natural interest in the modern world invites a host of topical themes that engage the adolescent's interest: world events, world cultures and the diversity of nations, languages and customs open up an understanding of differences and an enhanced sense of fraternity with others.

17. See note 15 above.

18. W. Von Eschenbach (approx 1200), *Parzival A Romance of the Middle Ages,* Vintage Books, New York 1961.

19. The Constantia Waldorf School in Cape Town runs a five-day camp where Grade eleven children (aged 17-18) journey through nature using the Parcival legend as a challenging rite of passage. Dramatic stage productions can be selectively utilized for the same purpose.

Projects consciously chosen allow the young student to go through a life process that can be deeply transformative. One highlight of the twelfth year of the Waldorf curriculum is the working on a project of one's own choice and its ultimate presentation to the Waldorf School community.

20. Batya Daitz an experienced Waldorf teacher in Cape Town has developed a course for young adults called *Quo Vadis? Where are you going?* in which these questions have a central place.

21. Quoted from a letter to F.H. Jacobi, where Johan Wolfgang Goethe describes his notion of the relationship of light and darkness – the central idea in his *Theory of Colour,* published in 1810.

22. In anthroposophical literature a number of authors have explored the sevenfold nature of the human soul: In his seminal work *Occult Science*, Steiner describes a vast cosmological picture that spans the evolution of the macrocosmic universe, the microcosmic human being and the earth. Originally the human being, the universe and the earth were a single united entity. In the evolutionary process the universal human being passes through a warmth stage called Saturn evolution, a light/air stage called Sun evolution, a watery stage called Moon evolution and a solid stage called Earth evolution. The human being undergoes a stepwise descent into matter and a progressive separation from his divine universal origins. Humanity is currently in this Earth phase of evolution and will in far distant time pass into the fifth (Jupiter), sixth (Venus) and seventh (Vulcan) evolutionary epochs. Steiner also describes seven planetary spheres through which the human individuality journeys in his sojourn after death and again in his journey towards birth on earth. These are named according to the seven primary planets recognized by ancient cultures and still accepted today by many esoteric circles: Saturn, Jupiter, Mars, Sun, Venus, Mercury, Moon. It is through these seven spheres that the human astral body is formed on its way to incarnation on earth. This results in seven aspects of the human soul that are named in accordance with these planetary spheres: the Saturn type, the Jupiter type, etc. Lievegoed describes the seven types as *the investigator, the thinker, the entrepreneur, the balancer, the carer, the innovator* and *the conserver.* Max Stibbe calls them the *ego-conscious, dominating, aggressive, radiant, aesthetic, mobile and dreaming* types. The influence of the seven planetary forces on the life processes and the formation of organ systems has been described in Chapter seven (page 183).

23. A number of authors have explored these themes:

W. Pelikan, *The Secrets of Metals*, Anthroposophic Press, Spring Valley, NY 1973; A Selawry, *Metall-Funktionstypen in Psychologie und Medizin*, Haug Verlag, Heidelberg 1984; U. Renzinbrink, *Die sieben Getreide* Rudolf Geering-Verlag Dornach, Switzerland 1981.

They all take their starting point from the broad universal picture that Steiner gives of the sevenfold nature of existence. Steiner was certainly not the first to speak about these seven principles. Many

cultures, mythologies and mystery centres throughout the ages are anchored in a knowledge that encompasses these seven principles. The connection between the seven grains and metals, and the planets, is generally considered to be as follows:
Grains:
   Saturn = maize / Jupiter = rye / Mars = barley / Sun = wheat / Venus = oats / Mercury =millet / Moon = rice.
Metals:
   Saturn = lead / Jupiter = tin / Mars = iron / Sun = gold / Venus = copper / Mercury = quicksilver, mercury / Moon = silver.

24. J. Kepler (1599), *The Harmony of the World,* translated into English and edited by E.J. Aiton, A.M. Duncan, J.V. Field, American Philosophical Society 1997.

25. B. Lievegoed, *Man on the Threshold. The challenge of inner development,* Hawthorn Press, Stroud 1985.

26. There are other planets such as Uranus, Neptune and Pluto but they are newcomers to our awareness (Uranus was discovered in 1781, Neptune in 1846 and Pluto in 1930), in contrast to the other planets that have been known to humanity since time immemorial.

27. A more detailed description of these relationships can be found in the following reference works: F. Husemann & O. Wolff, *The Anthroposophical Approach to Medicine. An Outline of a Spiritual Scientifically Oriented Medicine Vol 2,* Anthroposophic Press, Hudson, NY 1987; A. Selawry, *Metal-Funktionstypen in Psychologie und Medizin,* Haug Verlag, Heidelberg, 1985.

28. Alongside constitution and temperament, character is another useful typology. Typology is the study or systematic classification of types that have characteristics or traits in common. There are currently a number of typological schemes in vogue that are being used to classify knowledge in a wide variety of domains. Ken Wilber describes the 'four quadrants of existence', which summarize a wide field of information across developmental and evolutionary fields (K. Wilber, (1997) 'An Integral Theory of Consciousness', *Journal of Consciousness Studies,* 4 (1), February 1997, pp. 71–92). The Jungian types on which the Myers Briggs typology is based are used to identify personality types for educational, psychological, corporate and other reasons. Rudolf Steiner also made use of typological schemes to systematically characterize his view of the human being and the universe, but expressly warned against using them in a fixed and static way.

   It is evident that these different typologies all have their underlying philosophical and empirical foundations – which may be more or less appealing and convincing. In addition they all may be used, like any scheme, to label a person and box him into a rigid form. Can typologies be justified? If so how do we choose typological systems that can be useful as tools for understanding human nature and that do not lead to stereotyped fixing of the developing human individual?

I believe typology is justified when it is based on a universal principle that underlies the objective world of phenomena that we are investigating; and when it can be applied flexibly and intelligently.

If we consider the various typologies that we make use of in this book, they all reveal a higher universal principle that can be experienced by any unbiased person willing to explore her own vast potential of human experience. The typological scheme with its rigid structure then stands as symbolic representation of an eternal principle.

- *We can discover the universal principle of the threefold nature of the human being – body, soul and spirit, with the faculties of thinking, feeling and will, and organically in neuro-sensory system, rhythmic system and metabolic-limb system – by experiencing the contracting principle that hardens and draws in substance, the expanding principle that dissolves and frees substance, and the balancing, rhythmic principle that moves between the two polarities.*
- *Likewise we may arrive at the fourfold nature of the human being – the four elements of earth, water, air and fire, the four human sheaths (physical body, etheric body, astral body and I), the four ethers (life ether, chemical/sound ether, light ether and warmth ether) and four temperaments (melancholic, phlegmatic, sanguine and choleric) – through experiencing the distinctive nature of the four elements within us: earth that forms and solidifies us, water that enlivens and flows in us, air that activates, mobilizes and brings us to consciousness, and warmth that is all-pervasive and creates the power and will to drive our development and destiny.*
- *Similarly we can identify the sevenfold nature of the human being represented by the seven planetary forces in the manner described in this chapter.*

Chapter 10
The Body-Soul-Spirit Continuum In Childhood And Adolescence

1. R. Steiner, (1910), *A Psychology of Body, Soul and Spirit* GA 115 Anthroposophic Press, USA 1999. Desire arises from the sentient body which is the finer part of the etheric body.

---

2. *Recall any experience where feelings or emotions were strongly present and try to visualize the situation as vividly as possible. One quite easily becomes aware of a bodily sensation or feeling that arises in consequence.*

3. C. B. Pert, *Molecules of Emotions,* Pocket Books, USA 1997; C.B.Pert, M.R. Ruff, R.J.Weber, M. Herkenham, 'Neuropeptides and their receptors: a psychosomatic network', *Journal of Immunology,* 1985 Aug; 135(2 Suppl): 820s–826s

4. M. Irwin, K. Vedhara, *Human Psychoneuroimmunology,* Oxford University Press, UK 2005.

    Two meta-analyses of the literature show a consistent reduction of immune function in healthy people experiencing stress.

    • T. B. Herbert, S. Cohen, 'Stress and immunity in humans: a meta-analytic review', Psychosomatic Medicine; 55:364–379, 1993. Thirty-eight studies of stressful events and immune function in healthy adults were examined, including studies of acute laboratory stressors (e.g. a speech task), short-term naturalistic stressors (e.g. medical examinations), and long-term naturalistic stressors (e.g. divorce, bereavement, caregiving, unemployment). Consistent stress-related increases in numbers of total white blood cells, as well as decreases in the numbers of helper T cells, suppressor T cells, and cytotoxic T cells, B cells, and natural killer cells (NK).

    • Zorrilla et al., 'The relationship of depression and stressors to immunological assays: a meta-analytical review', *Brain Behaviour and Immunity,* 15(3), 199–226, 2001. This study replicated Herbert and Cohen's meta-analysis. Using the same study selection procedures, 75 studies of stressors and human immunity were analyzed, replicating the previous meta-analysis review.

5. There are nine sense organs that are anatomically and physiologically recognized by conventional medical science. These are the touch corpuscles (sense of touch), the autonomic nervous sytem (sense of life), proprioceptive organs (sense of movement), vestibular organs (sense of balance), taste buds (sense of taste), olfactory organs (sense of smell), visual organ (sense of sight), cold and warmth nerve receptors (sense of warmth), auditory organ (sense of hearing). The higher three senses – the sense of word or tone, the sense of thought and the sense of I, utilize organs of perception that are non-physical and exist at a spiritual level.

6. R. Steiner (1910), *A Psychology of Body, Soul and Spirit,* GA 115, Anthroposophic Press, USA 1999.
    Desire arises from the sentient body, which is the finer part of the etheric body.

7. Ibid. Feelings and deliberation are the core elements of soul life.

8. Ibid. Past mental images are induced by the I reflecting them through a mirroring activity of the etheric body. The child develops this ability to mirror past events only after self-awareness has occurred in the third year. Before this time, 'children absorb impressions unconsciously without the I being truly present in them... After this time, when a sufficient culmination and completion of the etheric body has taken place, the I enters the etheric body and acquires a mirroring capacity

through being able to reflect itself on the 'inner walls of the etheric body'. (R. Steiner, *Psychology of Body, Soul and Spirit lecture:* see note 5 above).

9. R. Steiner, *Riddles of Humanity*, GA 170, Rudolf Steiner Press, London 1990.
10. R. Steiner, *The Bridge between Universal Spirituality and the Physical Constitution of Man*, GA 202, Anthroposophic Press, Spring Valley USA 1979.
11. R. Steiner, I. Wegman, *Fundamentals of Therapy. An Extension of the Art of Healing through Spiritual Knowledge*, Rudolf Steiner Press, London 1983.

Chapter 11
Awakening To The I

1. In many books and lectures Steiner describes the natural sense of oneness with everything which the young child has before he names himself I. Examples are: *The Spiritual Guidance of the Human Being and Humanity*, GA 15, Anthroposophic Press, Spring Valley, New York 1961; *The Mission of the New Revelation*, GA 127, Rudolf Steiner Press, London 1987.
2. See note 1 above.
3. B. Lievegoed, *Phases of Childhood*, Floris Books, Edinburgh 1985.
4. R. Steiner, *The Foundation Stone*, Anthroposophical Publishing Company, London 1957.

Bibliography

Anthroposophy

Bockemühl, J., Lindenau, C., Maier, G., *et al.* (1985) *Towards a Phenomenology of the Etheric World*, Anthroposophic Press, New York.

Easton, S. (1982) *Man and World in the Light of Anthroposophy*, Anthroposophic Press, New York.

Gloeckler, M. (2008) *Knowledge Gained through Practical Engagement with Anthroposophic Research Findings, Illustrated by the Dual Aspect of the Human Being's Etheric Organization*, Dornach, Switzerland.

König, K. (1973; 1st edn 1959) *The Human Soul*, Floris Books, Edinburgh.

Marti, E. (1984) *The Etheric/The Four Ethers*, Schaumburg Publications, Illinois.

Shepherd, A.P. (1954) *A Scientist of the Invisible*, Hodder & Stoughton.

Soesman, A. (1990) *The Twelve Senses,* Hawthorn Press, Stroud.

Steiner, R. (1908) *The Influence of Spiritual Beings*, GA 102, Anthroposophic Press, New York.

Steiner, R. (1919) *Lucifer and Ahriman*, Rudolf Steiner, Canada.

Steiner, R. (1922) *The Human Soul in Relation to World Evolution*, GA 212, Anthroposophic Press, New York.

Steiner, R. (1957; 1st edn 1923) *The Foundation Stone*, Anthroposophical Publishing, London.

Steiner, R. (1961; 1st edn 1904) *Theosophy: an introduction to the supersensible knowledge of the world and the destination of the human being*, Anthroposophic Press, New York.

Steiner, R. (1966; 1st edn 1923) *Man's Being, His Destiny and World Evolution*, Oslo GA 226, Anthroposophic Press, New York.

Steiner, R. (1967; 1st edn 1916) *Menschenwerden, Weltenseele und Weltengeist*, GA 206, Rudolf Steiner Nachlassverwaltung, Dornach, Switzerland.

Steiner, R. (1967; 1st edn 1920) *Geisteswissenschaft als Erkenntnis der Grundimpulse sozialer Gestaltung*, GA 199, Rudolf Steiner, Nachlassverwaltung, Dornach, Switzerland.

Steiner, R. (1968; 1st edn 1912–13) *Life between Death and a New Birth*, Anthroposophic Press, New York.

Steiner, R. (1976; 1st edn 1917) *Von Seelenrätseln*, Rudolf Steiner Nachlassverwaltung, Dornach, Switzerland; translated as *Riddles of the Soul*.

Steiner, R. (1978; 1st edn 1909) *Rosicrucian Esoterism*, GA 109, 111, Anthroposophic Press, New York.

Steiner, R. (1979; 1st edn 1920) *The Bridge between Universal Spirituality and the Physical Constitution of Man*, Anthroposophic Press, New York.

Steiner, R. (1981; 1st edn 1907) *The Theosophy of the Rosicrucians*, GA 99, Rudolf Steiner, London.

Steiner, R. (1989; 1st edn 1922) *Knowledge of the Human Being According to Body, Soul and Spirit*, Lectures to the Workers of the Goetheanum, Rudolf Steiner, London.

Steiner, R. (1990; 1st edn 1916) *Riddles of Humanity*, GA 170, Rudolf Steiner, London.

Steiner, R. (1997; 1st edn 1921) *Die Gestaltung des Menschen als Ergebnis kosmischer Wirkungen*; English translation, *Cosmosophy* Vol 2 GA 208, Completion Press, Gympie, Australia.

Steiner, R. (1997; 1st edn 1923) *World History in the Light of Anthroposophy*, Rudolf Steiner, London.

Psychosophy

Steiner, R. (1990; 1st edn 1912) *Psychoanalysis and Spiritual Psychology*, Anthroposophic Press, New York.

Steiner, R. (1999; 1st edn 1910) *A Psychology of Body, Soul and Spirit*, Anthroposophic Press, New York.

Treichler, R. (1989) *Soulways: the developing soul life phase, thresholds and biography*, Hawthorn Press, Stroud.

Human Development and Human Consciousness

Lievegoed, B. (1985) *Man on the Threshold: the challenge of inner development*, Hawthorn Press, Stroud.

Steiner, R. (1972; 1st edn 1910) *Outline of Esoteric Training*, Anthroposophic Press, New York.

Steiner, R. (1986; 1st edn 1894) *Philosophy of Spiritual Activity*, Anthroposophic Press, New York.

Steiner, R. (2006; 1st edn 1904) *Knowledge of Higher Worlds*, Rudolf Steiner, London/*How to Know Higher Worlds: a modern path of initiation*, Anthroposophic Press, New York.

Wilber, K. (1997) An integral theory of consciousness, *Journal of Consciousness Studies*, 4(1), 71–92.

Human Anatomy/Physiology

Ayres, A.J. (1990) *Sensory Integration and the Child*, Western Psychological Services.

Doidge, N. (2007) *The Brain that Changes Itself*, Viking Press, New York.

Hoerner, W. (1978) Zeit *und Rhythmus*, Urachhaus, Stuttgart.

Mees, L.F.C. (1984) *Secrets of the Skeleton: form in metamorphosis*, Anthroposophic Press, New York.

Vogel, L. (1979) *Der Driegliedrige Mensch*, Philosophisch-Anthroposophischer Verlag, Dornach, Switzerland.

Psychology

Kaplan, H.I. and Sadock, B.J. (2003) *Kaplan & Sadock's Synopsis of Psychiatry*, Lippincott Williams & Wilkins, London.

Treichler, R. (1989) *Soulways: the developing soul-life phases, thresholds and biography*, Hawthorn Press, Stroud.

Wilber, K. (2000) *Integral Psychology*, Shambala Publications, Boston.

Body Mind Connection

Herbert, T.B. *et al.* (1993) Stress and immunity in humans: a meta-analytic review, *Psychosomatic Medicine*, 55, 364–79.

Irwin, M. *et al.* (2005) *Human Psychoneuroimmunology*, Oxford University Press.

Pert, C.B. (1997) *Molecules of Emotions*, Pocket Books.

Pert, C.B. *et al.* (1985) Neuropeptides and their receptors: a psychosomatic network, *J Immunol*, 135(2 Suppl), 820s–826s.

Zorrilla *et al.* (2001)The relationship of depression and stressors to immunological assays: a meta-analytical review, *Brain Behaviour and Immunity*, 15(3), 199–226.

The Child through History

Aries, P. (1962) *Centuries of Childhood*, Random House, Vintage Books, New York.

Garbarino, J. (1995) *Raising Children in a Socially Toxic Environment*, Jossey-Bass, San Francisco.

James, O. (2007) *Affluenza*, Random House, London.

Palmer, S. (2006) *Toxic Childhood: how the modern world is damaging our children and what we can do about it*, Orion Books, London.

Plumb, J.H. (1971) The great change in children, *Horizon*, 13(1), 5–13.

Postman, N. (1982) *The Disappearance of Childhood*, Vintage Books, New York.

Postman, N. (1986) *Amusing Ourselves to Death*, Heinemann, London.

Child Development

Aeppli, W. (1986) *The Developing Child*, Anthroposophic Press, New York.

Buzzell, K. (1998) *The Children of Cyclops*, The Association of Waldorf Schools of North America, Fair Oaks.

Cohen, D.B. (2006) Family constellations: an innovative systemic phenomenological group process from Germany, *The Family Journal: counseling and therapy for couples and families*, 14(3), 226–33.

Frommer, E.A. (1969) *Voyage through Childhood into the Adult World: a guide to child development*, Hawthorn Press, Stroud.

Goddard Blythe, S. (2004) *The Well Balanced Child*, Hawthorn Press, Stroud.

Goddard Blythe, S. (2008) *What Babies and Children Really Need*, Hawthorn Press, Stroud.

Hellinger, B. *et al.* (1998) *Love's Hidden Symmetry: what makes love work in relationships*, Zeig, Tucker & Theisen, Phoenix.

König, K. (1984) *Brothers and Sisters: the order of birth in the family*, Floris Books, Edinburgh.

Large, M. (2003) *Set Free Childhood*, Hawthorn Press, Stroud.

Lievegoed, B. (1987) *Phases of Childhood*, Floris Books, Edinburgh.

Louw, D.A. *et al.* (1998) *Human Development*, Kagiso Publishers, Pretoria.

Piaget, J. (1928) *The Child's Conception of the World*, Routledge, London.

Violato, C. *et al.* A meta-analysis of the published research on the effects of non-maternal care on child development, in Violato, C. *et al.* (ed.) *The Changing Family and Child Development*, Ashgate, London (in press).

Prenatal Existence and Development

Appenzeller, K. (1976) *Die Genesis im Lichte der menschlichen Embryonal Entwickelung*, Zbinden Press, Basel.

König, K. (1966) *Embryologie und Weltenstehung*, Verlag die Kommenden, Freiburg.

Weihs, T. (1986) *Embryogenesis in Myth and Science*, Floris Books, Edinburgh.

Wilmar, F. (1979) *Vorgeburtliche Menschwerdung*, J. Ch. Mellinger, Stuttgart.

Birth

Al Mufti, R. *et al.* (1997) Obstetricians' personal choice and mode of delivery, *Lancet*, 347, 544.

Behague, C.G. *et al.* (2002) Consumer demand for Caesarean section in Brazil, *BMJ*, 324, 942.

Bell, J.S. *et al.* (2001) Do obstetric complications explain high Caesarean section rates among women over 30? *BMJ*, 322, 894–95.

Drake, S. (1979) *The Path to Birth*, Floris Books, Edinburgh.

Efekhar, K. *et al.* (2000) Caesarean section controversy. Women choose Caesarisection, *BMJ*, 320, 1073.

English, J.B. (1985) *Different Doorway: adventures of a Caesarian born*, Earth Heart Publishers, Point Reyes Station.

English, J.B. (1994) Being born caesarian: physical, psychosocial and metaphysical aspects, *J Prenatal & Perinatal Psychol & Health*, 7(3), 215–29.

Enkin, M. *et al.* (2000) *A Guide to Effective Care in Pregnancy and Childbirth*, Oxford University Press.

Feher, L. (1981) *The Psychology of Birth: roots of human personality*, Continuum, New York.

Glazener, C.M. (1997) Sexual function after childbirth: women's experiences, persistent morbidity and lack of professional recognition, *Br J Obstet Gynaecol*, 104, 330–35.

Goldberg, R. (2002) *Caesarean Section: is the rising incidence a cause for concern?* Dreamcatcher Publications.

Hemminki, E. (1996) Impact of Caesarean section on future pregnancy – a review of cohort studies, *Paediatr Perinat Epidemiol*, 10, 366–79.

Hemminki, E. (1996) Long term effects of caesarean sections, *Am J Obstet Gynaecol*, 174, 1569–574.

Hollmen, A. *et al.* (1993) Influence of labour and route of delivery on the frequency of respiratory morbidity in term neonates, *Int J Gynaecol Obstet*, 43, 35–40.

Leboyer, F. (1975) *Birth without Violence*, Knopf, New York.

Lilford, R. *et al.* (1990) The relative risk of Caesarean section, *Br J Obstet Gynaecol*, 97, 883–90.

Oliver, R. (2000) The ideal caesarian delivery, *J Prenatal & Perinatal Psychol Health*, 14(3–4), 331–34.

Paxelius, G. *et al.* (1983) Catecholamine surge and lung function after delivery, *Arch Dis Child*, 58, 262–66.

Ray, S. *et al.* (1987) *Birth and Relationships: how your birth affects your relationships*, Celestial Arts, Berkeley.

Shapira, A.L. (2008) *The Emotional Ramifications of being Born in a Caesarian Delivery*, Santa Barbara Graduate Institute.

Snyman, L. (1999) Is the high Caesarean section rate a cause for concern? Review Article, Department of Obstetrics and Gynaecology, University of Pretoria.

Verny, T.R. *et al.* (2002) *Tomorrow's Baby: the art and science of parenting from conception through infancy*, Simon & Schuster, New York.

Early Childhood

Cook, P.S. (1999) Rethinking the early childcare agenda. Who should be caring for very young children? *Med J Australia*, 170, 29–31.

Glas, N. (1983) *Conception, Birth and Childhood*, Anthropsophic Press, New York.

Gross, T.F. (1985) *Cognitive Development*, Brooks/Cole Publishing, Monterey, California.

König, K. (1957) *The First Three Years of the Child*, Heil- und Erziehungsinstitut Bingenheim/Friedberg.

Linden, W. zur (1980) *A Child is Born*, Pharos Books, London.

Steiner, R. (1983; 1st edn 1911) *The Spiritual Guidance of Mankind*, Anthroposophic Press, New York.

Middle Childhood

Müller-Wiederman, H. (1973) *Mitte der Kindheit: Das neunte bis zwölfte Lebensjaht. Eine biographische Phänomenologie der kindlichen Entwicklung* (*Mid Childhood: the ninth to twelfth year of life. A biographical phenomenology of child development*), Verlag Freies Geistesleben, Stuttgart.

Steiner, R. (1996) *The Child's Changing Consciousness as the Basis of Pedagogical Practice*, Anthroposophic Press, New York.

Steiner, R. (1998) *Rhythms of Learning*, Selected Lectures, Anthroposophic Press, New York.

Late Childhood and Adolescence

Gädecke, W. (1998) *Sexuality, Partnership and Marriage from a Spiritual Perspective*, Temple Lodge, London.

Herman-Giddens, M.E. *et al.* (1997) Secondary sexual characteristics and menses in young girls seen in office practice: a study from the pediatric research in office settings network, *Pediatrics*, 99(4).

Lievegoed, B. (1979) *Phases: crisis and development in the individual*, Rudolf Steiner, London.

Louw, D.A. *et al.* (1998) *Human Development*, Kagiso Publishers, Pretoria.

Mattholius, H. (1997) Der Einfluss der Erziehung auf die Akzeleration des Menschen (*The Influence of Education on the Acceleration of Youth*), Beiträge zur einer Erweiterung der Heilkunst, issue 4.

Sleigh, J. (1982) *Thirteen to Nineteen – Discovering the Light*, Floris Books, Edinburgh.

General Education

Dewey, J. (1899) *The School and Society*, University of Chicago Press, Chicago.

Steiner, R. (1907) *Education of the Child*, Rudolf Steiner, London (1975)/ Anthroposophic Press, New York (1996).

Steiner, R. (1964; 1st edn 1924) *Kingdom of Childhood*, Rudolf Steiner, London.

Steiner, R. (1972; 1st edn 1923) *A Modern Art of Education,* Rudolf Steiner, London.

Steiner, R. (1976; 1st edn 1908) *The Four Temperaments*, Anthroposophic Press, New York.

Steiner, R. (1982; 1st edn 1924) *The Essentials of Education,* Rudolf Steiner, London.

Waldorf Education

Blunt, R. (1995) *Waldorf Education Theory and Practice*, Novalis Press, Cape Town.

Edmunds, F. (1992) *Rudolf Steiner Education*, Rudolf Steiner, London.

Harwood, A.C. (1974) *The Way of a Child*, Rudolf Steiner, London.

Harwood, A.C. (1975) *The Recovery of Man in Childhood*, Anthroposophic Press, New York.

Leber, S. (2002) *Kommentar zu Rudolf Steiner's Vorträgen über Allgemeine Menschenkunde als Grundlage der Pädagogik. Band III: Der leibliche Gesichtspunkt.* English Translation: *Commentaries on Rudolf Steiner's lectures – The Study of Man. Vol 3: The bodily viewpoint.* Verlag Freies Geistesleben, Stuttgart.

Maher, S. and Bleach, Y. (1998) *Putting the Heart back into Teaching*, Novalis Press, Cape Town.

Staley, B. (1988) *Between Form and Freedom*, Hawthorn Press, Stroud.

Steiner, R. (1975; 1st edn 1919) *Study of Man*, Lecture 4, Rudolf Steiner, London.

Steiner, R. (1986; 1st edn 1922) *Soul Economy and Waldorf Education*, GA 303, Anthroposophic Press, New York.

Steiner, R. (2008) *An Introduction to 'Waldorf Education'and Other Essays*, Anthroposophic Press, New York.

Nutrition

Glöckler, M. and Goebel, W. (2000) *A Guide to Child Health,* Floris Books, Edinburgh.

Goldberg, R. (2005) *Creative Nutrition for Healthy Children,* Nos 9 and10 in the series *Awaken to Child Health,* Dreamcatcher Publications.

Goldberg, R. (2005) *Creative Nutrition for Healthy Children,* Dreamcatcher Publications.

Hauschka, R. (1967) *Nutrition,* Stuart & Watkins, London.

Renzinbrink, U. (1981) *Die Sieben Getreide,* Rudolf Geering-Verlag Dornach, Switzerland.

Schmidt, G. (1975) *The Dynamics of Nutrition,* Vols 1 and 2, Biodynamic Literature, Pennsylvania.

Stories and Fairy Tales

Grahl, U. (1955) *The Wisdom of Fairy Tales,* New Know Books.

Grimm Brothers (1975) *The Complete Grimm's Fairy Tales,* Routledge, London.

Kingsley, C. (1985) *The Heroes,* William Clowes & Sons, London.

Mare, W de la (1977) *Stories from the Bible,* Faber and Faber.

Mellon, N. (2000) *Storytelling with Children,* Hawthorn Press, Stroud.

Querido, R. (1982) *Creativity in Education,* Dakin, San Francisco.

Steiner, R. (1937; 1st edn 1919) *Practical Advice for Teachers,* Anthroposophic Press, New York.

Streit, J. (1974) *Animal Stories,* Walter Keller, Dornach, Switzerland.

Streit, J. (1978) *And there was Light* (Bible Story companion for Class 3), Private publication.

Von Eschenbach, W. (1961) *Parzival: A Romance of the Middle Ages,* Vintage Books, New York.

Wilkinson, R. (1984) *Interpretation of Fairy Tales,* Henry Goulden Publications.

Eurythmy

Poplawski, T. *Eurythmy: rhythm, dance and soul,* pp. 80–84.

Steiner, R. (1955; 1st edn 1922–1924) *Eurythmy as Visible Speech/Eurythmy as Visible Sound,* Anthroposophical Publishing, London.

Stott, A. (2002) *Eurythmy: its birth and development,* Anastasi Ltd.

Parenting

Davy, G. and Voors, B. (1983) *Lifeways: working with family questions,* Hawthorn Press, Stroud.

Goldberg, R. (2002) *Enhancing Your Child's Potential,* Dreamcatcher Publications.

Salter, J. (1987) *The Incarnating Child,* Hawthorn Press, Stroud.

Health and Illness

Bühler, W. (1979) *Living with your Body: the body as an instrument of the soul,* Rudolf Steiner, London.

Glöckler, M. and Goebel, W. (2000) *A Guide to Child Health*, Floris Books, Edinburgh.

Goldberg, R. (2003) *Fever: a gift of health,* Dreamcatcher Publications.

Goldberg, R. (2004) *Infectious Childhood Illness: a developmental challenge for life*, Dreamcatcher Publications.

Goldberg, R. (2004) *Immunisation: should I vaccinate my child?*, Dreamcatcher Publications.

Newham, J.P. *et al.* (1993) Effects of frequent ultrasound during pregnancy: a randomised control trial. *Lancet*, 342, 887–891.

Stark, C. *et al.* (1984) Short- and long-term risks after exposure to diagnostic ultrasound *in utero*. *Obstet Gynecol*, 63, 194–200.

Anthroposophical Medicine

Bott, V. (1978) *Anthroposophical Medicine: an extension of the art of healing*, Rudolf Steiner, London.

Evans, M. (1992) *Anthroposophical Medicine: healing for body, soul and spirit*, Thorsons, London.

Fintelmann, V. (1987) *Intuitive Medizin Einfuhring in einer anthroposophisch erganzte Medizin*. English translation: *Intuitive medicine – An Introduction to an Anthroposophical Extended Medicine.*Hippocrates, Stuttgart.

Husemann, F. and Wolff, O. (1982) *The Anthroposophical Approach to Medicine: an outline of a spiritual scientifically oriented medicine*, 3 vols, Anthroposophic Press, New York.

Steiner, R. and Wegman, I. (1983; 1st edn 1925) *Fundamentals of Therapy: an extension of the art of healing through spiritual knowledge*, Rudolf Steiner, London.

Therapeutics

Kirchner-Bockholt, M. and Wood,(1969) *Fundamental Principles of Curative Eurythmy*, ISBN 0-904693-40-6.

Pelikan, W. (1973) *The Secrets of Metals*, Anthroposophic Press, New York.

Selawry, A. (1984) *Metall-Funktionstypen in Psychologie und Medizin*, Haug Verlag, Heidelberg.

Appendix

The Road Map

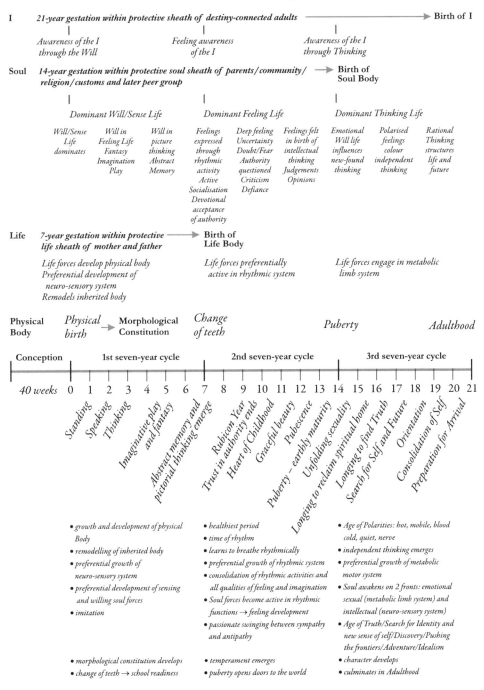

Index

Adam 108, 175, 177ff, 192, 198ff, 203, 204, 206, 239, 241ff, 258, 262, 267, 299, 310, 316, 323ff, 358ff
addiction 251
Ader, Robert 346
adolescence 273
adrenalin 284
aeriform
　element 36
　mode of observation 37ff, 40
　system 35
agape 291
Ahura mazdao 336
allantois 55, 58, 61
Alliance for Childhood viii, 6, 387
amniocentesis 67ff
amnion 55, 58, 61ff
amniotic sac 52ff
Ancient Moon 405
Ancient Saturn 323, 405
Ancient Sun 323, 405
animus/anima 292
Anthroposophic medicine x
Anthroposophy ix
antipathy 232, 238ff, 287, 293, 351
Aphrodite 333ff
Artemis 325
Arterial circulation 335
astral body 114, 254ff, 284, 287ff, 362ff, 365, 401
auditory apparatus 143ff
authority 202, 242ff,
autonomic nervous system 347

baby talk 155, 169
bedroom 170
bile 332
birth 72ff, 96ff
　astral/soul 79ff , 253, 274, 284, 316, 339, 402
　etheric 75ff, 316, 401
　four births 316, 344
　interventions 101
　of destiny 304ff
　of the I 316, 377
　options 98
　physical 73ff, 95,316
　three births 70ff
blastocyst 51
blood 280, 324
　embryonic 61
blue 323
body 31, 41, 85, 255
　awareness 23
　physical 41, 55, 114ff, 179, 259
　proportions 91ff
　soul connection 89ff, 362ff
　soul spirit 41, 90, 254
　systems 34ff
body–soul–spirit continuum 343ff
bones 280
bottle feeding 120
brain 328
　plasticity 163
breathing 217ff, 227ff
　in education 231
Bulani 191, 193, 203, 205, 205, 254, 264, 267, 311, 325ff
Buzell, Keith 163

Caesarian section 101ff
    rising incidence 101ff
    effects of 105ff
cardiac type 206
care
    of early childhood 166ff
    of middle childhood 269
    of newborn 116ff
    of late childhood/adolescence
        340ff
    of unborn child
    of young child 208ff
cell 46ff
central nervous system 182,
cerebral type 204
change of teeth 71ff, 76ff, 178,
    213ff, 375
character 319ff
    types 322ff
characterization 303
chest type 205
chi 24
child
    as sense organ 134
    earthly 204
    newborn 95ff, 126
    the first 111ff
    the second 112
    the third 112ff
    through history 3ff
    unborn child 96
    universal xiv, 1ff, 382, 3881ff
childhood
    early 175ff
    heart of 213
    illnesses 167ff, 189
    journey 15ff
    late 273ff
    middle 213ff
    verse 386ff
choleric temperament 265
chorion 54ff, 58, 61
Christ 33
Chronos 323
circulatory system 216, 228, 230,
    337
colostrum 119
colour 320
compassion 25
complementary medicine 347

concentration camp syndrome 222
concept 184ff, 300ff,
conception 48ff
conceptualizing 300
conclusion 302
constitution 203ff
copper 334
core picture
    of early childhood 166,
    of middle childhood 268
    of newborn 116
    of late childhood
    of unborn child 66
    of young child 207ff
cortisol 283
cosmic child 205
cow's milk 121
creative caring 379
creative resourcing 28ff, 379, 381
creche 199
curiosity 243

dance 236
Darwinism 5, 7
day care 199
definitions 303
deliberation 302, 352, 409
description 303
desire 133, 134, 286, 351, 352,
    353, 409
    unfulfilled 355
destiny 304ff, 377
Dewey, John 5
Diana 325
diary 296
digestion 277ff
digestive type 205
discerning 335
donkey's milk 121
Down's syndrome 68, 258
Drake, Stanley 64
drive 132ff

ear 128, 131, 144
earthly child 204
ectoderm 52, 60, 63
educational tasks 231ff
eighteen 312ff, 376
elemental organizations 34ff, 365
elements 35ff, 258ff, 365

airy 35ff, 259, 365
   fluid 34ff, 259, 365
   solid/earth 34ff, 259, 365
   warmth 35ff, 259, 365
eleven 249
embryoblast 51ff
embryological development 50ff,
   373
embryonic
   period 63
   sheathes 54ff,66
emotions 288
empathic listening 378ff
empathy 26ff, 378ff, 380ff
endoderm 52, 60, 63
enter–exit–behold 23
environment
   impact 114ff
   impressions 169
Erdenreife 253, 294
eros 290
etheric
   and memory 24, 220ff
   and time 219ff
   and thinking 185
   birth 75ff
   body/ life body 24, 41,47, 50,
      55ff 76, 82, 114ff, 150ff,
      179ff, 187, 218ff, 235,
      257, 259, 365
   and imagination 289
   and rhythm 219ff
   and thinking 185ff
   development of 343
   experiencing 183, 351ff
   forces 61, 77ff, 94, 115, 176,
      189 179ff, 188
   sheath 77
   stream 93, 202, 276, 343ff
ethers 187ff, 365ff
eurythmy 201, 237
evolutionary epochs 54, 405
excarnation 232
exercises 20ff, 390 (notes 4, 7),
   391(note 3), 392(notes 10, 19),
   392 (notes1), 393(notes 7, 1),
   396 (note 27), 397 (note 6), 398
   (note 19, 1), 399 (note 12),
   400 (note 1), 401 (note 20),
   402 (note 27), 403 (note 1),
      407, 408 (note 2)
experience 14 ff
   awareness 19
   literacy 22
   modes of 20
   original 16, 378
eye 128, 131, 141ff

fables 245ff
fairy tales 196ff, 244ff
fantasy 194ff, 288ff
father 382ff
feeding 120ff
feeling 20ff,184, 193ff, 211ff,
      226,238ff, 351, 409
   and rhythmic system 349
   in relation to time 344
female principle 44ff, 275
fertilization 48ff
fever 167ff
fifteen 305ff, 376
first moon node 314ff
fluid
   element 36
   mode of observation 37ff, 40
   system 35
foetal period 64
forceps delivery 107ff
formative forces 179ff
formula milk 121
foundation stone meditation 379
four bodily systems 34ff. 365
four cardinal organs 266ff
four elements 35ff, 259ff, 364
four ethers 187ff, 365ff
four fold
   births 316, 344
   child 55ff, 365
   embryo 58
   human being 55ff
   humours 260
   modes of observation 19, 365
   spheres 54
fourteen year 303ff
Freud, Sigmund 5

gap year 313
Garbarino, J. 8
gender 109ff, 292,
   identity 110, 292

reinforcement 110
    role 110
genital herpes 68
genome 47
gesture 22ff
Giovani da Bologna 226
Glöckler, Dr Michaela 121
goat's milk 121
Goddard, Sally 199
Goebel, Dr Wofgang 121
Goethe, J.W. 320
gold 336
green 333

Hahnemann, Samuel 223
Harwood, A.C. 243
Hauschka, Rudolf 223
head 85ff, 6
    type 204
healing 369
health 369
heart 86,218, 228, 268, 336ff
    primitive 61ff
Hellinger, Bert 395
heredity
    and individuality 188ff, 260ff
Hermes 329
HIV/AIDS 68
Hippocrates 260
historical perspectives 4
Hoerner, Wilhelm. 217, 218
home birth 99
homosexual 296
homunculus 129
horoscope 50
horse riding 252
Horus 336
Hypothalamic-pituitary - adrenal
    axis 347

I 57ff, 259, 365, 391
    activity 355, 366, 371
    and warmth 366
    and will 365ff
    as pure activity 371
    as source 371
    awakening 164ff, 194, 248,
        316, 342, 370ff, 381
    designation 370ff
    embodiment of 372ff

events 374
    expressions of 375ff
    Ich 391
    impact of environment on 116
    journey 372ff
    mission of 377ff
    nature of 370ff
imagination 162, 194ff, 288ff, 390
imitation 149ff
immunisation 120
incarnation 232
infancy 175, 177
infatuation 290
inflammation 225
inheritance 48, 109
inner child work 20ff, 390ff
Inspiration 390
instinct 133,
intellectual/mind soul 258, 364
integrative medicine 347
intention 396
International Association of
    Psychophonetics Practitioners
    390
Intuition 390
invoking 28
iron 331, 333

James. Oliver 8
John the Evangelist 377
Jonathan 97, 108, 126, 165, 191,
    192, 194ff, 205, 206, 327ff
journey 70ff
    down to earth 42ff
    on earth 70ff, 95ff, 126
judging 352
Jung, C.J. 292
Jupiter
    mythology 327
    planet, 327
    process 183
    thoughtful/organizing type 327ff

Kepler, Johann 235, 321
kidneys 268, 282ff
kinesics 146,
Know thyself 377
König, Dr Karl 54, 59, 111

Lamaze 98

Large, Martin 8, 163, 241
large-headed child 205
larynx 332
law of correspondences 88, 175ff, 182
lead 323
Leber, Stefan 236
Leboyer Method 100, 394
legends 245
Lievegoed, Bernard 258, 292, 322,
    375, 376
life
    forces 61, 77ff, 94, 115, 176,
        179ff, 188ff
    processes 183, 217ff, 363ff, 369
    stream 93, 202, 276
limb type 205
limbs 84
liver 268, 278, 328
Locke 5
love 289ff, 292
    friendship/philia 290
    romantic/eros 290
    spiritual/agape 291
lungs 228, 268, 330, 332
lymph 330

magic 245
male principle 44ff, 275
Mandela, Nelson 7
Maria 108, 191, 193ff, 206, 211,
    214ff, 239, 256, 258, 260, 263,
    267, 310, 329, 360ff, 364ff
Mars, 331ff
    active/masculine type 331ff
    planet 181
    process 183
Maslow, Abraham vii,
maternity hospital birth 99
melancholic temperament 261ff
Mellon, Nancy 247
memory 15ff, 25, 158, 353
    localized 158
    repetitive/rhythmic 159
    pictoral 159
menstrual cycle 220
menstruation 293
mental picture/image/representation
    159, 221, 241, 301, 350, 353ff,
    409
Mercury

metal 329
mobile/connecting type 328ff
mythology 226ff, 329
planet 328
process 183
staff of 226, 330
statue of 227
mesenchyme 53ff
mesoderm 60, 63
metabolic
    function 85
    organs 84, 182
    type 7
metabolic limb system 63, 225ff,
    231, 276ff, 349ff
    and will 350
metabolism 276ff, 393
    and will 281
Michael 333
model body 189
modes of enquiry /observation
    37ff, 131ff
Moon
    planet 180ff, 325
    process 183
    type/imitating/renewing 325ff
morning and evening forces 223
morphology 82, 177, 393
morula 51
mother 382ff
motivation 396
movement 23ff, 128, 235ff
muscles 280ff, 328
muscular type 205
music 169, 236
myths 246

natural childbirth 98
natural feeding 120
neural
    pruning 163
    tube defect 68
neuro-endocrine system 347
neuroplasticity 163,
neuro-sensory
    function 84,
    system 62, 84, 127ff, 224ff,
        31, 282, 348
        and sensing 348
        and thinking 348

nineteenth year 315
notocord 60
nursery school 199ff
nutrition 168

Odin-Wotan 329
Old Testament 246
Oliver, Dr Robert 106
Olympus 321, 327
orange colour 327
order of siblings 111
original experience 16, 381
Osiris 336
ovary 44
ovulation 49
ovum 45

Palmer, Sue 8
Paracelsus 182, 321
Parcival legend 318
pathology 368
  of warmth and cold 368ff
peer group 272
percept and concept 300
perceptions 300
Persephone 313
Persephone Institute viii, 389
personality 272, 319ff, 339
Pert, Candice 346ff
philia 290
philophonetics 389
Philosophy of Freedom
phlegmatic temperament 264
physical
  body 41, 55, 114ff, 179, 259
  constitution 203
  development
    first three years 127, 152ff
    first seven years 177ff
    second seven year cycle 213ff
    pubescence 249
    third seven year cycle 274ff
Piaget. Jean 5, 240
picture
  of Adam in tenth year 357ff
  of Maria as an adult 360
  of Rajan in sixteenth year 359
  of Thandi before third year
    355ff
  of Thandi after three 357

of Thandi at fifteen 346
placenta 62, 73ff
planetary types 322ff, 406
play 162ff, 194ff, 375
play group 199ff
pneumo-psychosomatic
  connections 346, 348ff
  experiencing 351
post traumatic stress disorder 222
prana 24
preschool 175, 178
primary planets 181, 183
psyche 21ff, 31, 56ff, 255, 259,
  347ff
psychoneuroimmunology 346
psychophonetics viii, 16, 221,
  389
psychosomatic 346
  connections 89ff, 362ff
  streams 93, 202, 276
psychosophy 351ff
puberty 71, 81, 249ff, 253, 274ff,
  294ff
pubescence 249, 293ff
pulse/breathing quotient 216ff

Ra 336
Rajan 191, 212, 272, 286ff, 303ff,
  311, 337ff, 359ff
Raphael 10ff, 329
reacting 21ff
reactions 21
Read, Dick 98
recollection
  autobiographical study 19
  body/soul connection 346
  feelings 238
  first love 289ff
  first three years 125
  first seven years 174
  I experiences 375ff, 378
  original experiences 378
  puberty 251
  rhythmic activities 234
  second seven years 174ff, 212
  seven to nine years 240
  sex 292
  sexual identity 292
  sexuality 291
  tenth year 19, 247

third seven years 273
red 331
regression therapy 16, 389
reflecting 21, 302
repetition 159, 193, 197, 201ff
reproductive organs 44ff
resolution 396
resonance 24
resourcing 28
respiratory
  system 216, 230
  type 206
rhythm 172ff, 193, 197, 201ff,
  216ff
  and life 223
  breathing 217, 230
  circulatory 230
  in home 233ff
  in homeopathy 223
  in school 233ff
  neuro-sensory 230
rhythmic
  activities 211
  function 85
  organs 84
  movement 235
  process 80, 216ff, 224
  system 63, 224ff, 349
    and feeling 349
rites of passage 272, 316ff
road map 71ff
  early childhood 127
  first seven years 177ff, 190ff
  second seven years 240ff,
  third seven years 303ff
romantic love 290
Rousseau 5
routine 172
rubella 68
rubicon year 9

Salter, Joan, 153
Sanguine temperament 262ff
Saskia 192, 204, 206, 272, 286ff,
  303ff, 334, 360
Saturn
  individuating type 323ff
  planet 323
  process 183
school readiness 79

sclerosis 225
search for meaning 309
secular trend 294ff
sensation 287ff, 352
senses 135ff
  higher spirit-based 148
  interoceptive 397
  lower body-based 138, 148
  middle soul-based 143, 148
  of balance 137
  of hearing 143ff
  of I 147ff
  of life 136
  of movement 137
  of sight 141
  of smell 139
  of speech 145
  of taste 138ff
  of thought 146
  of tone 145
  of touch 135
  of word 145
  of warmth 142
  proprioceptive 397
  tactile 397
  twelve 135ff, 148
  vestibular 397
sensing 19, 20ff, 124ff,175, 183ff
  and neuro-sensory system 348
sense organs 135ff, 182, 408ff
sensitivity 80
sensory type 20
sentient
  body 113ff, 362ff , 409
  soul 257ff , 362ff
sevenfold phenomena 320ff, 405
seven
  grains 406
  life/planetary processes 183,
  321ff
  metals 406
  primary colours 320
  primary planets 181, 183
seventeen 310ff
seven year cycles 70ff
  first 72, 173ff, 380
  second 72, 211ff, 380
  third 72, 272ff, 381
sex 292
sexual games 294

sexuality 252ff, 291ff
    development of 293
    factors determining 296ff
silver 325
Sivers, Marie 237
sixteen 308ff
skeleton 83, 324
skin 324
small-headed child 204
Soesman, A, 135, 141,
solid
    element 35ff
    mode of observation 37, 40
    system 34
song 236
soul 21ff, 41, 82ff, 254ff, 259,
    347ff
    birth 79ff
    body 79ff. 113ff, 150, 254, 362ff
    brain 88
    consciousness/spiritual 258, 402
    development 255ff, 344
        in first seven year cycle 127ff,
            90ff
        in relation to time 344
        in second seven year cycle
            237ff
        in third seven year cycle
            284ff, 303ff
    feeling 19, 88
    forces 94
    functions/activities 19, 88
        impact of environment on 115
    intellectual/mind 258, 364, 402
    mind/heart 402
    origin 42
    pictures 355ff
        of Adam in tenth year 357ff
        of Maria as an adult 360
        of Rajan in sixteenth year 359
        of Thandi before third year
            355ff
        of Thandi after three 357
    sentient 257ff, 362ff
    spirit interface 364
    stream 93, 202, 299, 344
    type 319ff
    will 99
sound 24ff
sounding 23ff,

speaking 24,154ff, 161, 165, 192
speech and movement 156ff, 192
sperm 45
spheres
    four 54ff
spirit 31ff, 41, 82,
spirit germ 43, 50, 58, 66
spleen 324
standing 152ff
Steiner, Dr Rudolf ix, 6, 89, 133,
    135, 142, 147, 158, 162, 182,
    188, 204, 205, 217, 220, 223,
    231, 237, 253, 257, 302, 322,
    353, 372, 379
stem cell research 131
stories 195ff, 244ff
substance abuse 251
sun
    harmonious/balanced type 336ff
    planet 180, 182, 336
    process 183
sympathy 232, 238ff, 287, 293,
    351
system 34ff, 259
    aeriform/gaseous 35, 259
    fluid 35, 259
    solid/earth 34, 259
    warmth 35, 259
syphilis 68

Tagar, Yehuda viii, 22
teenage pregnancy 67
teeth
    change of 71ff, 76ff, 178, 213ff
    permanent 393
temperament 258ff
    choleric 265
    melancholic 261ff
    phlegmatic 264
    sanguine 262ff
tenth Rubicon year 247ff, 375
television 163,169
testes 44
Thandi 191, 192, 206, 214, 239,
    254, 265, 267, 310, 311, 331ff,
    345, 355ff
Thor 321, 327
Thoth 329
three births 6
three fold 85ff, 90

cell 87
child 82ff
    embryo 59
    soul 87ff
    systems 89ff
three human capacities 151ff,
    165
thinking 19, 22, 157ff, 165, 184ff,
    198, 298ff
    and ethers 185ff
    and neuro-sensory system 348
    and speech 160
    body/will-based 157, 198, 298
    in relation to time 344
    intellectual/rational 298ff, 339
    pictoral or imaginative thinking
        159, 241ff, 298,
thirteenth year 253ff
tin 327
Tobias 10ff
toddler 124, 175, 177ff
toys 195
Treichler, Rudolf 286
trophoblast 51ff
twelve senses 135ff
twelfth year 252
twenty 315
typologies 406ff

ultrasound 67
umbilical cord 55, 73ff
union 48
universal
    adolescent 309
    child xiv, 1ff, 382, 388
    father 383, 385
    mother 383, 385
urogenital system 284
upright posture 152ff, 165

vaccinations 167
vaccuum extraction delivery 107ff
venous circulation 335
Venus 183, 333
    mythology 333
    planet 333
    receptive/feminine type 333ff
vernix 119ff
violet 325
visualization 23
visualizing 20ff

WALA 222ff
Waldorf method of education 4,
    243ff, 245, 318
Waldorf School viii, 6, 231, 237
walking 152ff
warmth 168, 170, 281, 366ff
    and will 366
    element 37, 39
    mode of observation 39ff
    system 35
water birth 100, 393
wet dream 294
Wilbur, Ken 245
will/willing 19, 22,132ff, 170ff,
    176ff, 190ff, 250ff, 276, 353
    and metabolic-limb system 350
    and warmth 366
    the sevenfold 133
    in relation to time 344
wish 396

XRays 67

yellow 328
yolk sac 52, 58, 62

Zeus 321, 327